W9-BLZ-318

HEALING NUTRIENTS

HEALING NUTRIENTS

The People's Guide to
using common nutrients
that will help you feel
better than you
ever thought possible

Patrick Quillin, Ph.D., R.D.

CB

CONTEMPORARY
BOOKS

CHICAGO · NEW YORK

Library of Congress Cataloging-in-Publication Data

Quillin, Patrick.
   Healing nutrients / Patrick Quillin.
      p.   cm.
   ISBN 0-8092-4796-8
   1. Diet therapy.   2. Nutrition.   I. Title.
RM 217.Q55 1987
615.8'dc 19   87-26484
                                    CIP

Published by Contemporary Books, Inc.
180 North Michigan Avenue, Chicago, Illinois 60601
Manufactured in the United States of America
Library of Congress Catalog Card Number: 87-26484
International Standard Book Number: 0-8092-4796-8

Published simultaneously in Canada by Beaverbooks, Ltd.
195 Allstate Parkway, Valleywood Business Park
Markham, Ontario L3R 4T8 Canada

To my bonnie valentine Noreen,
*   Confidante, multitalented helper, spiritual cheerleader, and*
sidekick par excellence. Thanks a nonillion.

                                                              Patrick

Contents

PREFACE

"We command Nature only by obeying her."   —Francis Bacon

A new era in health care is slowly emerging. We are beginning to work with nature to restore health, rather than antagonizing nature by subduing symptoms. We are starting to use substances that are inherent to the chemistry of the human body to treat a condition, rather than using foreign chemicals to muffle health warning signals.

For example; rather than taking risky drugs for the rest of their lives, many of the 50 million Americans who suffer from high blood pressure could be "cured" through healing nutrients. There are also 6 million heart disease victims, 12 million diabetics, and 20 million people with osteoporosis in the U.S., and many of them could be helped dramatically by the nutritional approach outlined in this book. Millions of other people suffer from cancer, allergies, kidney stones, gallstones, hemorrhoids, obesity, and other debilitating conditions. Optimal nutrition could prevent those conditions, support conventional therapy for them, or even cure some of them.

This book is for parents who want healthier babies and an easier delivery, for people who go through life at "half mast," never really feeling energetic or happy, for people who are sick, and especially for those who don't want to get sick. Nutrition offers an amazingly effective and low-risk approach to healing illness and achieving wellness. The alternative is to be slowly enveloped by the illness as the symptoms are treated but the condition continues to deteriorate. *Healing Nutrients* offers hope of safe and longlasting help.

For thousands of years, the brightest minds have had vague suspicions that what we eat has something to do with how we feel. It makes such perfect sense. The human body is entirely built from, fueled by, and repaired with substances found in our diet. Hence, nutrition has a huge role in health care. But these early thinkers could not quantify or prove any of their suspicions. Now we can. Nutrition scientists have provided a knowledge base that is so extensive that nutritional therapy can be tailored specifically to each individual's condition.

Modern medicine is permeated with the term *idiopathic*, meaning "no known cause" and usually followed by "no known cure." Physicians and patients are often left with a sense of helplessness as the capricious whims of fate randomly strike down certain people with "idiopathic" ailments. Hypertension, cancer, allergies, preeclampsia, gallstones, kidney stones, fatigue, and other common ailments often fall into the idiopathic category. But in many cases, there *is* a known cause and a cure: nutrition.

Nutrition is no longer shotgun-in-the-dark therapy. It is specific. And it works. The next step is to incorporate it into the health care system of America. Each day thousands die and millions suffer needlessly, because the facts found in nutrition science are not widely employed.

There are many challenges to living in 20th-century America, but there are many blessings too. Modern medicine has reached its crescendo in emergency medicine. Medical professionals can keep nearly anyone alive. But what they have often failed to do is prevent illness, cure many degenerative diseases, and make any efforts toward improving the quality of life. Nutrition can help there. With these two high-tech sciences combined, we have the option of experiencing more vigorous and longer lives than ever before. We can transcend mere survival and move on toward optimal health.

The science of nutrition is relatively new and hence surrounded by die-hard skeptics. Due to the controversy that envelops nutrition, I spent many months in the biomedical libraries and on the

Medline computer connection gathering valid scientific literature to support my statements. More than 1,500 scientific studies are listed in the bibliography of this book. The references support the validity of this book's point: that nutrition can prevent and even cure many ailments that are common in the U.S.

Caveat: Nutrition is most effective when used in concert with proper exercise, attitude, and body maintenance and when genetics and physical environment are taken into account. This book is intended to give you another choice in healing modalities, to improve your health and to support rather than replace modern medical practices. If you have unusual symptoms, see a physician. Take this book with you and discuss its contents with your doctor. Certain conditions demand immediate attention; delaying proper medical care can reduce your chances of survival. Do not randomly experiment with megadoses of nutrients. Although nutrients are very benevolent healers, they can be abused in extreme doses. More is not necessarily better.

The objective of this book is to prove that nutrition should be a viable alternative in the healing arts. Right now, nutrition is rarely considered and sometimes even scoffed at. But the allied health professions are merging, like Great Northern geese joining together. In classical V formation, all participants will be working efficiently together for the betterment of everyone.

We are very lucky to be alive in such exciting times and to have the potential for a long and vigorous life. This book is one of the key tools that will help you attain the goal of optimal health. The rest is up to you. May you apply the principles found in this book and live a long and exuberant life.

ACKNOWLEDGMENTS

"I couldn't begin to thank the many people who made this possible," says many an award recipient on television. Let me try. This project involved many willing and able hands. Thanks to Libby McGreevy for your amiable and competent molding of this book. Thanks to the publisher, Harvey Plotnick, for your confidence and support. Thanks to Harold Roth for your friendship and salesmanship. Thanks to my wife, Noreen, for handling the thousands of details that would have delayed the book's completion by a decade or so. And thanks to the unsung heroes of this book: the thousands of faceless dedicated brilliant scientists who painstakingly unravel the mysteries of our world and ourselves.

INTRODUCTION
How to Use This Book

You picked up this book because you think that there is room for improvement in your life. You may be seeking more energy, better thinking power, less sickness, prevention or healing of a disease, or, more generally, a longer and better life. *Healing Nutrients* can help you achieve those goals. This chapter will tell you how to get the most from this book, applying it to your specific needs and goals.

The overall theme of this book is that nutrition is at the very heart of the state of our health. The recommendations in the following chapters are based on these premises:

- Optimal nutrition could provide better health for nearly everyone in this country
- Many ailments are nutritionally related and hence could be nutritionally cured
- Much debilitation and early death is due to poor nutrient intake
- A large percentage of mental and physical disorders could be caused by suboptimal nutrition during the early, developmental stages of life

1

Since you did pick up this book, you are probably open to the idea that optimal nutrition can help improve *your* health. However, you may not be aware that Americans in general suffer from rampant poor health. How can this be? We spend the most money on health care of any nation on earth. Unfortunately, we are far from having the best health. Chapter 1 discusses the bottom line: our current health care system is not working. It treats symptoms, not problems. It is dehumanizing and often debilitating. We are not as healthy or as long-lived as we should and could be.

If there *is* a problem with our health, what is the solution? The solution is the interdisciplinary approach, with nutrition as a key ingredient. I am not going to tell you that nutrition will cure all health ailments. Yet nutrition is a *very* important factor in curing and preventing disease. Chapter 2 documents the great potential benefits and minimal risk in using nutrition as a preventive and healing force.

Even if it can be proven that our health care system is not working and that nutrition is a viable healing force, you might feel that the point is moot—surely no one is malnourished in a land of such agricultural abundance. Wrong. Using large dietary surveys and scientific studies and showing the changes that have taken place in the modern American lifestyle, we will see in Chapter 3 that the average American is poorly nourished and that some people are even blatantly malnourished. Poor nutrient status is common in America and leads to a large percentage of our health problems.

WHICH CHAPTERS RELATE TO YOUR NEEDS?

The first three chapters of *Healing Nutrients* lay the foundation. They explain why nutrition therapy is a very effective alternative to the poorly working system we now have in health care, why it is not being more widely used, and how so many Americans can be malnourished when we have so much food available. Read these chapters to gain a thorough understanding of the philosophy behind this book.

Chapter 4, on the Core Program, is for everyone. It enumerates the basic optimal nutrition program, including foods and supplements. If you are one of the few fortunate healthy young active people who are not subject to pollution, drugs, tobacco, alcohol, stress, and weight-loss dieting, and you have no family tendencies toward certain diseases, then all you may need from this book is to finish the first four chapters. However, for most people, several other chapters will be quite useful as well.

Common ailments like heart disease, osteoporosis, kidney stones, and cancer can run in families. You have four grandparents, two parents, and any number of siblings. If two or more of these people have contracted the same disease, then you might consider yourself to be at high genetic risk for that ailment. In that case, you should read the chapter that identifies the nutritional risk factors of that disease and recommends nutritional preventive measures; such as using nutrients to help prevent cancer.

You may also be interested in treating a disease you already have. All of the most common killers and cripplers in America— heart disease, hypertension, cancer, diabetes, obesity, osteoporosis, arthritis, infectious diseases, allergies, and others—are discussed in this book. Also covered are the many other health ailments that are rarely fatal but can limit your enjoyment of life substantially: irritability, impotency, poor appetite, kidney stones, prostate problems, asthma, gum problems, constipation, indigestion, acne, etc.

The chapters are categorized by the systems of the body and the problems that can occur with each system. Thus, hypertension is listed with the circulatory system, impotency with the reproductive system, behavior and intellect with the nervous system, and so on. Aging and eating disorders do not affect any one specific system of the body, but due to their relevance to American health, they merit their own respective chapters.

The chapters also are arranged in the order of prevalence of diseases in America. That is, the most common diseases—problems with the circulatory system—are discussed first. Cancer (a disease of the immune system) is the next most common killer in America and is listed second, and so on. See the table of contents and the index for clues as to where to find your particular problem.

You may be very healthy *and* want to have a healthy baby. If so, see the chapter "Making Healthy Babies" (under the reproductive system). You may want to become a serious competitive athlete. To use nutrition to help you achieve that goal, see the chapter on the muscular system. A growing number of Americans are justifiably concerned about the hazardous amounts of pollution that we face in our environment, our water, and our food supply. Certain nutrients can provide some protection against these deadly pollutants—see the chapter on pollution for more details. Decide what your particular needs and interests are, then find the appropriate section of this book.

It is, of course, possible to have more than one disease or condition. For example, it is not uncommon for an individual to be obese, while also having hypertension and low energy levels, as well as regular infections. Each of these conditions has its own separate chapter. Since obesity is a major risk factor toward hypertension, a primary concern for this individual would be to deal with the weight problem, which may then correct both the hypertension and the low energy levels. If you have a variety of health problems, find the chapters that apply to them and then start with the chapter that appears first.

In some cases, which chapter to consult may not be obvious. Skin problems are often the result of allergies, so you may also need to look under allergies rather than the obvious chapter on skin. Hearing can begin to fade due to plugged-up arteries in the head and neck region. Hence, instead of going to the chapter on the sense organs for better hearing, go to the chapter on the circulatory system. Each chapter contains a variety of possible cross references to help you find the right chapter for you. Add or subtract from the Core Program the nutrients and foods that are recommended for your specific condition.

Chapter 4 contains a chart indicating the supplemental ranges for various vitamins and minerals. Whatever your health problems, keep your total nutrient intake within this range, *below the toxicity levels listed.* If, upon consulting several chapters on several conditions, you find that each recommends supplementation of one particular nutrient, don't just add up the dosages given and take that amount. First, check the supplemental ranges and make sure the amount you have calculated falls below the toxicity level. In fact, in many cases it's best simply to take the largest dosage listed for any of the chapters consulted.

Ideally, you should change your eating habits as the foundation for optimal nutrition. With that goal in mind, Chapter 5 contains a chart showing food sources of all of the nutrients mentioned in the book. However, the nutrient levels needed to treat many ailments are beyond the amount that could be obtained from a normal American diet. Therefore, supplements (in pill and powder forms) become essential for some people.

Again, please use this program in conjunction with, rather than instead of, your current medical program. Share this information with your physician. Most health care practitioners want their patients to get better. Anything that will achieve that desired goal is to be encouraged. *Healing Nutrients* can help many people.

This book is based on the best scientific data available, not wild guesses, hopes, or unfounded claims. Each recommendation has at least one good scientific study to back it up, and most recommendations are supported by several studies.

In some cases, the study involves the use of laboratory animals. Some people might ask: "What does a rat study have to do with me?" Quite a bit, actually. For obvious humanitarian reasons, one cannot implant a tumor in a group of humans and then test various nutrients to see what happens to the tumor growth. One cannot deprive a group of pregnant women various nutrients just to see what might happen to the developing fetus. But all of this is and can be done with laboratory animals. (This is not a callous disregard for animal rights, but rather a choice for the better of two evils.) Although humans may appear to be very different from laboratory animals, our biochemistry and anatomy are quite similar to those of certain animals. There are differences, to be sure, but much can be learned from using lab animals in experiments that would be cruel or impossible to conduct with humans. For instance, most lab animals have been bred with their siblings for successive generations to achieve a more homogenous genetic strain. This reduces the possibility that genetic variance will throw off the study. It would not, however, be feasible to have five generations of human brothers and sisters produce infants, just to reduce the genetic diversity factor for a scientific study. Also, it is difficult to get humans to maintain a constant lifestyle of diet, exercise, stress, and physical environment. Changes in any of these factors in human studies can throw off test results. Using lab animals, researchers can obtain important data in less time, under more controlled situations, and for less money than it would require if they used humans. Results from animal nutrition studies can be quite valuable to the study of human nutrition.

WHAT IS MY PHILOSOPHY ON NUTRITION?

Where do I stand on the many controversial issues that surround the field of nutrition? My opinions (based on an abundance of good research by highly skilled scientists) are as follows.

Your body and mind are built from, repaired by, and fueled by nutrients that are supplied in your diet. It quickly becomes obvious that what you eat can influence your overall health and vitality, both now and later on. Nutrition is a logical explanation for how you feel today and how long you will live.

Poor diet is a factor in many health woes in America. For many Americans, poor diet contributes to poor health; in some cases, poor diet is the *sole* cause of disease and early death. The diet of most Americans provides for survival levels of health. *Survival health* means that people spend much of their lives far below their genetic potential for health, energy, disease resistance, and even happiness. In many people, marginal nutrient intake levels eventually lead to the degenerative diseases that are all too common among older adults in this country. Few people come near that elusive optimal health. Although we live amid agricultural abundance, the basic problem with our dietary intake is *poor choices.* Most Americans would have more physical and mental energy, be sick less often, be more productive, and live longer if they used the optimal nutrition guidelines presented in this book.

Nutrition is not a cure-all. Nor is any other form of health care. As mentioned earlier, modern medicine is quite effective at keeping patients alive in emergency situations, like accidents, heart attacks, serious blood loss, etc. Yet medicine treats only the symptoms of most health problems, which leaves the actual condition to deteriorate. For instance, if a high-fat/low-fiber diet caused plugged-up arteries, then bypass surgery may temporarily relieve the symptom of angina pain, but the underlying condition will continue. When nutrition is used in a balanced program that also addresses exercise, attitude, physical environment, and body maintenance, optimal health can be gained. Though nutrition is a very effective treatment tool and should be a regularly used healing modality in America, it currently is not only ignored by the medical community but often ridiculed as being impotent. This is grossly unfair to the millions of sick Americans who could profit from the applied clinical nutrition found in this book.

Ideally, most adults could attain good health by using just foods. This would mean living the "Tarzan" lifestyle of eating lots of healthy foods, exercising that food into a lean fit body, while avoiding drugs, pollution, tobacco, alcohol, and stress. In 20th-century technological America, however, the "Tarzan" lifestyle is quite rare.

More realistically, most Americans could probably gain measurable health benefits from using a high-quality, broad-spectrum nutrition supplement. That supplement should contain nutrient levels that approximate the Recommended Daily Allowances (RDAs). The RDAs are valuable guidelines that will maintain "normal" health in the average person. However, people who are sick or very active, those who are exposed to pollution and stress, pregnant and lactating women, rapidly growing teenagers, and older adults may need more than the RDAs. These "abnormal" situations often call for nutrient intakes that are far above what "normal" people would need to maintain "normal" health.

The "normal" American has precious little to boast about. That person has six colds per year; wears glasses; is overweight; suffers from constant indigestion, lethargy, and depression; wears dentures by age 45; becomes marginally functional somewhere in his or her seventh decade, and dies in the eighth decade. Thus, in order to transcend the "normal" health levels targeted by the RDAs, we may need above-normal levels of nutrient intake.

Nutrition is a potent tool in preventing many illnesses, in curing some, and in supporting conventional medical practices. Nutrition could probably "cure" half of the 50 million Americans with hypertension. Nutritional support could make drugs and surgery both more effective and less risky.

For the past three or more decades, American soil has been fertilized with only three or four nutrients—just enough to make the plants grow well. This can be deceiving. While humans require about 50 essential nutrients, plants need only about 15 nutrients. Hence, a plant could care less whether selenium or chromium is in the soil. If these minerals are there, fine. If not, that is fine also. This means that our land needs broad-spectrum fertilization with all nutrients that *humans* need, not just enough fertilizer to grow the plant itself. This lack of proper fertilization is one of the causes of marginal nutrient intake, poor health, and the need for supplemental nutrition in the United States.

Food should always be the mainstay of any nutrition program. Food provides *all* of the 50 essential nutrients plus other nutrients that are as yet undiscovered. Most broad-spectrum supplements contain only a dozen or so nutrients. Relying on supplements as a nutrition mainstay will result in malnutrition. It is the combined effect of foods and supplements that will elevate the health of most people.

Synthetic vitamins are identical to "natural" vitamins. It is the chemical structure of the vitamin that is important, not the source. Synthetic vitamins may even be better for supplement use, because synthetic vitamins are less expensive, more condensed, and less likely to carry "accessory" factors that could provoke allergic reactions in certain sensitive individuals. However, minerals from food are often better absorbed than minerals from supplements; e.g., iron from meats and calcium from yogurt. There may also be unknown "accessory" factors that improve the efficiency of absorbing and using vitamins from food. Vitamin C from plant foods often has bioflavonoids to assist in absorption of vitamin C. The superiority of nutrients from food is just another reason why supplements should be of secondary importance in a nutrition program, with food as the solid foundation.

Nutrition is a gentle healer. Although clinical nutrition can be abused, it is *much* safer than the typical drugs-and-surgery approach commonly used in American medicine. The risk/benefit ratio of nutrition says that nutrition should at least be tried before the other more invasive and draconian methods of medicine are employed. This book explains ways in which up to half of the 50 million hypertensive people in this country could be cured and discontinue their medication. Drugs and surgery have their values and their place in the American health care system, yet both carry major risks. *Most* medication has significant side effects. Surgery is very dangerous, quite expensive, and requires long-term recovery periods. For decades, women with lumps in their breasts or abnormal growths in their uterus region have had radical surgery to remove the defective part. That surgery was dangerous, irreversible, and perhaps unnecessary. This book contains nutritional approaches that should be tried before the dangerous and expensive surgical procedures are employed. Rather than placing a hyperactive child on a speedlike drug for the remainder of his childhood, why not try an optimal eating program first? The drug for hyperactivity can cause lethargy, headaches, and even growth retardation and merely sedates the child while doing nothing about the actual problem. At the very worst, the nutrition program will make the child healthier. At the best, nutrition may solve the hyperactivity.

It is ironic to see the malice that the medical profession—the same group that has employed widespread hysterectomies, mastectomies, and open-heart surgery, much of which has been shown to be of questionable value in recent years—extends toward nutrition. Nutrition has few limitations and many benefits. The risk/benefit ratio of nutrition is far superior to most conventional medical approaches.

WHY IS NUTRITION SO SPARSELY USED AND SO WIDELY CRITICIZED IN AMERICAN HEALTH CARE?

Some people have suggested that there is a conspiracy against the use of nutrition in health care. I don't think so. It is more like a stubborn blockade that is resistant to change. Many people resist change, even when that change can improve their lives. Other people resist change when someone is trying to eliminate their jobs. That is understandable. But the ideas in this book would create new positions in health care. With some retraining, no one would be unemployed because of the use of nutrition and preventive medicine. With blatant proof that our health care system is not working, the obvious conclusion is that we must try some other avenue for disease control. Nutrition is readily available, well researched, inexpensive, inoffensive, and viable.

When "miracle" discoveries in the medical sciences began during the 1950s, much of the commonsense practical medicine was forgotten. Baby formulas were considered to be superior to mother's milk. Today, there are dozens of known biochemical reasons why mother's milk is vastly superior to formula. Refined food was thought to be an improvement over Mother Nature's products—another misconception, which has now been proven to be false. During the same period, drugs were invented that could influence nearly any chemical pathway in the body. Their effect was often dramatic and instant. In only a few decades of growth, the drug industry in America has become an $80 billion-per-year business. That is a lot of momentum to try to change.

Physicians, who are still the focal point of American health care, do not study nutrition. Hence, many doctors do not believe in nutrition, and those that do are somewhat at a loss about how to use nutrition in the healing arts. It has been said that "what doctors are not up on, they are down on." Nutrition is a classic example of that. Ironically, many people in both the medical and dietetic professions insist that nutritional supplements should be used only under a physician's guidance and prescription. In light of the minimal risks involved in using nutrition, that argument loses any impact. Additionally, since physicians don't study nutrition, how can they be considered the experts in prescribing nutrition to heal the patient? Many physicians are still taught that the four food groups provide all the nutrients needed by the human body and (here's the stunning part) that a meal at a fast-food restaurant supplies all of the four food groups. Ergo, with these fast-food restaurants doing so well, Americans must be well nourished. Not so.

Time lags, obstinate people, lack of nutrition education in the medical community, vested interests, and a host of other factors are all responsible for delaying the widespread use of nutrition in American healing. But change is coming. And you can be a part of that change. If enough people use this book, are helped by it, and become convinced of the value of nutrition, then the obstacles previously mentioned will quickly dissolve.

FOR WHOM IS THIS BOOK INTENDED?

Everyone. If you eat, then you have an interest in putting nourishing food into your mouth so that food can improve your health rather than limit it. If you are sick, then nutrition could be a gentle healer for your condition. If you are at risk for getting an ailment, then nutrition can help you to prevent that disease. For people who are healthy and want to stay that way, or who have "normal" health and would like to pursue "optimal" health, or who are sick and would like to get well, or who are concerned about family tendencies toward certain ailments, this book offers invaluable information to improve the quality and length of your life.

I am assuming a nominal level of intelligence in the reader. You do not need a college degree to understand this book. You do need some common sense and at least a high school level of knowledge and comprehension. For instance, when I mention that up to half of all hypertensive patients could be cured of their high blood pressure through *Healing Nutrients*, be aware that you could be among the other half who are not helped. In that case, get to a doctor. Some people have the mistaken notion that "if a little is good, then more is better." Not so. If a certain amount of potassium, calcium, and magnesium is recommended to bring down blood pressure, that does not mean that doubling the dosage will cure it in half the time. Hence, common sense is an important assumption.

This is not a textbook; there are no prerequisites to understanding it. *Healing Nutrients* is a layman's guide to better health through nutrition. I purposely avoided the arcane language of the scientist; grandiose medical terms are either avoided or explained. If written for scientists, this book would be a convenient collection. Yet it is written for lay people and hence could save countless lives, money, and unnecessary suffering. That is the ultimate goal of this book: to improve the overall health of the people.

Please follow the recommendations. You have already shown a good deal of intelligence by reading this far. You are aware that nutrition has something to do with health, and you would like to know more. You are to be commended for that intelligence and curiosity. Follow the guidelines listed at the end of each chapter, and *Healing Nutrients* will become a landmark book in the lives of you and your family.

WHY SHOULD YOU BELIEVE ME?

That is a valid question. Sometimes the alleged expert turns out to be someone making unfounded claims simply to help promote his or her products. If I had a vested interest in any vitamin firm, my reasons for recommending certain amounts of nutrients could be seriously questioned. Rest assured that neither I nor any of my family members have any vested interest in selling vitamins. I buy my own vitamins, even from the companies that I recommend.

Also, I have considerable formal training in the field of nutrition, with a bachelor's degree (University of Notre Dame and San Diego State University), master's degree (Northern Illinois University), and doctorate (Kensington University) in nutrition. I also have considerable work experience in nutrition. I am a registered dietitian, have an active private practice, have worked with the world-famous Scripps Clinic and the La Costa Spa, have taught undergraduate and graduate-level nutrition for the past eight years at four universities, have been a hospital dietitian, am co-editor of a monthly newsletter that provides continuing education to licensed health care professionals, have contributed a chapter to a medical textbook, have worked with the USDA, and have written many publications for both lay and professional people.

An even better reason to believe me is the painstaking effort that I have taken to find credible scientific references to support my statements. This book is not conjecture and brow stroking, but rather a collection of the latest scientific data on nutrition.

I sincerely believe that the contents of this book can improve the vitality, longevity, and enjoyment of your life.

1
THE PROBLEM
Our Current Health Care System Is Not Working

"Let thy food be thy medicine and thy medicine be thy food."
—Hippocrates,
Father of modern medicine, circa 400 B.C.

This book provides the solution to a problem. The problem is our current health care system—a dehumanizing, outdated system that rewards illness and treats symptoms rather than causes. The solution is nutrition: to provide the "life forces" with all the proper nutrients to build, fuel, and repair your body. By combining the best aspects of modern health care with *Healing Nutrients* and the other important lifestyle factors, you should live a vigorous life of 8 to 12 decades.

Not even the wildest imaginations of yesterday could envision the lives that we are living today. We have lasers for communication, powerful lap-top computers, home TV satellite dishes, nuclear power plants, and the capability to create new forms of life with genetic engineering. Medical science has also been changing rapidly. There are surgery techniques using microscopes and lasers, CAT scan devices that allow detailed examination of live humans, and life support systems that can stave off death almost indefinitely. Emergency medicine can patch up almost any wound or injury. Yet all is not well in Camelot. The life expectancy of a 65-year-old man today is the same as it was in 1900,[1] when cowboys still roamed the West and the only thing that flew in the air

13

was birds. Today, as over 87 years ago, a 65-year-old man can expect to live another 13 years. Why? Our health care system is a lumbering dinosaur. It is doomed to extinction due to its awesome expense and poor results.

The United States produces more Nobel laureates than any other nation on earth. We spend more on health care and scientific research than any other country. Yet there are many other countries with a longer life span, including Japan and the Netherlands. Many other countries have a better record of infant survival, including the less developed nations of Venezuela, Sri Lanka, Mexico, and the Phillipines.[2] While fewer than 1 out of 10 American infants are born at home, the nation with the best record of infant survival (the Netherlands) has 1 out of 3 infants born at home. The World Health Organization has called American medicine "invasive, controlling, and sometimes disabling".[3] Another physician accuses Western society of "digging our graves with our teeth," due to the incredible relationship between rampant 20th-century ailments and poor nutrition.[4]

Health care costs now total $450 billion annually, which is over 12 percent of our gross national product. By contrast, England and Japan spend only 3 percent of their gross national product on health care.[5] Japanese citizens have a longer average life span, while the life span of a British citizen is similar to that of a United States citizen. Why does it cost the United States four times as much to get poorer results? A professor at Dartmouth College has estimated that poor health in the United States adds $100 billion to the cost of our products and services. This makes it very difficult to compete in the world marketplace.

In the last two decades, hospital costs have risen by 700 percent in the United States.[6] In 1980, 1 out of 3 health insurance policies had "no deductible" as an added benefit, meaning that the policy holder paid nothing out of pocket. Today, only 1 out of 14 health insurance policies is written with such a liberal attitude. Consumers have long since given up on trying to pay their own medical expenses. Most employees demand some type of medical coverage as a key "perk" in their benefits package. Only 1 out of 7 people is without any health insurance.

Yet not even the multibillion-dollar insurance companies can afford the cost of health care. They have begun Preferred Provider Programs, Diagnostic Related Groups, and Health Maintenance

Organizations in attempts to contain costs. When local governments could no longer afford health care for their needy, a federal program called Medicare was introduced. Medicare and Medicaid are scheduled to be cut by $90 billion over the next five years.[7] Medicare could be bankrupt by the year 1990.

The modern hospital can make impressive efforts to sustain nearly any critical patient, but these heroic efforts are costly. Struggling premature infants cost about $3,300 per day to keep in intensive care, excluding physicians' fees. Kidney transplant patients are charged about $2,100 per day, with an average stay of 13 days. Coronary bypass surgery costs about $30,000, yet only temporarily relieves angina pain and adds nothing to life span.[8] The average patient with acquired immune deficiency syndrome (AIDS) accumulates health care costs of over $100,000 and almost inevitably dies within a year. On a per-weight basis, many drugs now cost the same as or more than gold.[9] One arthritis medication costs 4 times that of gold, and another costs 100 times that of gold. And nearly all drugs carry with them an extensive list of side effects, including nutrient interactions that worsen a patient's nutritional status.

All of these opulent expenses would be easier to tolerate if they were bringing us closer to a healthy population. They aren't. There are virtually no diseases that can be treated better today than they could be 30 years ago.[10] That includes such common killers as heart disease, cancer, and diabetes, as well as common cripplers such as arthritis and osteoporosis. In addition, a Harvard professor has compiled statistics to show that we have lost the war against cancer.[11] In spite of expensive and spectacular therapies, the cancer incidence and death rate continues to climb in America.

The data above are not meant to imply that we should pull the plug on these sick people or ignore them. But our system is working at the wrong end. We currently spend only 3 percent of federal health money on preventive public health measures, with 92 percent of the funds going to critical health care.[12] We need to spend more time, money, and expertise to prevent these catastrophes. Optimal nutrition offers us hope that we *can* prevent many of these ailments.

Not only is nutrition an excellent tool for preventing disease, but it can also heal or improve certain conditions. Instead of using drugs and surgery to remove the *symptoms,* nutrients can often clear up the problem itself. There are some cases when drugs and surgery are the definite treatment of choice. Yet, Dr. Eugene McCarthy, Director of the National Second Opinion Program, has estimated that two out of three surgeries could be avoided by using nonsurgical alternatives. Dr. Sidney Wolfe, Director of the Public Citizen Health Research Group, claims that at least $100 billion yearly is wasted on needless and dangerous medical procedures. And the Health Benefits Research Center has found that 51 percent of all hysterectomies were considered unnecessary by a second opinion. This book provides options for the risky and expensive methods of surgery and drugs.

Let's say that your car engine started making a loud noise, and a red light began flashing on the dashboard. You take the car to your mechanic, who says, "We'll wrap the engine with sound-proofing insulation and then put tape over that bothersome red light on the dashboard." Doesn't make sense, does it? In many cases, drugs and surgery do just that: treat the symptoms rather than the cause, leaving the condition free to deteriorate until it is beyond anyone's control. You can always buy a new car. You cannot buy a new body.

Healing Nutrients takes a different approach. Your body is an incredible coordinated effort of 60 trillion cells. The human organism is built from, fueled by, and repaired by the nutrients found in your diet. If something goes wrong, there is a good chance that nutrient supplies from the diet are not meeting nutrient needs in the body. Although medical science has made some significant advances and helped millions of people, 9 out of 10 deaths in America are due to degenerative diseases. Modern health care is largely an expensive and wasted effort against most of these conditions. A renowned physician has reported in the prestigious *New England Journal of Medicine* that current methods of curative medicine are not pragmatic but rather "dramatic, invasive, and expensive. . . ."[13]

Our domestic pets and rare zoo animals get the best of nutritional care. Read the contents on a package of dry dog food and notice the broad-spectrum vitamin and mineral supplementation that our pets get on a daily basis. Veterinarians know the irreplaceable value of proper nutrition. A sign in the world-famous San Diego Zoo warns people near the vending machines: "For human consumption only. Do not feed this to the animals, or they may get sick and die." The same refined food that millions of American children eat daily could deteriorate the health of a 400-pound ape. Some humans think that they can eat for sensory pleasure only and disregard the fact that all creatures on earth must get their essential nutrients from their diet. Rats cannot survive on white bread, which is the most commonly eaten food in America. In many biochemical ways, humans and other animals are quite similar: we are dependent on our food supply for the raw materials to fuel and repair the body.

We can no longer continue with our current health care system. The decadent cost combined with low health returns make our current approach unacceptable. What improvements are offered by using nutrition? Treating the cause, rather than just the symptoms. Preventing the problem, rather than wrestling with these formidable diseases once they are firmly implanted in the body. A longer and more vibrant life, rather than a decade of semiambulatory existence before death in the eighth decade. A more rational approach to healing. A less expensive and much less risky modality of health care. Personal involvement in your health rather than complete, naive reliance on others. Working with your personal biochemistry, rather than trying to jam warning signals. Nutrition has been scientifically proven to be a major preventive, supportive, and curative tool in health care. It only waits to be used.

2
THE SOLUTION
Nutrition Makes Sense

"It is what we think we know already that often prevents us from learning."   —Claude Bernard

Few of our current health predicaments—heart disease, hypertension, diabetes, cancer, arthritis, osteoporosis—were serious problems until the second half of the 20th century. Could 20th-century lifestyle be the cause of some of our health woes? Let's look at diabetes as an example.

Researchers in Australia wanted to see how diabetes relates to lifestyle. They selected 10 full-blooded adult male Aborigines who had adult-onset (type II) diabetes and asked them to return to the hunter/gatherer routine that they had practiced as youths in northwestern Australia.[1] All subjects were middle-aged and overweight. Seven weeks after returning to their native lifestyle, all had lost weight (an average of 16 pounds, in spite of making no effort to reduce), and all had markedly lowered their blood fats (serum triglycerides) and improved their glucose tolerance until their diabetes was basically "cured." This seemingly miraculous cure stemmed from returning to their native lifestyle and diet; no fancy medicine was involved. Regular activity, a low-fat diet (wild game is very low in fat), and large amounts of fresh plant food provided the "cure" that modern medicine couldn't.

Another group of scientists examined the diet of primitive hu-

18

mans by analyzing the remains of early human gathering grounds.[2] The foods that humans have evolved to thrive on are most likely to contain the nutrients that will keep us in good health. Therefore, knowing what early humans ate can give us a better idea of our "factory specification" diet. The "factory specification" diet for cows, for example, is grass, and for squirrels it is nuts. The health of these animals would deteriorate rapidly if they were fed milk, meat, or fish. Our "factory specification" diet gives us insight into the foods and nutrients that the human system needs.

Humans have been on the planet earth for the past 5 million years or so, and we cannot ignore the diet that got us this far. It is always best to use any instrument (including the human body or even a car) the way that it was built to be used. Hence, the "factory specification" diet is important in understanding how our 20th century diet has deviated from our native food pattern and may be responsible for our health dilemma. Food intake in the past 50 years is radically different from the diet of our first 5 million years. And today's lifestyle, including poor nutrition, is killing us.

Many millions of years ago, the earliest mammals ate insects. Shortly thereafter, plant foods, including roots, beans, nuts, tubers, fruits, flowers, and gums, were introduced into the diet. Five to seven million years ago, the earliest humans were primarily meat eaters, but the wild game that these early humans consumed was very low in fat (about 4 percent fat compared to 30 percent fat for today's domestic beef), contained about five times the level of polyunsaturated fats, and provided considerably more eicosapentaenoic acid (a.k.a. *EPA*, a fat that is very valuable in keeping blood vessels healthy and immune systems functioning). Seafood was introduced about 20,000 years ago. Then, about 5,000 years ago, when these hunter/gatherers settled down to farming, grains became popular. The primitive diet at this point had an overall polyunsaturated-to-saturated-fat ratio of about three to one. Ours is about one to three, which is a nine-fold deterioration in the "factory specification" for fat intake. These early humans consumed 16 times more potassium than sodium. We consume four times more sodium than potassium. That's a 6,400 percent deterioration in this critical balance of electrolytes. They consumed 1,500 mg of calcium per day, while most adults today consume one-third that amount. These primitives ate 10 times the vitamin C and three times the fiber that the average American consumes. With this "factory specification" diet in mind, it becomes more understandable why the unique 20th-century diet has brought with it epidemic proportions of ailments that were once rare.

Over the course of thousands of years, our ancestors adapted to a certain food intake pattern which contained a set of nutrients. Our ancestor's dietary intake might be considered our "factory specification" for keeping our bodies in decent health. This "caveman diet" is a guideline, but probably not an optimal diet. Hence, when we change the "factory spec" nutrient intake from 16 to 1 (potassium to sodium) to 1 to 4, we have invited serious health problems. That 16 to 1 potassium to sodium ratio may not be optimal, but it is definitely a rough guideline to follow. From our ancestor's diet, we learn general guidelines of nutrient intake. From 20th-century science, we learn how to "fine tune" the caveman diet into an optimal nutrition program.

A more recent example of "factory specification" diet comes from a study involving a group of herdsmen (called the Turkana) living in Kenya. For hundreds or perhaps thousands of years, these people have used the dairy products from their herds as their dietary staples. About 20 years ago, a splinter group from the Turkana left the main tribe and settled on the shores of a lake that abounded with fish. This splinter group began subsisting on fish, rather than their usual dairy products. Soon thereafter, many fish-eating Turkana developed a wide range of ailments that had been uncommon in their past, such as infections, warts, and diarrhea.[3] Although fish is, generally speaking, good food, it is not what these people evolved to thrive on. By deviating from their prescribed food intake, they created a host of new health problems.

Americans did not evolve to thrive on a continuous stream of refined sugar, hydrogenated fat, salt, pastries, bleached white flour, soda pop, and high-fat beef, yet these are true staples of the modern American diet. Humans evolved as active omnivorous grazers, primarily suited to a semivegetarian diet. We survived for millions of years because our diet provided extensive nutrients and minimal pollutants. In contrast, today we consume a highly refined, nutrient-depleted diet rich in animal fats, salt, additives, and sugar. When you consider the fact that we need even higher nutrient levels because of drugs, alcohol, tobacco, fad dieting, continuous stress levels, and exposure to frightening amounts of pollution, it is amazing that *more* people are not sick.

But you can do something about this health dilemma. Nutrition makes sense.

RISKS AND BENEFITS OF
DRUGS VERSUS NUTRIENTS

The concept of risk/benefit is central to this book. In any decision that you make in life, the risks are compared to the benefits. The risks of getting into an accident on the way to work are weighed against the benefits that you get from your job. You make a decision based upon the risk/benefit ratio. In medical science, these judgment calls do not come easily. Most surgical procedures and drugs carry with them an extensive list of hazards and side effects that must be measured against the possible benefits. Thus, most medical scientists and physicians have developed the habit of thoroughly scrutinizing proposed healing methods for possible dangers. Unfortunately, they bring the same preconceived notions of major risks into the analysis of using nutrients. "Sure," they say, "selenium might prevent cancer. But if it is that potent, then there must be some side effects. We need more time to evaluate the risks." This is like comparing darts to softballs. Children play with both, but it is much more likely that people will get hurt playing with darts than with softballs. Similarly, both drugs and nutrients have their place in the healing arts; but it is much more likely that people will get hurt using drugs than using nutrients.

The "powers that be" in the American health care system find it hard to believe that anything can be beneficial without doing any harm. They hesitate to accept the healing principles of nutrition, suspecting that there *must* be some risk in using nutrients.

Our health care system revolves around the $80-billion-per-year drug trade. All drugs have side effects, and many can be quite harmful or lethal in anything beyond the recommended dosage. As the dosage increases, most drugs have an "effective" level followed immediately by a toxic level. The fact that nutrients do not follow this paradigm is a key obstacle to the medical profession's and the Food and Drug Administration's acceptance of nutrition as a healing modality. The FDA cannot shift mental gears and understand how something can help the body without creating a serious hazard at a slightly higher level, as drugs do.

An example of this "if it doesn't hurt, then it can't help" idea took place in 1959, when Dr. Henry Turkel developed a nutritional supplement that he proved could help the symptoms and appearance of Down's syndrome victims.[4] Down's syndrome is an inherited genetic defect that is incurable and leaves the person with mental and physical retardation, yet the possibility of living a normal life span. Dr. Turkel filed a new drug application with the FDA on his discovery, calling it the "U" series, from the Greek word meaning to "normalize an abnormal situation." The FDA denied his drug application on the basis that his product had no toxicity level, even though it did work.

In order to be accepted for drug patent protection, a substance must have valid scientific data showing its effective *and* its lethal range. The "U" series of nutrients had no lethal range and therefore could not be considered for drug patent protection. Even when consuming thousands of times the recommended levels of intake for this product, the best researchers could do was to get the lab rats to vomit up the "U" formula. No other side effects were observed. The "U" series died an ignominious death, since few investors are willing to market a product that has no protection from competition, as is provided for unique drugs.

Obviously, the mentality of certain medical and government authorities must change before nutrients will be used widely to heal people in America. First, they must understand that nutrients are *not* drugs. In the last few decades, scientists *have* begun using nutrients to treat certain ailments, but this field has been called *nutritional pharmacology*,[5] which is misleading, because *pharmacology* refers to drugs. There is a major difference between drugs and nutrients. Drugs are usually chemicals that have been created in the laboratory and are completely foreign to the body's biochemistry. In contrast, nutrients are natural substances, which the body's "blueprints" of DNA need to build and maintain the human body. Nutrients are found in foods in varying levels and are essential for life. There is *no* biochemical need for drugs; in fact, the body only conditionally tolerates drugs. There *is* a need for nutrients. Drugs often work quickly and forcefully. Nutrients usually work slowly and subtly but are still effective. Drugs often jam or block certain chemical pathways in the body. Nutrients supply the raw materials to promote normal chemical pathways in the body. Drugs are often addictive and must be provided in escalating doses to get the same effect, since the body attempts to adjust to the drug. Nutrients are not addictive and need not be taken in increasing amounts over time to maintain the same effect. If taken in extremely high dosages for long periods of time, some nutrients (like vitamin C) can instill a high physiological need in the body. By slowly withdrawing the nutrient one avoids any possibility of untoward effects. Drugs usually have side effects and nearly always have a narrow range between a useful and a lethal dose. Food nutrients and supplemental nutrients (i.e., pills) rarely have any side effects. With respect to nutrients, there is a wide range between useful doses and harmful doses. (See Chapter 4 for the chart that shows useful versus harmful levels of nutrient intake.) While a 10-fold increase in the normal dosage of a prescribed medication could be fatal, a 10-fold increase in nutrient intake would probably either be beneficial or go completely unnoticed. Nutrients are rarely harmful and almost never fatal. If only drugs and surgery had the same track record!

Another issue that confounds the FDA regarding nutrients as healing agents is that, according to FDA reasoning, if nutrients do improve health, then they should be considered drugs, should be regulated by the FDA, and should be restricted to a physician's prescription. In the early 1970s, in the midst of the Watergate scandal, Congress attempted to pass legislation that would make it necessary to obtain a physician's prescription in order to purchase supplements that contained anything more than 150 percent the RDA of any nutrient. The problems involved in enforcing this law were immense. For instance, a person would need a prescription to buy a bag of carrots or a serving of liver, since these foods contain more than the RDA of several different nutrients. If someone wanted to defy this law, all he or she would need to do is to take several vitamin pills at once. At a time when the stability of our federal government was in peril, there was more mail on this issue than on the Watergate scandal. The American people were overwhelmingly in favor of defeating this bill. The whole idea was dropped, and the FDA has since considered nutrients a confusing issue. The FDA's mentality is: "If nutrients work, then they should be a prescribed drug. If they do not work, then who cares?" Neither stance is valid. Nutrient healing is in a class all by itself.

When the sedative thalidomide was offered to pregnant women in the early 1960s, it was thought to relieve some of the discomfort of pregnancy. A woman gynecologist in the U.S. fought the approval of the drug, and due to her efforts thalidomide was used much less widely in the U.S. than in Europe. Soon thereafter, it was found that thalidomide produced dramatic birth defects. There is no bodily need for thalidomide. There is a need for the B vitamin, folacin. Supplements of folacin have been shown to nearly eliminate certain types of birth defects with no risks whatsoever when taken by pregnant women. Yet somehow, scientists refer to the thalidomide disaster when they continuously post cautions about using supplements to treat or prevent ailments, especially during pregnancy. There is a major difference between giving an elective drug (thalidomide) and giving an essential nutrient (folacin) to a pregnant woman. As you will see in the chapter "Making Healthy Babies", there is good evidence to show that widespread use of multiple vitamin and mineral supplements for pregnant women would markedly improve the health of both mother and child with no risk whatsoever.

If you don't believe that nutrition has enormous potential benefits with very few risks, consider some facts about malpractice insurance. Insurance companies calculate the risk of selling insurance to those in a particular profession. The greater the chances that an insurance company will have to pay a claim against a policyholder, the higher the insurance premiums. Malpractice insurance for physicians averages about $20,000 per year. For chiropractors, it is $1,200 per year. And for registered dietitians it is $50 per year. According to these numbers, conventional medicine is roughly 400 times riskier than nutrition therapy. Yet many scientists still approach nutrients as though they were dispensing dangerous experimental drugs. For instance, there is substantial evidence to indicate that supplemental calcium could prevent hypertension, eclampsia (hypertension of pregnancy), osteoporosis, and colon cancer. There are no known risks in taking 1,500 milligrams of calcium daily, which would be enough to prevent many of those conditions, yet professors of nutrition at the University of Wisconsin have asserted, ". . . calcium must be viewed as an experimental drug."[6] One of these people is on the panel that designed the RDAs. Again, you cannot compare the risk/benefit paradigm of drugs and nutrients.

HOW DO NUTRIENTS
IMPROVE HEALTH SO EFFECTIVELY?

1. In some cases, nutrition therapy merely provides what you should have gotten from your diet but didn't. If you have normal nutrient needs, proper nutrition may cure your disease by providing your body with the raw materials (essential nutrients) that you are currently not getting from your food intake.

2. Nutrition can also prevent future disease by elevating you out of a long-term state of subclinical deficiency into a healthy saturation state for all nutrients. In other words, while you may not be obviously ill now, you may be suffering a nutrient deficiency that will cause you problems later. Subclinical deficiencies are difficult to detect, as compared to clinical deficiencies such as scurvy and rickets. Avoiding these long-term subclinical deficiencies can prevent both infectious and degenerative diseases.

3. You also could be one of those people whose nutrient requirements are far above what could be obtained from a good diet. Genetic defects, stress, pollution, age, superactivity, pregnancy, and other factors can elevate your nutrient needs.

4. Certain nutrients, when taken in high doses, develop new "supernutrient" powers. For instance, 20 mg of niacin per day (the RDA) will keep most people reasonably healthy and maintain proper energy release. But take anywhere from 5 to 150 times that amount, and niacin also becomes an effective dilator of blood vessels.[7] These large doses of niacin improve the levels of fats in the blood so impressively that niacin can help to prevent recurring heart attacks in people who have heart disease and help to prevent plugged-up arteries in people with a genetic vulnerability to that condition.[8] High doses of vitamin A help to gird the body against the destructive (but potentially helpful) effect of chemotherapy. As another example, high doses of vitamin E reduce breast tenderness in premenstrual syndrome patients and also thin out the blood to improve circulation in a variety of conditions. And high doses of zinc bolster immune function and wound healing. Thus, "normal" amounts of these nutrients help to maintain "normal" health, while above-normal amounts develop supernutrient abilities and help to treat abnormal situations.

5. Nutritional support can increase the effectiveness of drugs, surgery, cancer therapy, and other techniques. Many conventional medical techniques are less effective than they could be because these aggressive procedures create stress in the body and elevate nutrient needs at a time when the patient is less likely to eat well. Malnutrition then reduces the benefit of the therapy and retards healing while increasing the risk of complications. Optimal nutrition allows the patient's own natural healing forces to assist in the medical treatment.

6. Finally, optimal nutrition raises many people above "normal" health into a far more desirable level of physical and mental vigor. Instead of just getting along, they get along well.

When researchers fed "normal" levels of vitamin C and folacin to pregnant guinea pigs, they produced normal litters of pups. When more vitamin C and more folacin were added to the diet of the pregnant guinea pigs, there were fewer aborted fetuses, more pups per litter, and larger pups.[9] Above-normal nutrient intake yielded above-normal success in pregnancy. A variety of studies in the chapter "Making Healthy Babies" show that this principle applies to humans as well. How intelligent, strong, fast, durable, disease resistant, and emotionally tranquil can we be? Whatever these vague and undefined optimal limits are, you can be sure that we have not achieved them yet.

NUTRIENT NEEDS:
AN INDIVIDUAL MATTER

It is important to understand at this point that each individual has different needs for the 50 essential nutrients. In fact, a single individual's needs will vary during his or her lifetime. Think of your body as having a reservoir for each nutrient. In some life situations (e.g., pregnancy, stress, and wound recovery), the reservoir is drained more quickly than usual. Optimal nutrition makes sure that each nutrient reservoir in the body is filled, in order to provide tissue saturation for all of the needed raw materials.

Stress increases the need for the amino acid tyrosine and the vitamins C and pantothenic acid. Stressed animals respond to tyrosine supplements with improved behavior,[10] but tyrosine supplements have little value to nonstressed animals. Hence, stress empties certain nutrient reservoirs more quickly than lack of stress.

Infection and wound healing can markedly increase the need for vitamin C and zinc. Sick people are able to tolerate up to four times the amount of vitamin C that normal healthy people can tolerate before diarrhea sets in.[11]

There are other examples when above-RDA nutrient levels may be needed. For instance, the RDA for vitamin B_6 for lactating mothers is 2.5 mg daily. Yet a study done at Purdue University found that mothers had to consume 20 milligrams of B_6 (eight times the RDA) before enough B_6 was in their milk to properly nourish their babies.[12]

Sometimes, these elevated nutrient needs cannot be satisfied merely with food. Supplements can help keep the nutrient reservoirs full, which then lowers the effects of stress, pregnancy, wound recovery, and other abnormal states.

As mentioned above, some people are born with a higher need for certain nutrients.[13] An undetermined percentage of the population is born with errors in metabolism that increase their need for nutrients beyond what can be supplied by the best of diets.[14] According to the prestigious panel that wrote the RDAs, at least 2½ percent of the American population (or about 6 million people) would be deficient in each one of the essential nutrients, even if they were consuming 100 percent of the RDA.[15] Through statistical probability, we can calculate from our 6 million people per nutrient that are deficient, that about 30 million Americans would be deficient in at least one of the 50 essential nutrients. This means that, even if all of us were consuming 100 percent of the RDA for all the essential nutrients, 30 million Americans would still be deficient in one or more nutrients. Genetically endowed higher nutrient needs (a.k.a. *genetotrophic diseases*) are one reason why nutrition therapy is essential to treating certain individuals.

Since Nobel laureate Dr. Linus Pauling first published his theories on "orthomolecular" nutrition, many other studies have found his "chin stroking" to be true. The theory is that some people have inherited a biochemistry that requires very high nutrient intake.[16] Without that high nutrient intake, sickness of mind and/or body sets in.

Schizophrenia is an example of a disease that has been linked to unmet, elevated nutrient needs. In one study, a group of schizophrenics were found to have abnormal metabolism of vitamin C.[17] In another classic case, Mark Vonnegut, son of novelist Kurt

Vonnegut, experienced debilitating schizophrenia until Carl Pfeiffer, M.D., Ph.D., found he had an unusually high need for certain ingredients, including protein, vitamin B_6, and zinc. Only weeks after Mark began following a nutrition program, his condition improved dramatically. He later graduated from Harvard University medical school and is now a practicing physician.

THE LONG-TERM EFFECTS OF MARGINAL NUTRITION

Blatantly bad nutrition brings about serious (clinical) symptoms quickly. Yet, more commonly in America, it is our marginal diet that encourages subclinical deficiencies—deficiencies that do not really surface as a diagnosed problem until years have passed. We know this to be true of osteoporosis, cancer, and heart disease. A person with no symptoms yet abnormally high serum cholesterol is at risk for eventually developing heart disease. A person with no symptoms but abnormally high platelet aggregation (stickiness of blood cells) is at great risk for suffering a stroke or some other circulatory disorder. A person with a low selenium or vitamin A level in the blood is at greater risk for contracting cancer.

What people eat today may not affect them drastically today, but it will likely come home to roost in the future. This is another explanation for the effectiveness of healing nutrients. Cumulative poor nutrition creates diseases that are not recognized as nutrition-related disorders. But they are.

Even if symptoms are not immediately present, subtle problems become monumental problems if allowed to continue for years or decades. Long-term subclinical deficiencies of vitamin C are known to produce anything from heart disease to gallstones.[18] Since a large number of Americans are consuming less than the RDA for vitamin C (60 milligrams) and far below tissue saturation levels (at least 200 milligrams), long-term subclinical deficiencies of vitamin C could be responsible for a wide array of diseases in older Americans. As another example, long-term subclinical deficiencies of chromium may bring about heart disease and poor glucose tolerance in later life.

For instance, the average intake of vitamin E in this country is 12 international units (i.u.).[19] The RDA for vitamin E used to be 30 i.u., but was lowered to 15 i.u. since no blatant deficiency diseases could be found in the general public. Yet, heart disease, lung damage from air pollution, cancer, premenstrual syndrome, and premature senility have been on the rise for several decades. There is abundant evidence that vitamin E helps to prevent each of these conditions. Long-term subclinical deficiencies of vitamin E among Americans probably surface as common diseases (such as heart disease, cancer, senility, allergies, cataracts, PMS, and premature aging) rather than a neat and concise vitamin deficiency disease. Early work in nutrition showed that a nutrient deficiency caused a specific problem, such as thiamine* deficiency leads to beriberi. Most nutrients do not have their own personal deficiency condition, such as beriberi, but instead surface as a variety of seemingly unrelated diseases.

HOW MUCH EVIDENCE IS ENOUGH?

How much proof is necessary to convince the science and lay communities of the value of nutrition? Chronic disease has often been linked to poor nutrition, yet carping intellectuals continually point out pedantic limitations in the research. Meanwhile, innocent people suffer and die needlessly because some people refuse to admit that they have been wrong about nutrition.

A Harvard professor says that most "facts" today are actually only accepted theories.[20] Although evolution is still only a theory, it is accepted as fact by most scientists. What will it take to prove irrefutably the value of nutrition? How much evidence is enough? Many scientists are looking for an extreme degree of proof before they move themselves into the nutrition camp. A crime does not need to be committed in front of a crowd at Yankee Stadium in order to obtain a conviction, but that is what the medical community seems to be demanding in the way of proof that nutrition has healing and preventive powers.

Let's look at one case in which the evidence of nutrition's efficacy gradually mounted up. Autism is an incurable mental aberration that is usually detected in a child when he or she is quite young, is usually found in males, and causes the child to withdraw from the outside world. One mother whose son was diagnosed as autistic was, understandably, quite distraught and sought help

*Thiamine may also be spelled "thiamin"

from various doctors and clinics. She got nowhere, so she began reading in earnest on the subject. She tried every treatment she could find, even the most bizarre. She found that her son's condition improved somewhat after she gave him large doses of vitamin B_6. This is considered *anecdotal evidence*. She then wrote to a famous author and researcher on the subject of autism, telling him of her discovery. The researcher, being open-minded and personally involved in autism, kept the letter. More letters from mothers began to filter in to this researcher with the same report: that large doses of vitamin B_6 significantly improve the symptoms of (but do not cure) autism. When enough letters arrived, the researcher began to wonder about the potential value of this treatment. Since he is a trained professional, this gathering of anecdotal evidence under his scrutiny could now be considered *clinical observations*. The evidence was getting stronger. He then obtained research money and designed a double-blind experiment (in which neither the subjects nor the researchers giving out the pills knew who was getting the tested substance) using humans to test the theory. Vitamin B_6 worked. The researcher now had a controlled *scientific experiment* to support the use of B_6 to treat autism. Now the evidence was very strong. This is an actual example of how the separate effort of many mothers gradually evolved into a well-documented treatment that was published in a scientific journal.[21]

Some scientists would then demand to do it all again, or have *reproducible evidence*. Yet half of the papers published in even the prestigious *New England Journal of Medicine* are merely anecdotal case studies.[22] It seems that anecdotal evidence is adequate for many physicians and scientists, but only if the viewpoint expressed is compatible with theirs. They do not provide or demand reproducible and irrefutable evidence for many of the treatments that they use. Yet one out of five people in American hospitals gets an infection while in the hospital (called *nosocomial*, or hospital-induced) and somewhere around 300,000 deaths per year (estimates vary considerably) in America may be iatrogenic, or caused by a physician's treatment. In several instances, physicians and hospitals were chagrined when a doctors' strike resulted in much lower death rates in their area.

The conclusion? Given the risk/benefit ratio of conventional medicine versus nutrition, nutrition is vastly preferable if it has any chance of being effective for a given condition. Since they are not trained in nutrition, many physicians express little more than sarcasm for nutrition. Since most government authorities who set the rules and pay the Medicare bills are strongly influenced by the medical community, they too deny the value of employing nutrition in the health care system.

With the great genetic diversity of the human species and the incredible biochemical individuality that has been found, scientists are lucky to be able to "prove" anything while using human subjects. Allergy specialists practice such widely diverse techniques that it is hard to believe they are all in the same field. And there are precious few reproducible double-blind experiments proving the safety and efficacy of many drugs, elective surgery procedures, psychiatric approaches, and other "mainstays" of modern medicine. Still, many scientists want to avoid making any recommendations involving nutrition until all possibility of error is excluded.[23]

We may all be dead by then.

Each recommendation in this book is supported by at least one valid scientific study, with some recommendations based on several studies. A great deal of meticulous library and computer research was conducted to gather all of the available scientific data from credible journals and to reference each major statement. People who are looking for irrefutable, double-blind, reproducible scientific evidence from large-scale human studies for all statements made may have to wait another few decades. Given the potential benefits and the minimal risks of nutrition, waiting may be foolish.

RISKS OF USING NUTRITIONAL THERAPY

There are risks in using nutritional supplements, but they are slim ones. For example, excessive mineral intake can create an imbalance. Excessive intake of vitamins A, D, and the mineral selenium can be toxic. Check the chart in Chapter 4 for specific amounts that are toxic.

Supplements also can foster an attitude of pill dependence, and some people who take inordinately high amounts of vitamins can develop high needs (physiological dependence) so that ceasing nutrient intake could create a rebound deficiency. Other individuals use supplements as an excuse to avoid necessary medical attention. It is also possible to waste money on overpriced or poorly designed supplements. Finally, some people can have an adverse reaction to the fillers and excipients used in vitamin manufacturing. All of these are, however, extreme cases.

No sane pharmacist would dispense cortisone (a drug used to reduce inflammation, among other purposes) to everyone, since few people would benefit and many would be harmed. Yet a well-designed, broad-spectrum vitamin and mineral supplement would help most Americans and hurt none. Again, there is a big difference in the risk/benefit ratio of drugs and nutrients.

NUTRIENTS ARE OFTEN MORE EFFECTIVE THAN DRUGS

Not only are nutrients less toxic than most drugs, but often they are also more effective. Throughout this book, you will find many examples of nutrients that are more effective than the expensive and dangerous drug alternatives. I briefly mentioned some examples earlier, and here is just a hint of what you will find in chapters to come:

- Postoperative patients who did not receive vitamin E and calcium supplements had 200 percent more blood clots in the legs, 600 percent more cases of blood clots in the vessels of the lungs (pulmonary embolisms), and 900 percent more fatalities from pulmonary embolism than the patients who did receive vitamin E and calcium.[24] No drug can match such a benefit to postoperative patients.
- Although numerous multinational drug companies are in the chase for a "cure" for heart disease, nutrients that come close to being a "cure" already are available. Large doses of niacin were found to reduce serum cholesterol by 22 percent and triglycerides by 52 percent. The researchers were so impressed that they commented, "To our knowledge, no other single agent has such potential for lowering both cholesterol and triglycerides."[25] EPA, garlic, and other nutritional approaches to heart disease are more effective than potent prescription drugs, with a near-zero risk.
- Nearly 10 percent of all people who receive blood transfusions from anonymous donors end up with hepatitis, which is a serious crippler of the liver. While no drug can control these

viral infections, large intravenous doses of vitamin C (7 grams daily) were able to almost completely eliminate hepatitis incidence in a controlled study.[26]

- Potassium, calcium, magnesium, and the essential fatty acid (linoleic acid) can each individually lower blood pressure more safely and effectively than the most potent prescription drugs for hypertension.
- Gingerroot is more effective in treating motion sickness than the favorite prescription drug.[27]
- Vitamin B_6 cures carpal tunnel syndrome (a tingling sensation in the hand) in 27 out of 28 patients tested in double-blind fashion.[28] Medicine's answer to this problem is surgery.
- Folacin prevents neural tube defects in infants.
- Vitamin A mops up destructive free radicals more effectively than any prescription drug made.
- The amino acid tryptophan has been shown to treat insomnia without side effects, even when potent prescription drugs failed.[29]
- EPA fish oil reduces tissue swelling, such as occurs in arthritis, more effectively than prescription drugs in some people and without any side effects such as occur with long-term use of cortisone.
- Premenstrual syndrome can often be treated effectively with broad-spectrum nutrition. The alternative for the PMS victim is to take potent hormones, like estrogen and progesterone, or to submit to serious sedatives.

The list goes on, as you'll discover in the rest of this book.

WHY AREN'T HEALING NUTRIENTS MORE WIDELY USED?

Simply stated, nutritional therapy is different, and change is difficult for people. When New England missionaries moved to Hawaii in the 19th century, they continued their custom of bringing out their long wool underwear every October. To these people, change was more uncomfortable than wearing wool underwear in a tropical climate.

Proven new concepts always take years or decades to implement. Although Europeans had been eating tomatoes for centuries, it was not until the early 20th century that Americans considered tomatoes a food, rather than a poison.[30] In the late 19th century, one New England fellow ate several tomatoes on the town courthouse steps in order to encourage tomato consumption. Still no one would eat tomatoes. Explorers of the 17th century brought the potato to Europe from its native Andean highlands. Royalty was disgusted. Scientists reviewed the matter thoroughly and finally pronounced potatoes to be adequate for animal feed, even though these people were told that an advanced civilization in South America had thrived on potatoes for centuries. In the earlier part of this century, gold and aspirin were effective and accepted treatments for arthritis. Then someone pronounced arthritis to be an infectious disease, which obviously ruled out gold and aspirin as acceptable treatments, even though they were effective. This nonsense continued for decades until just recently, when both treatments were reaccepted. Two thousand years after the Greek astronomer Eudoxus discovered that the sun was at the center of our solar system, that "fact" was finally accepted. Fifty years after an English physician discovered that limes cured and prevented scurvy, the English navy mandated the carrying of limes aboard ships. Twenty years after niacin was proven to treat pellagra, it was finally accepted as *the* treatment. Dr. Goldberger, who discovered that pellagra was a nutritional and not an infectious problem, even swallowed a capsule full of sputum from a pellagra victim to prove to his peers that pellagra was not contagious. Still no one was convinced.

Change is painful and stressful for many people, probably in part because it requires us to admit that we were wrong in the past.

If a cure existed for your health problem, how long would you like to wait before having access to it, especially if the risks were almost nonexistent and the potential benefits great? *This book is composed of scientifically proven facts about nutritional therapy.* They may not be totally accepted by the conservative core of the scientific community yet. But tobacco kills, niacin cures pellagra, the earth revolves around the sun, potatoes and tomatoes are quite edible foods, and healing nutrients work.

Another obstacle to incorporating nutrition therapy into our health care system is the painful transition period the system will have to undergo. Doctors, hospitals, pharmacies, drug companies, and other core members of the health community would have to reorient themselves to using new therapies. Granted, some professions would be lost. But others would be gained. The net result would not be unemployment, but some retraining.

After World War II, both Japan and Germany were banned from having an armed force. Economists say that a capitalistic society basically focuses its efforts toward making either "guns" (meaning defense military spending) or "butter" (meaning items for lay consumption, like computers, medicines, and services). With no alternative, Japan and Germany entered the world market as makers of "butter." Over the past three decades, the United States has gradually become a major manufacturer of "guns." The government spends nearly $400 billion per year on defense, and our system seems to be committed in this direction. In order to change over to "butter" production, some people would have to be retrained, some jobs would be lost, other positions would be gained, and a painful growing experience would have to take place. But, as witnessed by the affluence that Japan and Germany have enjoyed, a country can be successful at making "butter."

Our health care system is in a similar bind. We are in a self-perpetuating rut that may be difficult to escape. We have spent most of our time, money, and talent dealing with sickness. And certain vested interests don't *want* that to change. Since nutrients cannot be patented like drugs, the profit picture for nutrients is much less enticing than for drugs. Currently, the hospital, physician, and pharmacist will be reimbursed for most procedures done to a patient, regardless of the prognosis for the patient or the danger of the procedure used. Yet it is difficult for a registered dietitian to get paid by Medicare or private insurance carriers to do even the most basic nutritional consultation on a patient. Private and government health insurance will pay $20,000 and up for an operation with few hesitations. In contrast, it is nearly impossible for a nutritionist to get paid to do a basic evaluation of that surgical patient so that complications and risks can be avoided. A dietitian with a master's degree earns less money than a dockworker, garbage collector, or supermarket clerk. The nutritionist is given little respect, authority, credibility, or pay in American health care. So doctors, hospitals, drug companies, and many other participants all benefit from sickness. We have spent almost no time or effort attempting to bring about wellness. A move from sickness to wellness would be a painful but most rewarding shift in the health care system in America, and nutrition would be a primary component of that shift. Due to the major changes in money, jobs, and authority that would be necessary, I do not foresee that shift occurring in the immediate future—unless enough people, like you, demand that it happen.

A final, and very difficult, obstacle to nutrition's incorporation into American health care is the medical community's long-standing resistance to change. That is, to some extent, understandable. The specter of quackery has always loomed large over physicians. And the Hippocratic oath binds doctors to "abstain from all intentional wrongdoing and harm," so it is not surprising that they feel they must exercise extreme caution in treating their patients, especially with a new form of therapy. But that does not excuse the medical community from drifting toward a position of self-protection that has become an impediment to improved health care. A professor from the University of Chicago accuses the medical community of being harsher on the irregular physician than the inept physician.[31] Neither is encouraged, but a maverick doctor runs a greater risk of license revocation than an incompetent one. How can we progress unless we are willing to accept something different? Nutrition *is* different, but it works. Yet physicians who admit to including nutrition in their medical practices are charged as much as 50 percent extra in their malpractice insurance premiums. The fear of quackery is unfounded here. Although nutrition quackery was widely practiced in the early part of this century, today there are thousands of scientific studies proving the healing value of nutrition.

Until scientists, physicians, politicians, dietitians, and others can alter their thinking on the relative risks of drugs versus nutrients, healing nutrients will be relegated to a minor role in health care. But the inevitable change is coming. When? Based on public and professional moods, the time could be soon. The general public no longer blindly accepts conventional medicine as it once did. And neither the government nor private insurance carriers can afford our current health care system. Major financial cuts and structural changes are already under way. Most health care practitioners are becoming increasingly disenchanted with the poor results that they get by using the healing methods that they have been taught. All of these forces indicate that a change is imminent and that the people would be receptive to a change in our health care system *now*.

THE INTERDISCIPLINARY APPROACH TO HEALTH

Nutrition is an important factor in determining how well and how long you will live. But it is not the only factor. Long ago, psychologists, exercise physiologists, physicians, pharmacists, and nutritionists each thought that their subject was the only worthwhile one. Today, these health care professionals are beginning to make a cooperative effort. Wellness (a.k.a. *preventive medicine, interdisciplinary health, multifactoral health*, or *holistic health*) takes a multifaceted approach to your health. These are the forces that shape your health and longevity:

GENETICS

Father's sperm and mother's egg each carry genetic material (DNA) that will dictate many of your features. Skin color, eye color, and genetic diseases are nonnegotiable and inflexible traits. Many other features, such as intellect, emotions, disease resistance, talent, and stature, are based on both a genetic framework and the other five factors mentioned below. You must have at least decent genes, or you would not be alive and reading this. But you probably do have some genetic vulnerabilities, and you need to be wary of them, like a ship steering clear of a rocky shore. You cannot move that dangerous shoreline, but knowing it's there can help you avoid it.

For example, Jim Fixx was the guru of the running world for nearly a decade. When Jim was 36 years old, he was an obese, chain-smoking, highly stressed executive. His father had died at age 36 of a heart attack, and Jim realized that his genes were vulnerable to heart disease and that his lifestyle was doing nothing to stop the onset of vascular problems. He quit smoking, found a less stressful position, improved his diet, and started running. Although he died of a heart attack at age 52 while running, his shift in lifestyle had added 16 years to his life beyond his father's life span. If Jim had changed his lifestyle earlier, he could have added even more years to his life.

If diabetes, cancer, arthritis, or other common ailments run in your family, then do something about that vulnerability now, before you are face to face with the disease. Proper use of nutrition, exercise, and attitude can lower your risk of contracting many diseases.

EXERCISE

Humans evolved as active creatures, but we are now primarily sedentary. This change has greatly eroded our health. Scientists have shown that the "dis-eases" of old age may be caused by the "dis-use" of the body.[32] Regular exercise lowers blood pressure, fats in the blood, and pulse rate, while improving blood glucose, kidney function, absorption of nutrients, and life span.

Not only does exercise help the body, but it is probably *the* simplest and most effective healing therapy for the mind. Scientists find that regular exercise lowers depression, stimulates intellect, improves self-image, and stimulates alertness, among other beneficial effects.[33] Exercise allows people to eat more without having weight problems, improves the function of the gastrointestinal tract, and has other interplays with nutrition. Exercise improves your attitude toward life, so it relates both directly and indirectly to health.

ATTITUDE

Your mind is a potent determinant of the quality and quantity of your life. Social networking, or the extent of your friends and relationships, is a major predictor of life span.[34] In other words, loneliness kills. Researchers have a hard time separating the actual effects of a drug or nutrient from the *belief* that it should help that person. This "placebo" effect can cause up to half of the people receiving inert sugar pills to experience the same benefit as the person who receives the active ingredient.[35] Investigators even found that, given identical hospital talent and equipment, the patients who were confined to a hospital with a friendly and communicative staff environment had a much lower death rate than those who were not.[36]

The burgeoning field of "psychoneuroimmunology" has well documented the relationship between your attitude and your disease resistance.[37] Your mind (psyche) influences your nervous system (neuro), which directly affects your level of disease resistance (immunology). Priests, shamans, and mystics have used this concept for thousands of years. Now, overwhelming scientific evidence proves that your thoughts can directly affect your health, your disease resistance, the accumulation of fats in your blood, and your life span. And there are other connections between attitude and health:[38]

- Women's cancer survival after 5 years was found to be related to their psychological reaction to their diagnosis.
- A 17-year study involving over 2,000 men found that depression doubles the risk for death from cancer.
- Military cadets under great stress were more likely to get mononucleosis.
- Rheumatoid arthritis in women often followed a stressful period in their lives.

Your attitude also influences whether you will make exercise fun and whether you are amenable to changing your diet.

As mentioned earlier, psychological stress can increase your need for certain nutrients. Nutrition can influence emotions, intellect, and behavior. The mind plays a strong role in what you eat, how often, how much, how quickly, and in what mood. Attitude, like exercise, relates both directly and indirectly to your overall health and longevity.

PHYSICAL ENVIRONMENT

Until this century, the primary cause of human death was infectious disease, which is caused by microbes from the surrounding physical environment. Half of the known world was killed in the bubonic plague of the 14th century. Thanks to improved hygiene and inoculation programs, epidemics no longer inflict such mortality.

Yet our environment is now infiltrated with other hazards, primarily from 20th-century pollution. And exercising in polluted air can bring in even more pollutants than sedentary people would encounter. Sunlight, electromagnetic radiation (from computer screens, color television, FM transmitting towers, high-voltage power lines, etc.), smog, noise, bacteria, viruses, pollutants, and other factors in our environment can seriously affect your health. Chapter 16 in this book specifically addresses how nutrients can help protect you from the dangers of our polluted environment. Breathing in asbestos particles would be disastrous, regardless of how much protective nutrition you use, but in some cases optimal nutrition can buffer the effects of pollution on the body. For instance, optimal selenium intake can reduce the amount of lead that your body absorbs from polluted air. Aluminum accumulation may cause Alzheimer's disease in some people while fluoride intake reduces aluminum absorption. Many pollutants are carcinogenic, yet certain nutrients can lower this cancer risk. *Anything* that gets to you from your surrounding environment can strongly influence your health.

BODY MAINTENANCE

Teeth, gums, back, feet, skin, eyes, ears, hair, and other bodily parts need proper care. Abuse or neglect of the body may not shorten life, but it will make some people wish that their life *was* shorter. By exercising with supportive footwear, you get the benefit of the exercise without the risks of ruining your feet, ankles, knees, and back. Although tryptophan has been used to treat certain types of pain, if the back pain is a result of a worn-out bed, or poor posture, or lack of muscle tone in the back region, then tryptophan will be of little value. Nutrients can help to keep your skin, hair, and nails in attractive, healthy condition. Proper body maintenance, like the use of mild shampoos, gentle brushes, etc., can further enhance your health.

NUTRITION

Your body is, in the most literal sense, a product of your nutrient intake. The rest of this book shall be spent emphasizing this point.

All of these factors relate to your health and each interrelates to the others. Proper nourishment improves your ability to think and exercise, while regular exercise improves digestion and attitude. The big package of interdisciplinary health has the potential to bring a long and zesty life to most people. Keep in mind that nutrition is just one part of the package. Using nutrition therapy alone will not solve most problems. If you live in a polluted environment; or if you smoke; or if you don't like yourself, your neighbors, or your job; and you are sedentary, then following this book to the letter will still leave you far short of good health.

THE BOTTOM LINE

In spite of megabillions of dollars spent, degenerative diseases are still on the increase in America. They shouldn't be. Using proper nutrition, many of these diseases are preventable, and some are curable. Let's look at an example.

Although about one million Americans die annually from cardiovascular diseases (heart disease and high blood pressure), the *actual* cause of death would more accurately be stated as one or more of the following:

- *Diet* (high intake of fat, sodium, and cholesterol and/or low intake of fiber, vitamin C, vitamin E, vitamin B$_6$, calcium, magnesium, selenium, and chromium)
- *Sedentary lifestyle* (very little movement)
- *Stress* (too much tension, worry, depression)
- *Pollution* (including environmental toxins such as smog, pesticides, and industrial wastes found in water and food; also includes voluntarily induced pollutants such as tobacco, drugs, and alcohol)

With this in mind, my estimates of the actual causes of death in America are somewhat different from widely available statistics. My reasoning is based on some well-known facts. For instance, the Environmental Protection Agency estimates that up to 20 percent of all deaths in America are due to pollutants and environmental hazards.[39] It is also well accepted that poor diet is a major risk factor in heart disease and cancer, our nation's primary killers (see the chapters on those diseases for documentation of this and for more information). In addition, loneliness, depression, and tense behavior all contribute to heart disease, cancer, and early death. Based on all the data I have collected, I have arrived at these estimates of the actual causes of death and disease in America:

- *Stress level and attitude—25%*
- *Nutrition related—25%*
- *Pollution—11%*

- *Poor hygiene and poor medical care—10%*
- *Sedentary lifestyle—10%*
- *Infectious diseases—3%*
- *Genetic—3%*
- *Accidents—2%*
- *Others—11%*

As you can see, nutrition is a primary component in interdisciplinary health. Keep in mind all of these factors and use the whole picture of interdisciplinary health to increase your chances for a long and vigorous life!

3
MALNUTRITION
IN AMERICA

". . . for purple mountains majesty, above the fruited plains."
—from the song, "America"

For millions of years, all creatures on earth have spent most of their waking hours in search of food. Not for variety or flavor do they eat, but for mere survival. Only a few civilizations in human history have transcended this hand-to-mouth existence. Americans have eclipsed all of these previous advanced cultures with an agricultural prosperity such as the world has never seen. We grow enough food to feed ourselves, make half the population overfat, throw away food that would feed another 50 million people daily, and ship massive amounts of food overseas. We have literally mountains of government surplus food that is slowly spoiling. We eat as much red meat as mainland China, a nation of four times our population. Two-thirds of all grain exports on the world's marketplace are from the United States.[1]

What possible nutritional deficiencies could a nation of such productive farmers experience? Many. Put simply, we often make the wrong choices at the dinner table.

While 10 percent of Americans are still underfed, many of the remaining 90 percent are overfed or improperly fed. This seeming contradiction can be explained by our sedentary lifestyle. We eat less, yet we have considerably more overweight people, because our

43

modern lifestyle involves precious little movement. And many of us are improperly fed because not only do we eat less overall food than our great grandparents did, but what we eat is much lower in nutrient density. This means that both the quality and quantity of our food intake have deteriorated in recent decades. Coincidentally, many ailments that were once unheard of have flourished amid Western lifestyle. The Framingham study from Harvard University introduced the phrase "our way of life is related to our way of death."[2]

Government surveys show extensive malnutrition among Americans. Stress, tobacco, drugs, alcohol, and chemical pollutants from the environment can elevate the need for certain nutrients. In addition, rampant fad dieting usually involves eating nothing or a seriously imbalanced diet. We do not eat enough of various essential nutrients, including calcium; potassium; magnesium; zinc; iron; chromium; selenium; vitamins A, D, E, C, and B_6; riboflavin; folacin; pantothenic acid; fiber; and complex carbohydrates. We eat too many calories, salt, and additives and too much fat in general and saturated fat in particular, sugar, cholesterol, alcohol, and polluted water.

In many underdeveloped nations, malnutrition is not being able to get enough food to survive. For other, more prosperous groups, malnutrition means a subclinical (difficult to detect) deficiency. Yet, because the U.S. has the capacity to seek out "optimal" health rather than just settling for "survival," not achieving optimal nourishment could also be considered malnutrition. Malnutrition does not just encompass being borderline dead; it can also mean not achieving one's genetic potential due to nutritional limitations. For a wide variety of reasons, many Americans are malnourished.

OUR MODERN LIFESTYLE INDUCES MALNUTRITION

Over the course of millions of years, humans evolved as active omnivorous grazers. In this last century, we have deviated significantly from that "factory specification" lifestyle. As we drift from our inherited food intake pattern, our nutrient status deteriorates.[3] Almost all residents of the original 13 American colonies were farmers, and they had to rely on their own vegetable gardens, fruit trees, and fresh animal products for food. They also had minimal access or funds to buy nutrient-poor food, which has become an American staple. Today, less than 3 percent of Americans farm, and our rural-to-urban movement has lead to more processed foods and less fresh produce. In addition few of us get the exercise that our great grandfathers did, so we need many fewer calories. It took roughly 8,000 calories to cut and stack a cord of firewood to keep a pioneer family warm, but to adjust the automatic thermostat on the wall to keep a modern house warm takes roughly 3 calories. Yet the overwhelming incidence of obesity today indicates that we have not adjusted our calorie intake accordingly.

Most of our grandmothers worked in the home and spent considerable time preparing meals. Until recently, the mother was the traditional "nutritionist" in the American home. But many women now work out of the home, and both mother and father often return from work too tired to cook. This usually results in fewer home-cooked meals and less supervision of meals for children. Unfortunately, children are not the most sensible eaters. One study found that 30 of the 800 schoolchildren examined were consuming over 300 milligrams of caffeine daily from colas and candy.[4] That would be equivalent to five cups of coffee; yet it is even more concentrated in small bodies with higher metabolic rates. One-third of these children with a high caffeine intake were considered to be hyperactive.

It could be said facetiously of Americans that our favorite recipe is "heat and serve." Or, husband or wife asks the other, "Honey, what are you going to make for dinner?" and gets the answer "Reservations." Restaurant food is not necessarily bad, but most restaurants use an abundance of fat, salt, sugar, MSG (a flavor enhancer with a variety of health detriments to its credit), and metabisulfite (a produce preservative that can cause allergic reactions in many sensitive individuals). Restauranteurs and food companies understand your taste buds better than you do—they know that Americans have developed a penchant for certain flavorings, in spite of their dubious health credentials. The food processor removes valuable nutrients in an effort to extend food shelf life and to create a specific texture and flavor of food. The net result is that restaurant and processed food often provides abundant calories, fat, salt, sugar, cholesterol, additives, and alcohol while short-changing the diner in vitamins, minerals, and fiber. Scientists have found that highly refined foods are more digestible (instigating overfatness), more absorbable (amplifying the "highs" and "lows" of blood glucose levels), and more usable by the cariogenic bacteria in the mouth (instigating cavities).[5]

The stressful lifestyle of modern society also has taken its toll on our nutrient status. First, psychological stress increases nutrient needs while decreasing the efficiency of intestinal absorption. Second, stress often provokes drug, tobacco, and alcohol use, which also increases nutrient needs. Third, stress almost always changes people's eating patterns: some people eat too much, some eat too little, and many develop obsessive binge eating patterns as emotional outlets.

Another development new to the 20th century is the number of people living alone in America. Families were once spoken of as "nuclear" and "telescoping." *Fragmented* would be a more appropriate term today. Rampant divorce combined with an independent group of senior citizens has created a nation of loners. In case you haven't experienced it lately, cooking for yourself is no fun. Many people who live alone suffer extensive malnutritive conditions due to their diet of canned soup, crackers, and beer. Elderly men living alone are so inattentive to their diet that they are at risk for developing scurvy,[6] something you would expect more among the ragged ship crew of a 17th-century vessel.

In short, society has undergone numerous changes in lifestyle as we near the end of the 20th century, and few of them have been for our nutritional betterment. This does not, of course, mean that we need to return to Stone Age routines. You can eat good food *and* use your computer, digital watch, high-tech racing bike, turbocharged auto, and VCR. Modern nutritional and agricultural science give us the knowledge we need to nourish the mind and body optimally for a vigorous life and to eat almost any food that we want year-round. We can take the best of both the caveman era and the 20th century to enjoy ourselves and nourish our health. So far, however, most Americans have not exercised this "best of both worlds" option.

GOVERNMENT SURVEYS FIND WIDESPREAD MALNUTRITION

Inspired by the 1960 presidential campaign of John F. Kennedy, the Ten State Survey was conducted by the Department of Health,

Education, and Welfare to determine the nutritional status of low-income Americans. The findings, published in 1970, found that many people were deficient in iron, calcium, vitamin A, thiamine, riboflavin, and vitamin C. Growth retardation due to malnutrition was common. One-third of the children were low in serum vitamin A, while 4 percent had scorbutic gums.[7] That's right, in the "land of plenty," 1 out of 25 children had scurvy, or blatant vitamin C deficiency. Sixteen percent were low in body protein levels, while 5 percent had severe protein deficiencies (kwashiorkor), which were thought to exist only in drought regions of Africa or Asia.

Yet this survey examined primarily poor people. Researchers wondered how well the "average" American would compare in such a survey, so they began the HANES (Health and Nutrition Examination Survey), which was published in 1974. HANES examined many different strata of the population. The results were equally disturbing. Fourteen percent of the whites and 29 percent of the blacks were clinically low in thiamine. Fifteen percent of whites and 29 percent of blacks were low in iron. Protein, vitamin A, and riboflavin were also commonly deficient in American diets. The data was beginning to mount that perhaps Americans were not as well fed as was once thought.

In 1978, the third and most extensive survey of all, the Nationwide Food Consumption Survey, revealed even more widespread malnutrition than the former studies. One-third of Americans were low in vitamin A, vitamin C, and iron, while one-half were low in vitamin B_6, calcium, and magnesium.[8] Wealthy people were just slightly better nourished than the lower-income groups. In order to be considered deficient in a nutrient, a person must be consuming less than 70 percent of the RDA. Thus, there were untold legions of other people who consumed less than the RDA but not low enough levels to be considered deficient. Only 3 percent of the 20,749 subjects examined in this study were free of the 48 most common symptoms of malnutrition.[9]

The most frequently consumed foods in America are coffee, white bread, and sugar, in that order.[10] White flour is definitely a staple in this country. To produce white flour, the processor removes the better part of 24 nutrients from whole wheat and replaces 4 of these nutrients to call it "enriched." Only 2 percent of the flour consumed in America is whole wheat, with the remainder being "enriched" or even unenriched, highly refined pastry flour.[11]

White flour has about 1 percent of the chromium, 14 percent of the vitamin E, 50 percent of the pantothenic acid, and 28 percent of the vitamin B_6 that was once found in the original whole wheat kernel.[12] Literally all of the zinc is lost in wheat milling.

Half of all foods eaten in America are processed convenience foods,[13] and processing generally wreaks havoc on the nutrient content of foods.[14]

Even conservative food preservation techniques can inflict major damage on nutrient content. For example, canned salmon loses more than half of its vitamin B_6. Canned spinach loses 80 percent of its pantothenic acid and 82 percent of its manganese. Even frozen vegetables lose up to 44 percent of their B_6. Orange drinks are seriously lacking in the fiber and bioflavonoids that are found in the original orange.

The four food groups have long been considered the ultimate guide to good eating. Yet studies show that following the four food groups does not ensure adequate intake of the vitamins E, B_6, and folacin or of the minerals iron, zinc, and magnesium.[15]

Also, our affluence seems to work against us in our nutrient intake. As income increases, fewer nutrients are obtained per dollar spent on food.[16] High-fat meats, pastries, alcohol, and snack foods are expensive, yet almost comically low in their nutrient density.

I was recently behind a grocery store shopper whose purchases seemed to summarize the halfhearted awakening of Americans toward nutrition. This portly and pale-looking middle-aged gentleman with blotchy skin bought hot dogs, buns, chips, vodka, beer, cigarettes, and canned olives. As an afterthought, he added a bottle of the cheapest generic vitamins from the checkout display. He apparently had a vague suspicion that nutrition might have something to do with health and was willing to make a meager compromise. Unfortunately, the odds are that this fellow's health will deteriorate markedly within the next decade in spite of his minor concession to nutrition.

Malnutrition can be a subtle long-term condition that persistently hacks away at one's health and energy levels. As mentioned earlier, decades of subclinical malnutrition can eventually bring on degenerative diseases, such as heart disease, diabetes, cancer, arthritis, osteoporosis, gallstones, kidney stones, and other ailments.[17] Severe malnutrition in infants can permanently and irremedially retard growth, of both the brain and the body. Even in adults, severe malnutrition can have long-standing implications. A group of neurologists from London examined 898 men who had been prisoners of war in the Far East during World War II. These scientists found continued symptoms of nerve damage in these former POWs, even 36 years after being malnourished.[18]

Based upon many well-conducted surveys, Americans are commonly deficient in these nutrients:

- *Vitamins:* A, E, D, C, thiamine, riboflavin, pyridoxine, folacin pantothenic acid
- *Minerals:* calcium, potassium, magnesium, zinc, iron, copper, chromium, fluoride, selenium
- *Macronutrients:* protein, complex carbohydrates, fiber, polyunsaturated fats, and clean water
- *Quasi nutrients:* (substances that may be essential for some people during certain stages of life, such as stress, pregnancy, sickness): bioflavonoids, carnitine, eicosapentaenoic acid, taurine, coenzyme Q, and lipoic acid

The American diet commonly contains excessive amounts of these substances:

- Calories, which can come from too much carbohydrate, fat, protein, or alcohol
- Fat in general; saturated fat, hydrogenated fat, and cholesterol in particular
- Phosphorus (found in meats, colas, and most processed foods via the phosphoric acid added)
- Sodium (primarily from salt that is added to the food by the food processor, restaurant chef, home chef, and diner, at the table)
- Sugar (added to nearly all bottled, canned, packaged, or frozen foods)
- Additives (there are over 2,800 FDA-approved additives with another 10,000 additives being "incidental" to the agriculture and food-processing business)
- Alcohol (which contains calories, reduces the consumption of nourishing food, and creates deficiencies by using up many different nutrients)

Is there malnutrition in the United States of "Abundance"? Does this malnutrition lead to many of our health ailments? Can proper nutrient intake prevent and even cure some diseases while supporting the medical treatment of others? The answer to each question is an unqualified yes.

SURVIVING VERSUS THRIVING

The law of nature is "survive to reproduce." All else is optional. Dr. Roger Williams found that both laboratory animals and plants exist at less than ideal levels of nutrient status. With an effort at optimizing the nutrient supply, both plants and animals grow better and are healthier. For example, wild corn barely produces enough corn kernels to be able to reproduce and certainly not enough to feed any number of people. When corn is cultivated and kept relatively free of weeds, it produces 5 to 10 bushels of corn per acre of land. Yet, under ideal conditions, the same breed of corn plant can yield 250 bushels per acre.[19] This is still not considered the upper limit of productivity.

Animals follow the same pattern—few live at ideal nutrient intake levels. Various groups of pregnant guinea pigs were given varying amounts of folacin and vitamin C. At the Recommended Daily Intake (RDI, a nutrient guideline for animals used in experiments) for folacin and vitamin C, there was a certain average size of litter, size of pup, and numbers lost during uterine development. When researchers upped the intake of vitamin C and folacin to four or five times the RDI, there were more pups, larger pups, and fewer aborted fetuses.

Humans are no different. Twenty-one pairs of human siblings in rural Louisiana were enlisted for a long-term study to see if there are shades of health above "normal" in humans. For the first set of infants, the mothers ate normally and produced normal infants that grew into normal children who tested out to be "normal." Nothing surprising about that. But next, the researchers provided additional foods through the WIC (women, infants, and children) government feeding program to the same 21 women, who were now pregnant. For this set of infants, mothers were provided with nutrient-dense foods in addition to their normal diet. Oatmeal, oranges, cheeses, and nuts were part of this additional nutrient intake. The same foods were offered to the nursing mothers once their infants were born and to the kids throughout early childhood. At age six, these children were tested. They were superior to their older brothers and sisters in every physical, emotional, and intellectual test used. Apparently, above-normal nutrition had produced above-normal children.

In spite of all the odds, millions of people around the world survive their poor nutrition and other challenges. Yet how much better would health, intellect, emotions, disease resistance, and longevity be if we were all nourished optimally? Undoubtedly, most people would experience measurable improvements, and some would make quantum leaps in health.

The goal of health care professionals used to be to "normalize" their sick patients. Yet "normal" is not that desirable a condition. A "normal" serum cholesterol level in an older adult male is indicative of a high risk for heart disease.[20] Suddenly, "normal" does not sound that enticing.

But going beyond "normal," what is "optimal"? Can anyone quantify just how healthy and long-lived a human being could be? Not exactly and not yet, but we are getting closer to understanding "optimal" human health. One researcher has discovered an enzyme system that would allow medical technologists to compare your vitamin C level to "optimal" levels, rather than the conventional "normal."[21]

One thing is quite certain: very few people today are at optimal levels of nourishment. In some cases, healing nutrients improve health by bringing the "normal" person out of a subclinical deficiency and closer to "optimal" nutritional status.

And what is this "normal" standard that all nutrient intake is compared to? It is the RDAs, defined by the scientists who established them as "the levels of intake of essential nutrients considered, in the judgment of the Committee on Dietary Allowances of the Food and Nutrition Board on the basis of available scientific knowledge to be adequate to meet the known nutritional needs of practically all healthy persons."[22] Researchers, medical specialists, and food labelers needed something as a reference point, and the RDAs are just that: a reference point—not to be inscribed in stone, nor to be ridiculed or ignored.

One Harvard professor who sits on this blue-ribbon panel of scientists has admitted that many of the RDAs are merely "guesstimates of unknown reliability."[23] The RDAs provide for "normal" health in most nonstressed people. Those who fall below the RDA intake levels are not necessarily guaranteed to develop a deficiency, and those who go significantly above the RDAs are unlikely to develop a toxicity.

Very little is known about the nutrient needs of the very young, the very old, the sick, and the superactive individual. Preliminary evidence indicates that older people probably need greater than RDA levels of certain nutrients.[24] Very little is known about human requirements for trace minerals, such as molybdenum and selenium. There are also substances known as *quasi-nutrients* that certain groups of people may need during certain stages of the life cycle. For instance, infants may need taurine (a substance found in mother's milk but not in infant formulas), alcoholics may need carnitine (a substance that helps the body to burn fats more efficiently), and certain adult diabetics may need Glucose Tolerance Factor (GTF, a substance found only in brewer's yeast that assists in insulin and glucose metabolism).

The RDA board readily admits that its values are not meant to create "optimal health" since it is difficult for scientists to quantify the upper limits of human potential. Scientists are hesitant to approach this subject of "optimal" because there are no table values in books for it. You cannot weigh it or measure it. It is some vague better health state that most people admit exists but aren't real sure how to describe. But the fact that we don't know our limits should not prevent us from concluding that we are not there yet. There is significant room for improvement in human health, physique, endurance, disease resistance, wound-healing capacity, intellect, emotional stability, and longevity.

The bottom line here is that about 20 percent of Americans are clinically and obviously malnourished. Another 40 percent are subclinically malnourished, with the malnutrition eventually surfacing as some disease, marginal health, or early death. And another 30 percent are measurably below optimal nutrient status. This means that at least 90 percent of Americans would be considered malnourished with respect to optimal standards. Why settle for anything less than the best of nourishment levels, when we have that option available to us for the first time in history?

4
THE CORE PROGRAM FOR OPTIMAL NUTRITION

This chapter provides the foundation for the rest of the book. Here you will learn what constitutes a nourishing diet and which supplements are considered baseline for protection against various common diseases. The Core Program is designed to provide you with better disease resistance and higher energy levels and should elevate you out of any possible subclinical deficiency.

Healthy, young, active people who are exposed to minimal stress and pollution and have no family history of any particular ailment can consider the Core Program to be their guide. Most people, however, are faced with less than ideal health situations. If you want to prevent a disease that runs in your family, help heal an ailment, an injury, or another condition you now have; or maintain optimal health in the face of special circumstances such as pregnancy or exposure to pollution, check the table of contents and the index to find the chapters that apply to your needs. Each of those chapters lists the foods and nutrients to be subtracted from or added to this core program. If you need to incorporate several chapters into your total supplement program, merely select the highest nutrient intake level recommended for any given nutrient.

To make nutrition your ally rather than your lifetime adversary, you should, at the very least, follow the Core Program of both foods and supplements. Supplements take most people beyond the nutrient intake level that will ensure survival and closer to "optimal" health. Supplements fill in the nutrient gaps that are created by depleted foods, dieting, food storage and processing, marginally nourished soil, stress, pollution, occasional alcohol intake, and other factors that increase nutrient needs.

FOOD:
THE PRIMARY SOURCE OF NOURISHMENT

The Core Program is based on food. Supplements are valuable but of secondary importance. Vitamin pills are very helpful in improving the nutritional status of most people, but pills cannot take the place of proper eating. Scientists of the past thought they knew exactly what was in mother's milk and proceeded to create an infant formula that they thought was superior. In the last two decades, however, nutritionists have found a variety of factors that make mother's milk far superior to the ersatz version. As nutrition scientists learn more about the nutrients in foods, it becomes more obvious that there are unidentified factors in foods that are essential for health. So, although supplements are an important "insurance" part of this Core Program, it is the food that is the mainstay of proper nourishment. To encourage good eating, a chart in this chapter provides food sources of all nutrient factors mentioned throughout the book.

Eating properly in America can, of course, be a real challenge. Friends and family tempt you. Television advertisements seduce you with your favorite fast food. Food manufacturers know exactly how to "push the buttons" on the consumer's taste buds, with fat, salt, sugar, and coloring agents. As people eat more salt and sugar, their taste buds become "habituated," meaning that the sensory nerves in the tongue and nose continuously adjust and more stimula is needed each time to get the same response. In other words, salters usually get worse and complain of no taste in their food when asked to avoid using the salt shaker. Yet when these flavorings are withdrawn slowly, in a gradual weaning process, the change is unnoticeable and painless.

Once you have firmly rooted yourself in this new and healthy way of eating, you will find it easy to comply with. Many of the people who have made the transition from processed to wholesome, nourishing food say that their old foods now taste artificial, obnoxious, cloying, and unsatisfying. This chapter shows you how to select foods that are inexpensive, tasty, and invigorating to your body.

Some people say that they have no time to worry about food—they eat whatever is quickest and easiest to prepare. Well, there are many nourishing foods that do not require extensive preparation. In addition, those people who do not take the time for wellness (including good nutrition) will have to make the time for sickness.

Other people say that they cannot afford to eat these nourishing foods. Actually, quite the opposite is true. An average family of four people would save approximately $1,400 per year by switching to these nutritious foods. And disregarding these savings, you cannot afford *not* to eat well. Even if 100 percent of your medical expenses are covered by an insurance policy, you still cannot afford to ignore good nutrition. There must be some way of placing a value on the lost time and talent along with the needless suffering and early death that often accompany a lifetime of poor eating.

No book can tell you exactly what to eat for the rest of your life. But you can be taught how to choose foods wisely for yourself. Sailors cannot be shown all around the world. But they can be taught how to use a sextant, a compass, and a map and thus find their *own* way. This chapter should be considered your navigating instruments to steer you toward nourishing foods and away from the rocky shoals of nonfoods. The object of this food section is to teach you good nutritional judgment.

You *can* eat properly without having to become a professional nutritionist, as long as you understand a few simple concepts that years of study have yielded. Though there is no one perfect food—even the lowliest of foods usually provides at least fluids or energy—one is usually preferable to the other when you compare two foods. Here are some guidelines for making such comparisons:

NUTRIENT DENSITY

Nutrient density refers to the amount of vitamins, minerals, protein, and fiber found in 100 kilocalories of any given food. The more nutrients per kilocalorie, the greater the nutrient density and the more desirable the food. An orange has more nutrients per kilocalorie than peanuts. And peanuts are more nutrient-dense than candy. With nutrient density in mind, liver outranks steak, and steak outranks bologna. In any given situation, choose the food that has a greater nutrient density. It is amazing how many people who are not schooled in nutrition seem to have an intuition for guessing which food would be more nutrient-dense. Anyone can fill up on kilocalories. It takes guided discretion to fill up on nutrients. But your body will thank you for it.

RISK/BENEFIT RATIO

The risk/benefit ratio of a food is a look at the pros and cons of eating that food. Let's look at some examples:

- Peanuts are high in fat and kilocalories, yet they are a decent source of niacin and protein. For a growing child or an active adult, the benefits may outweigh the risks.
- Liver is high in cholesterol, yet it is also one of the most nutrient-dense foods available. For an active person with no serum choleterol problems, the benefits outweigh the risks: liver could be a valuable item on the menu once each week.
- Ice cream is high in fat, cholesterol, and sugar, yet it is also a nutrient-rich dairy product. For active children, ice cream is a viable alternative to nutrient-poor pastries, soda pop, and "junk food." But for the overweight, sedentary adult, the risks of ice cream outweigh the benefits.
- Eggs are high in cholesterol, yet they are also high in protein, vitamin A, and iron. Eggs are also inexpensive, easy to cook, and easy to chew for people with dentition problems. For many people, including older adults, who have healthy levels of serum cholesterol, eggs might be considered good food.
- A glass of wine with dinner seems to improve digestion for many older adults and encourages better sleep. However, a glass of wine taken by a pregnant woman may interfere with the healthy growth of her unborn infant.

Try to look at foods as being somewhere in between "perfect" and "terrible." Weigh the benefits against the risks for your stage of life and make a decision as to whether that food is good for you.

OCCASIONAL VERSUS REGULAR USE

If you go to the ballpark a few times each summer for a baseball game, you probably have the typical beer-and-hot-dog feast while there. Eating that only a few times each year will not harm the average healthy person. If unwise food choices become a weekly or daily routine, however, they can tarnish your health. Every once in a while, each of us has to visit a well-intentioned friend's house for dinner, or eat on a plane, or stop for a quick meal at a restaurant. These meals are usually not the nutritional ideal. Yet, if they are the rare exception to your normally fantastic eating habits, they will not be destructive. It is your nutritional *habits* that will influence your quality and quantity of life, not the sporadic detours from good eating. This understanding helps to curb the "puranoid" (a cross between a purist and a paranoid) who lurks at many parties, preaching contemptuously of the vile foods that you are putting in your mouth. The puranoid alienates others toward nutrition. The rational, nutritionally oriented person sees that a 98 percent excellent diet is not going to be thwarted by the 2 percent that is less than good.

EAT WHAT YOUR CULTURAL TRADITION DICTATES

Oh, what a fantastic collage is the human species. Some cultures are long-standing vegetarians. Others survive almost entirely off dairy products. Some eat much fat. Others eat very little fat. There is a rich and varied tapestry of human life on earth. Cultural diets are equally varied. Greenland Eskimos eat a diet with very little fiber and vitamin C and 50 percent more fat than even Americans consume. Yet the protective value of fish fat, combined with the Eskimos' long-standing ability to tolerate such a diet dictates that this program is the best for them. Orientals who change their dietary habits to more Western ways, with fewer vegetables and more animal products, are experiencing even a higher incidence of heart disease than Westerners. Why? Because their new diet is so different from their evolutionary cultural diet. You may recall the group of nomadic herdsmen from Kenya mentioned earlier. These Turkana switched from dairy to fish as their dietary staples and suffered marked deterioration in their health.[1]

But what if your parents and grandparents had a predisposition toward a certain disease, and you know that their diet may have contributed to it or even caused it? Obviously, you'd hesitate to follow the same diet. Well, in many instances, people today are several generations removed from their cultural diet. Whatever your ancestors ate to get them through the last millennium is probably more compatible with your system than what 20th-century processed foods provide. You may have to go back a few generations to find your real food "roots," but the investigation may prove worthwhile. More simply stated: Eat what your cultural heritage dictates. (Many Americans are from mixed ancestry, in which case this recommendation becomes difficult to apply.)

The more narrowly restricted your ancestors' diet was, the more important it is for you to follow your cultural food pattern. Certain groups, like the Eskimos (with their high-fat fish) and the Masai tribe in Africa (with their high dairy intake), are extreme examples of cultures that have evolved from a narrowly restricted diet. If your cultural diet is one of diverse foods, then you do not need to be as concerned with this point.

THE EIGHT PRECEPTS OF NUTRITION

After you take into account the general guidelines above, you should adhere to the following set of easily understood rules, which summarize thousands of pages of complex biochemical facts regarding nutrition. Once again, these guidelines help you to become your own nutritionist and develop good judgment in food selection. They may seem simple, as they are intended to be, but they are derived from the most current data about human nutrition.

1. Eat foods in as close to their natural state as possible. Refining foods (whether done at a food-processing plant or at home by the cook) usually does one or more of the following:
- Removes valuable nutrients (e.g., vitamins, minerals, fiber)
- Adds questionable agents (e.g., additives, fat, salt, sugar)
- Markedly increases the cost (potato chips are 1,000 percent more expensive per pound than potatoes)
- Needlessly increases industrial energy expenditure
- Creates packages that must be disposed of in our already crowded dumps

Therefore, a baked potato is better than mashed potatoes, which are better than french fries, which are better than potato chips.

2. Eat a wide variety of foods. People who eat a more varied diet have a better nutrient intake.[2] A wide variety of foods will help you to include known essential nutrients as well as those essential nutrients that are not yet recognized, to avoid excess toxins (both natural and synthetic), and to minimize the risk of allergies due to a buildup of a particular food in the bloodstream.

Although there are about 20,000 varieties of edible plants on earth, and at least 2,000 of the 20,000 are found in America, the typical American consumes only about a dozen of these plant types. One reason is that only about three dozen plant types are available commercially. Even so, there is still plenty of room to expand your food horizons, as long as this rule is compatible with what your cultural tradition dictates.

3. Eat small, frequent meals. Humans evolved as "grazers," eating small amounts as they moved, not the "gorgers" we have become. This concept (periodicity) has been proven to reduce the likelihood of heart disease, diabetes,[3] overfatness,[4] and intestinal problems; stabilizes blood sugar and serum lipids;[5] and quite possibly increases life span. Instead of eating two or three large meals each day, try eating the same amount of food and calories in five or six smaller snacks. By eating a small, healthy snack every two or three hours, you will find marked improvements in your mental and physical energy levels. Do not eat large, high fat meals late in the day since the fat will be absorbed while you sleep (instead of being burned off through daily exercise) and is more likely to be deposited along the blood vessel walls than is fat obtained through earlier meals.

4. Avoid or minimize your intake of common "saboteurs." Restrict your consumption of fat in general and hydrogenated fat, saturated fat, and cholesterol in particular and of salt, sugar, alcohol, caffeine, and most food additives. In small quantities, these are probably harmless to most people. Yet in normal American quantities, these substances can become saboteurs from within.

Avoid processed meats (e.g., lunch meats, salted meats, and smoked meats), food colorings, MSG (a flavor enhancer), and nitrites. Eating none of these would be preferable to eating small amounts of them.

5. Maximize your intake of fresh vegetables, fruit, whole grains, legumes, low-fat dairy, clean water, fish, and poultry. These foods should be the staples of most diets.

6. Get your nutrients with "a fork and spoon" if at all possible. Foods are your best proven source of nutrients.[6] Only foods can provide all essential nutrients; pills contain an incomplete set of nutrients. Yet, realistically, supplements probably are useful for most people and essential for some people. Take supplements in divided dosages, at mealtimes, and in well-designed formulas. Poorly designed supplements can bleed the wallet with little benefit to your health. Consult the chart in this chapter to identify the ideal amounts of vitamins, minerals, and other nutrient factors that should be included in a useful supplement program.

7. Balance calorie intake with expenditure. For a rough idea of calorie needs for healthy adults (assuming that you are already at your ideal weight), multiply your weight in pounds by 10 if you are sedentary, by 17 if very active, or any number in between 10 and 17, depending on your activity level. Thus, a moderately active person (using a factor of 14) weighing 180 pounds would need 2,529 kilocalories per day ($14 \times 180 = 2520$) to maintain his or her body weight.

8. Maintain adequate protein intake. Protein is a very crucial macronutrient. A protein shortage can be disastrous to health in general. To roughly calculate protein needs in grams, divide weight in pounds by 2.2. Thus a 150 pound adult would need 68 grams ($150 \div 2.2 = 68$) of protein per day to stay healthy. Pregnancy, lactation, growth, and wound recovery have higher needs for both energy and protein.

You also need to maintain ideal body fat composition, so you should be more concerned about the *quality* of body weight than about the *quantity* of weight, which is revealed by the bathroom scale. Grab your skin just above the hipbone. If the thickness of the skinfold is one inch or less, then you are in good shape (or possibly starving yourself via anorexia). If the skinfold thickness is one to two inches, then you could turn up your fitness program a notch or two. If the skinfold thickness is more than two inches, then you are in serious need of catching your obesity before it becomes a self-perpetuating vicious cycle.

THE EXCHANGE SYSTEM

Humans need about 50 different nutrients in their diet to maintain health. Different food groups provide different nutrients. Decades ago, scientists realized that they would have to boil down this complex nutrition business into some simple eating guide that everyone could follow, and the "four food groups" guideline was born. Meat, breads and cereals, fruits and vegetables, and dairy products comprised this tidy little system. It is easy to learn and provides a decent spectrum of nutrients. Yet this system has its limitations. The four food groups emphasize high-fat animal products. Also, they do not stipulate portion control. A "serving" could mean anything from ½ cup to a mountain of mashed potatoes, depending on the person. Nor does the system adequately provide for the option of vegetarianism. Fruits and vegetables certainly contribute different nutrients, but the four food groups system does not separate them. For instance, cabbage and apricots each make unique nutrient contributions to the diet, although in the four food groups they would be considered identical. The four food groups system does not separate the meat group into various fat content categories, either. There is a big difference between the risk/benefit ratios of low-fat fish and high-fat bologna. The four food groups also allow people to ignore the calorie content of the butter on their bread or the fat used to fry their chicken. And even if you were following the four food groups exactly, you could still be deficient in a variety of vitamins and minerals.[7] Considering all of these weaknesses, a new system had to be designed.

Enter the exchange system of meal planning. It is more accurate than the four food groups and much easier to use than the USDA Table of Nutrient Values, which is a scientific table listing the nutrient content for most foods commonly eaten in America. The exchange system is easy to learn, flexible enough to allow you to select foods wisely in any setting, and more likely to provide you with all the nutrients you need. It is sanctioned by every major health organization in the United States. *Exchange* means that you can substitute any member in a group with any other member and still have nearly the same calories, protein, and other macronutrients. For example, a six-inch corn tortilla could be exchanged for a slice of bread, which could be exchanged for half of a bagel, which could be exchanged for ½ cup of cooked rice. All are similar in nutrient values. The following table shows examples of selections from each of the six groups. For a more detailed list of members in each group and how to use this system, consult any cookbook or nutrition guide for diabetics. Although you do not need to be a diabetic to benefit from this eating program, diabetics are forced into good eating habits through their erratic blood sugar levels.

The exchange system consists of six food groups from which to select:

- Vegetables (such as asparagus, beets, cabbage, peppers, greens, onions, tomatoes, and zucchini)
- Fruits (such as apples, apricots, bananas, cherries, oranges, pineapple, plums, and watermelon)
- Fats (such as margarine, butter, avocado, nuts, salad dressing, cream cheese, bacon, and olives)
- Breads and starches (such as bread, bagel, muffin, tortilla, cereal, grits, rice, popcorn, crackers, beans, corn, peas, and potatoes)
- Protein (such as meat, fish, poultry, cottage cheese, beans, and eggs)
- Milk (such as milk, buttermilk, and yogurt)

There is also a free group, the members of which contribute so few calories that they can be used freely in normal quantities without having to be counted. Chicory, endive, lettuce, parsley, radishes, vanilla, artificial sweeteners, vinegar, coffee, and tea are a few examples of these freebies.

Quantities allowed are different for each group and for each member within that group. Yet you are undoubtedly not interested in memorizing an exact quantity for every food. Unless you are a brittle diabetic (with difficult-to-control blood sugar variations), there is no need to be so particular about exact measurements. Thus, the exchange system can be simplified tremendously by groupings.

QUANTITIES ALLOWED FOR ONE EXCHANGE

Vegetables: Basically, ½ cup, but see the explanation under "fruits."

Fruits: Up to 1 cup if the fruit is low in sugar and high in fluid content (such as watermelon) or as little as ¼ cup if the fruit is more concentrated in sugar content (such as grape juice and prune juice). Use your taste buds to provide you with good judgment. The sweeter the fruit, the higher the calorie content. Use ½ cup as a rough guideline for each fruit exchange. Thus 2 small apricots, 12 grapes, or 10 cherries would each make up one fruit exchange, since they are each about ½ cup in volume.

As a general rule, if you are hungry, then consider the fruit and vegetable groups to be fair snacking territory. With the exception of brittle diabetics, most people should be able to eat all the fresh fruits and vegetables that they want. Both fruits and vegetables are sufficiently high in fiber and water and low in calories that normal servings will fill people up with valuable nutrients and make no major contribution in calories.

Fats: One fat exchange is 1 *teaspoon* of concentrated fat, such as margarine, butter, or oil; or 1 *tablespoon* of high-fat food, such as nuts, bacon, avocado, or salad dressing.

Breads and Starches: Basically, 1 ounce of starchy food. One slice of bread, ½ cup of rice or cereal, 3 cups of popcorn, and ¼ cup of wheat germ each provide about 1 ounce of starchy food and equal one bread exchange.

Protein: A protein exchange equals 1 ounce or ¼ cup of most members, but this group is also subdivided according to fat content:

- Low-fat (lean cuts of meat, clams, oysters, scallops, shrimp, cottage cheese, beans, peas, lentils)
- Medium-fat (organ meats, eggs, and fattier cuts of meat)
- High-fat (marbled meat, most luncheon meats, most cheeses)

Be realistic. If your hamburger keeps a raging fire going on the barbecue grill, then that beef is high-fat. A low-fat protein exchange is merely a protein exchange. A medium-fat protein exchange is counted as a protein plus half a fat exchange. A high-fat protein exchange constitutes a protein exchange plus a full fat exchange.

Milk: Basically, 1 cup of nonfat milk products, including buttermilk and nonfat yogurt. Low-fat milk would equal one milk exchange plus a fat exchange. Whole milk would constitute a milk exchange plus two fat exchanges.

GUIDE TO THE EXCHANGE SYSTEM

The table below shows the number of kilocalories and the number of grams of protein, carbohydrate, and fats found in one exchange of each group. Once you know the exchange system, you can use this information to calculate your total daily calories. Thus, dieters do not need to carry calorie counters; they need only learn the basics of the exchange system.

The importance of the percentage of your food calories that are coming from carbohydrate, fat, and protein was established by the Senate Dietary Goals. These goals were established by a blue-ribbon panel of congressionally appointed experts who analyzed the American diet in 1977 and made nutritional recommendations that would improve our health. The goals recommend that we eat 58 percent of our calories from carbohydrates (primarily complex and naturally occurring), 30 percent from fat, and the remaining 12 percent from protein. In the typical American diet, 46 percent comes from carbohydrates, 42 percent from fat, and 12 percent from protein. So, if you want to, you can even get into some sophisticated nutritional analysis with this easy-to-learn exchange system. The sample exchange guide listed below has already had these Senate Dietary Goals (12 percent protein, 58 percent carbohydrate, 30 percent fat) built in to its (the guide) formulation.

GUIDE TO THE EXCHANGE SYSTEM

	Protein	Fat	Carbohydrates	Kilocalories
Vegetables	2g	0	5g	25
Fruits	0	0	10g	40
Fats	0	5g	0	45
Breads	2g	0	15g	70
Protein	7g	3g	0	55
Milk	8g	0	12g	80

SAMPLE EXCHANGE PATTERN

The following sample exchange pattern shows you how to customize the exchange system to come up with that elusive "balanced" diet. Calculate your daily kilocalorie needs from the seventh precept of nutrition and then consult the table to see how much of each food group you can have for a day's worth of optimal eating.

SAMPLE EXCHANGE PATTERN

	1,000 Kcal/Day	1,200 Kcal/Day	1,900 Kcal/Day	2,400 Kcal/Day
Vegetables	4	4	7	7
Fruits	3	4	7	10
Fats	3	3	8	10
Breads	3	5	8	11
Protein	5	5	5	5
Milk	2	2	3	4

A SAMPLE MEAL FROM THE EXCHANGE SYSTEM

Let's use the exchange system to analyze a sample meal:

- 3 ounces broiled salmon = 3 low-fat protein exchanges
- 1 cup cooked brown rice = 2 bread exchanges
  with ½ cup soy sprouts = 1 protein exchange + 1 bread exchange
  with 1 teaspoon butter = 1 fat exchange
  with seasonings = free group
- 1 cup cooked carrots = 2 vegetable exchanges
  cooked with 1 tablespoon honey = 1 fat exchange ("empty" calories are always categorized under the fats group)
- 1 cup tossed salad of sprouts, cabbage, tomatoes = 2 vegetable exchanges
- Mint tea = free group
- 1 cup whole-milk yogurt = 1 milk exchange + 2 fat exchanges
  with whole banana cut up into the yogurt = 2 fruit exchanges

This meal managed to use up 4 vegetables, 2 fruits, 4 fats, 3 breads, 4 proteins, and 1 milk for a total of 870 kilocalories. We obtained 50 grams of protein and complied with the seven precepts of nutrition. If you were to follow the 2,400-kilocalories-per-day guide, then you still have 3 vegetables, 8 fruits, 6 fats, 8 breads, 1 protein, and 3 milk exchanges to procure before the day is out. Work with these numbers until you understand how this simple yet effective system functions. It's much like typing. Using the exchange system requires some conscious thought at first but soon settles into a simple and subconscious healthful way of eating.

SUPPLEMENT PROGRAM

While foods provide all the nutrients needed by humans, supplements provide only a few. Yet, considering America's stressful lifestyle and ubiquitous pollution, our eat-on-the-run nutrient-depleted foods, our penchant for bizarre diets, and the possibility that many of us need greater-than-RDA levels of nutrients for optimal health, supplements are an essential part of the core nutrition program.

If you are a healthy, active adult who is eating an excellent diet, not genetically prone to any particular ailments, not exposed to pollution, not using any drugs or alcohol, and not living a stressful lifestyle, then the supplement amounts recommended in the following table would keep your health and nutrient intake at optimal levels. Besides the amounts recommended, the percentage of the RDA, normal supplemental ranges, and possible toxic doses for various nutrients are also listed. For many nutrients, there are no known toxicity levels, so they are quite safe when taken in the supplemental ranges that are listed. A question mark near a toxicity number indicates that there is some, though not substantial, evidence to consider that intake level to be toxic. The supplemental ranges are taken from the hundreds of studies found throughout this book that show measurably enhanced health in some people at these nutrient intake levels.

CORE PROGRAM SUPPLEMENTS

Nutrient (Form Used)	Amount Recommended	Percentage of RDA	Supplemental Ranges	Toxicity
A (beta-carotene)	10,000 IU	200	5,000–50,000 IU	unknown
D (cholecalciferol)	400 IU	100	200–1,000 IU	2,000 IU
E (d-alpha tocopherol)	200 IU	666	30–800 IU	1,500 IU ?
K (phytonadione)	100 mcg	*	30–600 mcg	1,000 mcg
B$_1$ (thiamine–HCl)	4.5 mg	300	1–100 mg	unknown
B$_2$ (riboflavin)	5.1 mg	300	1–100 mg	unknown
B$_3$ (niacinamide)	40 mg	200	5–1,000 mg	3,000 mg
B$_6$ (pyridoxine–HCl)	6 mg	300	1–100 mg	500 mg ?
B$_{12}$ (cobalamin)	12 mcg	200	6–1,000 mcg	unknown

CORE PROGRAM SUPPLEMENTS (continued)

Nutrient (Form Used)	Amount Recommended	Percentage of RDA	Supplemental Ranges	Toxicity
Folacin (folic acid)	400 mcg	100	400–3,000 mcg	15,000 mcg ?
Biotin (biotin)	300 mcg	100	100–3,000 mcg	unknown
C (ascorbic acid)	500 mcg	833	50–5,000	20,000 mg ?
Pantothenic acid (Ca-pantothenate)	30 mg	300	5–1,000 mg	unknown
Choline (as bitartrate)	250 mg	*	100–5,000 mg	unknown
Calcium (as carbonate)	400 mg	40	200–1500 mg	4,000 mg
Potassium (K-chloride)	300 mg	*	100–5,000 mg	10,000 mg ?
Magnesium (Mg-oxide)	200 mg	50	100–1,000	2,000 mg
Zinc (Zn-gluconate)	15 mg	167	5–60 mg	400 mg
Iron (ferrous fumarate)	18 mg	100	2–60 mg	100 mg

Copper (Cu-gluconate)	1.5 mg	125	2–20 mg	50 mg
Iodine (potassium iodide)	150 mcg	100	50–3,000 mcg	unknown
Manganese (Mn-gluconate)	8 mcg	*	2.5–15 mg	30 mg ?
Chromium (from yeast)	200 mcg	*	50–2,000 mg	unknown
Molybdenum (Na-molybdate)	150 mcg	*	100–1,000 mcg	2,000 mcg
Selenium (from yeast)	200 mcg	*	50–1,000 mcg	3,000 mcg
Silicon (Mg-trisilicate)	10 mg	*	1–20 mg	unknown
L-carnitine ($) (as HCl)	500 mg	**	100–10,000 mg	26,000 mg ?
EPA ($) (eicosapentaenoic acid)	1,000 mg	**	500–3,000 mg	10,000 mg ?

* is established as essential for all humans but no RDA is given.

** is not yet established as essential for all humans.

If you were to purchase these supplements separately, they would be prohibitively expensive. Yet there are now several vitamin companies that make high-quality, broad-spectrum supplements that include all or almost all of the above-mentioned nutrients for a reasonable price. Both carnitine and EPA are preceded by a dollar sign because they are expensive and rarely found in multivitamin tablets. You may consider these two nutrients optional if the rest of your nutrient intake is good and you have a limited budget. Otherwise, the remaining nutrients should not cost more than $20 per month. (If you consult other chapters in addition to the Core Program, however, the amount of nutrients taken probably will go up, depending on the risk factors involved.)

I do not want you to spend a lot of money or take handfuls of pills on this program. Spending less than $20 per month and taking only two or three tablets per meal, you can markedly enhance your nutrient intake and health while substantially reducing the likelihood of encountering the common degenerative diseases in America. There are numerous vitamin firms that sell through the mail. If you are in doubt about whom to buy from, I have listed two reputable mail order vitamin companies in the Endnotes.[8] These company names are listed for your benefit, not for mine or theirs.

FOOD SOURCES OF NUTRIENTS

Since foods are so important to your total nutrition program, the last section of this chapter lists the best food sources of *all* of the nutrients that are mentioned in this book. If you read about a nutrient and would like to see what foods contain that substance, then check back to this chart. The nutrient often may have an alternate name, which is listed in parentheses. The food sources are listed in descending order of prevalence, with the richest source first and so on. Some foods are highlighted with an asterisk, since they are notably high in that particular nutrient.

VITAMINS

A (beta-carotene is the plant version): Liver,* fish liver oil,* dark green vegetables (like broccoli, peas, kale, spinach), yellow vegetables (like squash, carrots, pumpkin, sweet potatoes), vitamin A-fortified milk, butter, margarine, egg yolk, orange fruits (like apricots, cantaloupe, papaya, peaches), watermelon, cherries. Generally speaking, the more intense the green or yellow color in the fruit or vegetable, the higher the beta-carotene content. Animal versions of vitamin A (preformed A) can be toxic in continuously high doses. Plant version is unlikely to be toxic. Although some people do notice a slight yellowish coloration to their skin when their beta-carotene consumption is high, this is not harmful. When the coloration reaches the whites of the eyes, then you are definitely eating too much beta-carotene.

D (cholecalciferol): Fish liver oil,* fortified milk, certain high-fat fish (like salmon, herring, sardines), sunshine on skin (15–30 minutes/day), butter, eggs.

E (tocopherol): Wheat germ oil,* wheat germ, most vegetable oils (like corn, soy, cottonseed, safflower, sunflower), mayonnaise and margarine (both of which are made with these vegetable oils), egg yolk, butter, liver, nuts. Most commercial oils are heat-processed, which destroys some of the vitamin E content. Most margarine has been hydrogenated, which further reduces the vitamin E content. White flour has almost no vitamin E, while whole wheat flour has decent amounts.

K (menadione): Produced by bacteria in the human intestines. Therefore, yogurt and other cultured food products help to stimulate vitamin K production by encouraging the growth of helpful bacteria in the intestines. Also found in liver and dark green leafy vegetables. (Phytonadione is the synthetic version of vitamin K used in supplements.)

*C (ascorbic acid): Terminalia ferdinandiana,** (a fruit that is native to Australia and is similar to an English gooseberry yet contains about 20 times the vitamin C concentration of citrus fruits), Barbados cherry* (from the Caribbean area), rosehips,* kiwifruit,* sweet peppers, broccoli, cauliflower, kale, lemons, strawberries, papaya, asparagus, spinach, cantaloupe, oranges, grapefruit, tomatoes. Most fruits and vegetables contain some vitamin C, while liver is the only appreciable animal source of vitamin C. The vitamin C content in mother's milk will be a reflection of the vitamin C found in mother's diet.

B_1 *(thiamine):* Brewer's yeast,* pork, kidney, liver, peas, wheat germ, macaroni, peanuts, whole grains, beans, nuts.

B_2 *(riboflavin):* Brewer's yeast,* kidney,* liver,* heart,* milk*, broccoli, wheat germ, almonds, cottage cheese, yogurt, tuna, salmon, macaroni, brussels sprouts, asparagus, eggs, green leafy vegetables.

B_3 *(niacin):* Brewer's yeast,* liver*, peanuts, poultry, fish, meat, whole grains, eggs, milk, and other high-quality protein foods. Niacin is found in both a preformed state and as the raw materials (precursor) to make it in the body from the amino acid tryptophan. Therefore, diets that are low in protein are at great risk for niacin deficiency. See the section on protein later in this chapter.

B_6 *(pyridoxine):* soybeans,* liver,* bananas,* lamb,* kidney, chicken, steak, poultry, tuna, fish, legumes, potatoes, oatmeal, wheat germ.

B_{12} *(cyanocobalamin; also cobalamin):* Liver,* oysters,* poultry, fish, beef, pork, clams, eggs. Although the richest sources of B_{12} are animal foods, plant foods that are intentionally fermented or are composed of micro-organisms also have decent amounts of B_{12}. Thus, spirulina (blue-green ocean algae), certain seaweeds, miso (fermented soybean paste), tempeh (fermented whole soybeans), and brewer's yeast grown in a B_{12}-rich environment are all good sources of B_{12} for the vegetarian.

Folacin (folic acid, folate): Liver,* eggs, asparagus, whole wheat, green leafy vegetables (such as kale, spinach, parsley), salmon, beans, broccoli, sweet potatoes.

Biotin (vitamin H): Liver,* kidney,* produced by bacteria in the healthy intestines, egg yolk, milk, yeast, whole grains, cauliflower, nuts, legumes. Excessive intake of raw egg whites can create a biotin deficiency due to a binding factor (avidin) in the egg white.

Pantothenic acid (pantothenol): Royal bee jelly,* liver,* kidney,* heart, egg yolks, bran, fish, whole grain cereals, cauliflower, beans, nuts, cheese, sweet potatoes.

MINERALS

These are listed in descending order of prevalence in the human body. Thus, the mineral listed first is the one that is found the most abundantly in the normal adult body. The last minerals listed are trace elements that are found in almost imperceptibly small amounts.

The amounts found in the body are important, since this gives us a clue regarding relative amounts that should be in the diet. "Bulk" macro-minerals found in the body need to be included in bulk amounts in the diet. Trace microminerals found in the body should be included in trace amounts in the diet. Some trace minerals in the body are actually impurities or toxins and should be avoided in the diet.

Calcium: Cooked bones (such as in fish flour, canned salmon and anchovies, and old-fashioned homemade soup stock), collards, yogurt, turnip greens, broccoli, milk and dairy products, kale, tempeh and tofu (soybean products), hard water (contains dissolved salts of magnesium and calcium). Calcium absorption is increased with vitamin C, lactose (milk sugar), and acid foods (such as citrus, pineapple, and tomato).

Phosphorus: Meat,* soda pop* (from the phosphoric acid), fish, poultry, eggs, cereal, processed foods (from the many phosphorus compounds that are added). Most Americans get too much phosphorus, which creates an imbalance with other minerals, such as calcium and magnesium. For that reason, supplements of phosphorous are not recommended.

Potassium: Dried apricots,* cantaloupe,* lima beans,* potatoes, avocados, bananas, broccoli, liver, milk, peanut butter, citrus, fruits and vegetables in general. Much potassium can be lost when a food is boiled, such as with boiled potatoes.

Sulfur: Egg yolks,* garlic, onions, beans, high-protein foods (from the sulfur-containing amino acids like cysteine and methionine), asparagus. Little is known about sulfur deficiency states. It is rarely added to supplements.

Chloride: Table salt,* salted foods, soy sauce. Chloride basically comes from table salt (sodium chloride). Since most Americans eat too much salt, chloride is unnecessary in supplements.

Sodium: Salt,* salted foods, soy sauce, monosodium glutamate (MSG), cheese, meat, milk, most animal foods. Look for the sodium on food labels, such as sodium nitrite, sodium monophosphate, etc. Most Americans eat too much salt; therefore, adding sodium to the diet is not recommended. For people who perspire regularly, or with repeated vomiting or diarrhea, sodium levels in the body can become depleted. Strict vegetarians eat considerable amounts of potassium from their plant foods and would probably benefit by adding some sodium to their diet to balance the important electrolytes of sodium and potassium. Note that grazing vegetarian animals (like deer and cattle) will seek out a salt block and visit it regularly to balance their potassium and sodium intake.

Magnesium: Soybeans,* buckwheat, shrimp, wheat germ, almonds, cashews, Brazil nuts, whole grains, molasses, clams, cornmeal, spinach, oysters, crabs, peas, bananas, potatoes, oatmeal, salmon, milk, liver, beef, green vegetables (chlorophyll contains magnesium), hard water (has dissolved magnesium and calcium salts in it, which are removed by a water softener). Magnesium intake should be balanced with other minerals. A 2:2:1 ratio of calcium, phosphorus, and magnesium would be ideal. Vitamin D aids in the use of calcium and magnesium.

Zinc: Oyster,* herring,* clams, wheat germ, bran, oatmeal, liver, nuts, beef, lamb, peas, chicken, carrots. The amount of zinc in plant food varies considerably with the soil region, since zinc is not a normal part of fertilizing efforts.

Iron: Pork liver,* cast-iron cookware (using acid foods, such as tomato and pineapple, in cast-iron cookware dissolves a thin lining of iron and can double or triple iron intake without any change in the diet), cream of wheat, clams, beef, pork, veal, chicken, fish, spinach, asparagus, prunes, raisins, nori seaweed. Iron absorption increases with animal food that contains a chelated version of iron, called heme iron, and with vitamin C intake. Chelated (pronounced key-lated) minerals are bound in the middle of a larger molecule and are often better absorbed by the body than nonchelated minerals.

Copper: Shellfish (such as shrimp, lobster, abalone, oyster), liver, cherries, nuts, cocoa, gelatin, copper water pipes (homes built with copper water pipes provide some copper to the residents via their drinking water), whole grain cereals, eggs, poultry, beans, peas. Copper should be balanced with zinc in a 1:10 ratio of copper to zinc.

Iodide: Iodide tablets (used to purify drinking water when bacteria may be present), iodized salt, ocean seafood (not commonly found in freshwater seafood), food grown on high-iodide soil, milk (since iodide-based detergents are used to cleanse the machinery in dairy farms).

Manganese: Rice bran,* wheat bran,* corn germ, whole grains and cereals, green vegetables, nuts, legumes, tea, ginger, cloves.

Chromium: Brewer's yeast,* liver, meat, cheese, legumes, beans, peas, whole grains, black pepper, molasses. Brewer's yeast is the only source of GTF (glucose tolerance factor) yeast. GTF is better absorbed and more potent than elemental chromium. In some people, GTF yeast may be essential, if they are unable to make their own GTF from dietary chromium. Whole grains and cane sugar contain some chromium, while refined white flour and sugar contain almost no chromium.

Fluorine: Naturally fluoridated water (from underground sources), artificially fluoridated water (added to the city water supply), crops raised on fluoridated water, food cooked in fluoridated water, mackerel, salmon.

Selenium: Brazil nuts* (one nut can supply up to 50 mcg of selenium), food grown in selenium-rich soil, soybeans, tuna, seafoods, meat, whole grains.

Molybdenum: Buckwheat,* lima beans, soybeans, wheat germ, liver, barley, oats, lentils, sunflower seeds. Much molybdenum is lost in food refining.

Cobalt: Liver, kidney, oyster, clams, meat, fish.

Nickel: Widely distributed, especially in fruits and vegetables.

Silicon: Whole grains.

Vanadium: Black pepper, vegetable oils (like soy, corn, olive oils), olives, gelatin. Vanadium is lost in refining.

Tin: Unknown.

Other minerals that are found in the human body include: cadmium, aluminum, arsenic, barium, boron, bromine, gold, lead, mercury, and strontium. It is not known whether these minerals are toxic in any amount, essential in tiny amounts, or harmless trace impurities from the environment.

QUASI VITAMINS

A few other substances may be essential to some people during certain periods of their life. Though they aren't essential for all humans, and are unlikely to be promoted to the rank of "vitamin" in the near future, some scientists are calling this group "conditionally essential" nutrients. For instance, very young and sick people may need taurine (an amino acid) in their diet. People who have a hard time keeping their blood pressure down may need eicosapentaenoic acid (EPA, from fish oil) as an essential nutrient. "Conditionally essential" nutrients are a whole new area of nutrition that resides precariously between the known essential nutrients and the many nonessential dietary factors.

Choline: Lecithin,* egg yolks, liver, soybeans, fish, whole grain cereal, legumes, most fatty foods.

Myo-inositol: Oranges, grapefruit, tangerines, most citrus (except lemons), cantaloupe, heart, fruit in general, meats, milk, nuts, vegetables, whole grain cereals.

Carnitine: Sheep,* lamb, beef, chicken. Almost totally restricted to animal foods. Humans can produce some carnitine internally from lysine (an amino acid), vitamin B_6, vitamin C, and iron. Alcohol consumption increases the need for carnitine. Some people with high blood fats may not be able to produce optimal amounts of carnitine to handle their body fats properly.

Bioflavonoids: There are over 500 different bioflavonoid compounds, which are all basically substances that help plants in the photosynthesis process. Found in fruits (especially the white rind in citrus), vegetables, whole grains (especially buckwheat), legumes, and honey.

Coenzyme Q (CoQ, ubiquinone): Some CoQ can be made internally from tyrosine and phenylalanine (amino acids), vitamin E, niacin, folacin, pantothenic acid, B_6, and B_{12}. CoQ food sources include beef heart and muscle, organ meats, egg yolk, liver and heart of codfish, milk fat, wheat germ, and whole grains.

Lipoic acid (thioctic acid): Liver,* brewer's yeast.* Some lipoic acid can also be manufactured internally.

Nucleosides: These substances include the blueprints in the cell nucleus (DNA) and the helper substances that allow protein synthesis to occur (RNA), plus the "gold currency" of energy exchange (ATP) and all the intermediate steps that the body takes to make these vital end products. Inosine and adenosine are intermediate steps. These substances are of unknown value when taken internally, but have some useful functions when given intravenously. These substances are found in the metabolically active parts of foodstuff, like seeds and nuts, green leafy vegetables, liver, foods that could be sprouted (like whole grains, beans, peas, alfalfa seeds). Orotic acid (orotate) is a favorite nucleoside for nutrition therapy. Food sources of orotic acid are unknown.

Glucose Tolerance Factor: GTF is a substance made in the body from dietary chromium that helps insulin get glucose into the cells of the body. Some people may not be able to make enough GTF from the chromium in their food supply to maintain good health. GTF is found only in specially cultured brewer's yeast.

Taurine: This is an unusual amino acid. Amino acids are usually the building blocks of protein and prefer to participate in building tissue. In contrast, taurine promotes many chemical reactions, as opposed to becoming construction material. Most people can make some taurine from methionine and cysteine (sulfur-bearing amino acids) and vitamin B_6. Taurine is found in mother's milk, but not found in most infant formulas. There is some taurine in certain animal foods (e.g. shellfish and muscle tissue), but none in plant foods.

Chondroiton sulfate: Found in the cartilage tissue of most animals.

PROTEIN

Protein provides the bulk building blocks to form much of the human body, including muscle, organs, portions of brain tissue, skin, parts of blood, disease resistance factors, and most enzymes that are responsible for getting things done in the body.

Foods are generally categorized by the *quality* of protein that they contain. Protein is composed of amino acid building blocks. The closer the amino acid pattern in a given food comes to satisfying the ideal amino acid needs of the human body, the higher the "biological value" of that food protein.

High-Quality Proteins (can sustain both growth and adult life): Egg whites, dairy products, fish, meat, chicken, spirulina (blue-green algae), wheat germ (and the germ from other grains), brewer's yeast. Or, by mixing grains (such as wheat, rice, oats, corn, millet, etc.) with legumes (such as soybeans, garbanzo beans, lentils, peas, other beans), you can form a protein of equal quality to that of steak. Therefore, smart vegetarians can be well nourished with respect to protein intake. Chili (made with kidney beans) and corn bread form a high-quality protein when consumed at the same meal. A peanut butter sandwich is another example of this grains-with-legumes combination.

Medium-Quality Proteins (can sustain adult life, but may not be able to provide optimally for rapid growth stages): Grains (such as wheat, oats, barley, rice, millet, sorghum, corn), legumes (most beans, peas, lentils, peanuts), nuts (walnuts, cashews, Brazil nuts), seeds (sesame seeds, sunflower seeds).

Low-Quality Proteins (probably cannot sustain human life without some other food protein assistance): Fruits, vegetables, gelatin.

FATS

Dietary fat can be categorized for both quality and quantity. With respect to quantity:

Foods That Are Very High in Fat: Oils, margarine, butter, bacon fat, lard, mayonnaise, many salad dressings.

Foods That Are High in Fat: Nuts, seeds, olives, avocados, thick dairy products (like cream cheese and ice cream), luncheon meats, most cheeses, high-fat meats (like hamburger, duck, prime rib).

Foods That Contain Some Fat: Most of the remaining high-protein foods (like fish, poultry, pork, organ meats, shellfish), soybeans, other legumes.

Foods That Are Low in Fat: Most grains, fruits, and vegetables.

Different types of fats have amazingly diverse effects on the human body. Cholesterol is a type of fat that is essential in the body, yet it can become a prime cause of vascular disease if it accumulates along the vessel walls. Cholesterol is found only in animal foods. The richest sources are brains, egg yolks, liver and other organ meats, followed by red meat, and high-fat dairy products.

The different effects that fats exert on the body depend primarily on the chemical structure of the fatty acids that make up the fat. Fats in the diet normally contain three fatty acids that are attached to a glycerol molecule and hence are called triglycerides (or triacylglycerols). The fatty acids in foods vary considerably. Most animal fats are higher in saturated fats. Most plant fats (except coconut oil) are higher in unsaturated fats. Saturated fats are solid at room temperature, while plant fats are liquid at room temperature. This makes perfect sense in nature's routine, since an animal could not be sloshing around with liquid fats within. The solid saturated fats inside humans provide a foamlike cushioning that could not be obtained from liquid fats.

Within the category of unsaturated fats, there are:

Polyunsaturated fats: From safflower oil, soy oil, cottonseed oil, corn oil, sunflower oil, and other plant oils. These foods contain the known essential fatty acid, linoleic acid.

Monounsaturated fats: Found primarily in olive oil, with some in dairy products. Olive oil is becoming more convincingly the oil of choice for cooking due to its nutritional value (explained in Chapter 5).

Omega-3 fats: These special fatty acids are longer and contain more double bonds than normal polyunsaturated fats. They have special health values that are explained throughout this book. Eicosapentaenoic Acid (EPA) and docosahexaenoic acid (DHA) are two of the better known omega-3 fatty acids. The best sources are fish oil, especially from high-fat fish (like salmon, haddock, sardines, tuna). In fish that has a low fat content in its flesh, these valuable fatty acids are usually stored in the liver. This is where industry taps concentrated sources of EPA and DHA, such as is found in cod or menhaden liver oil. DHA is found primarily in brain tissue, fish oil, and mother's milk, providing yet another valid argument in favor of the superiority of breastfeeding to ensure optimal brain growth.

Other types of omega-3 fatty acids can be found in linseed oil (from the flax seed that was traditionally used for weaving) and purslane (which is a salad vegetable common to the Mediterranean region). The evening primrose plant that is native to cool climes of North America contains oils that are high in gamma-linolenic acid (GLA). GLA is a unique fatty acid that is somewhere between linoleic acid and EPA in its length and degree of unsaturation. Evening primose oil is discussed in several sections of the book.

CARBOHYDRATES AND FIBER

Fiber is a basically indigestible carbohydrate, so carbohydrates and fiber are lumped together in this section. Carbohydrates are categorized as either simple (as sugars) or complex (as starches).

Simple: From fruits, lactose (milk sugar), honey, and some vegetables. Refined carbohydrates (table sugar or sucrose) are absorbed rapidly into the bloodstream. Your tongue is an accurate detector of simple carbohydrates. The sweeter the food tastes, the higher it is in simple carbohydrates.

Complex: From whole grains, legumes, most vegetables, seeds, and nuts. Refined complex carbohydrates, like white flour and white rice, have had the outer bran and inner germ removed. Many nutrients are lost in this process. Also, these refined foods are absorbed more rapidly into the bloodstream.

Fiber: Fiber is categorized by soluble fibers, including pectin, gums, and mucilages, which are provided by apples, grapes, prunes, carrots, seaweed, and other plant foods. Insoluble fibers include cellulose, hemicellulose, and lignin, which are provided by bran, whole grains (including wheat bran and popcorn hulls), many vegetables (including celery strands), and legumes. Although most seeds and nuts are rich in fiber, they are also high in fat and calories and hence are not considered ideal sources of fiber. Cruciferous vegetables (cabbage, cauliflower, broccoli, brussels sprouts) contain *indoles*, which have a special ability to prevent problems of the gastrointestinal tract.

5
THE CIRCULATORY SYSTEM
Heart Disease, Hypertension, Clots, Etc.

More Americans will die this year from circulatory disorders than died in all of our wars combined.[1] Circulatory ailments have been called the "bubonic plague" of the 20th century, since half of all deaths in America are caused by them. The "average" blood cholesterol level in America is indicative of a high risk for heart disease.[2]

The circulatory system is an amazing and complicated network of a pump and its connecting tubes. Over the course of an average lifetime, your heart will pump 55 million gallons of blood through your 60,000 miles of blood vessels. The whole purpose of the circulatory system is to deliver needed supplies to the body's 60 trillion cells and then to remove waste products. In other words, the circulatory system brings "groceries" and takes out the "trash." The blood vessels near the heart can be up to one inch in diameter. The capillaries, where the actual exchange of goods takes place, are so small that blood cells must squeeze through one at a time, like people moving down a narrow hallway. This system is as impressive as it is vulnerable. The deterioration of the circulatory system is the main cause of death in the Western world.

Medical science has not been idle on the subject. Heart transplants, artificial pacemakers, bypass surgery, artificial hearts, and a medicine wagon full of different drugs have been developed to treat problems of the circulatory system. Bypass surgery was performed on 100,000 people in 1982 at a total cost of $5 billion. As mentioned earlier, bypass surgery, for most patients, can temporarily relieve angina pain but does nothing to improve survival rate and life span.[3]

Much money and brain power has been spent on solving the heart disease riddle, yet these efforts have fallen short. The healing focus has, once again, been directed toward drugs and surgery. The death rate from heart disease has steadily fallen over the last decade. Yet this is a deceptive statistic. The *incidence* of heart disease has not lessened, but the *death rate* has fallen due to the spread of CPR (cardiopulmonary resuscitation) classes and the preparedness of emergency medicine. Once again, this is like applying ointment to the blister, but not removing the friction that brought about the blister.

Still, there is hope. Optimal nutrition can prevent most forms of circulatory problems and even cure some. Working with nature provides amazing results without the cost and side effects found in the conventional drugs and surgery approach. Patients with continuous angina pain often submit to a variety of surgical procedures designed to open up the blood vessels that are blocked. These techniques are dangerous, expensive, quite temporary, and require a long convalescent period. As an alternative, L-carnitine,[4] Coenzyme Q,[5] EPA,[6] and other nutrient factors have each been shown to improve angina pain in human patients. These nutrients begin to reverse the fat deposition process so that, ultimately, nutrients can increase survival rate and life span. There is a myriad of drugs available to treat hypertension, but many of them have side effects including irregular heart rhythm, impotence, deterioration of glucose tolerance, and so on. There are various nutrients, including EPA,[7] linoleic acid (the essential fatty acid found in certain plant oils), magnesium, potassium, calcium, garlic, and other nutrient factors, that have been shown to reduce blood pressure in humans *without side effects*. Which makes more sense? The simple low-risk nutrition approach or the use of invasive and risky surgery and drugs to treat circulatory disorders?

There is no question that proper nutrition can prevent or at least slow the progression of heart disease and hypertension. For people who already have circulatory disease, nutrition still offers hope of a low-risk solution to the problem. All of these nutrition approaches to vascular disease will be discussed in this chapter.

In the most conservative of studies, nutrition was found to be a major factor in the incidence of circulatory disorders. A study of nearly 17,000 Harvard alumni found that heart disease risk could be cut by 23 percent with regular exercise, another 13 percent by eliminating smoking, another 11 percent by maintaining the ideal percentage of body fat, and another 10 percent if hypertension were controlled.[8] That totals a 57 percent cut in the risk of heart disease when you are willing to take charge of your lifestyle. Another group of researchers analyzed over 1,500 men and found diet to be at least as important a risk factor in heart disease as is smoking.[9] Thus, if we assign the same risk factor to diet as to smoking (above), we can add 13 percent to our previous total of 57 percent. You now have cut your risk for heart disease by 70 percent with some easy preventive measures. Three semirural communities in northern California were selected by Stanford University to determine if simple lifestyle changes could lower heart disease risk. Using only the most conservative data on lowering blood cholesterol levels, these researchers were able to cut heart disease risks for the community by 20 percent.[10] And none of these large-scale studies have explored the *proven* healing powers of certain individual nutrients.

The bottom line is that your risks for getting vascular diseases can be cut by 90 percent if you follow the guidelines that are found in this chapter. If you already have vascular diseases, this chapter gives you a decent chance of reversing the problem.

Can circulatory disorders really be "cured"? In many cases, yes. In some cases, diet alone can be the effective healing agent. Nathan Pritikin had a major heart attack in 1958 at age 42. His vessels were clogged, and his serum cholesterol level was 280 milligrams per deciliter. His autopsy 27 years later showed *no* blockage of blood vessels and a serum cholesterol level of less than 100 milligrams per deciliter.[11] His basic anti–heart disease program was a high-fiber, low-fat diet and regular, brisk walking. Although his diet was considered too austere for all but the most motivated heart disease victims, he died with blood vessels that were as clean as those of a 20-year-old marathon runner. And the Pritikin diet isn't essential; there are less severe but equally effective nutritional means of obtaining the same or better results. All of this background information was meant to introduce you to the concept that you do not have to accept heart disease as an inevitable byproduct of living in 20th-century America. You can do something about it, yourself, at home, with very little expense and taking very little time from your schedule. By using the diet and supplement program described in this chapter, you can eat appealing foods and probably outlive your peers by a decade or more.

WHAT CAN GO WRONG WITH THE CIRCULATORY SYSTEM?

Before we discuss the healing powers of nutrition, let's explain some basic facts about the heart and vascular network and the common malfunctions of this important system. We can compare the vessels in your body to the water pipes in your house. There are three major things that can go wrong with your vascular network:

1. "Plugged up plumbing," such as from fatty blockages or clots forming, more formally called *atherosclerosis* and *thrombosis*, respectively.

2. "Brittle plumbing," from hardening of the vessels (a.k.a *arteriosclerosis*), which can lead to bursting of these hard and brittle "pipes."

3. "Weak pump," from a worn-out heart or unbalanced electrolyte solution that helps to regulate heartbeat. These problems could lead to the implantation of a pacemaker or to an erratic heartbeat (ventricular fibrillation).

These problems can be caused by:

1. Fatty blockage (plaque). Fats, though essential for health, do not mingle well with the water medium of the blood. All fat-soluble substances (including cholesterol, triglycerides, vitamin A, and others) must have an escort in the blood to make sure they stay in solution. When most of the cholesterol is carried by HDLs (high-density lipoproteins) through the bloodstream, the cholesterol is less likely to collect along the blood vessel walls. When more of the cholesterol is carried by LDLs (low-density lipoproteins), it tends to sediment along the vessel walls and create fatty obstructions.

Though most areas of the body favor carbohydrates for fuel, the heart favors fats. This preference for fats provides the heart with a dependable fuel supply yet also is often the demise of the heart, since the vessels near the heart can plug up with fatty occlusions. As the passages in the vessels narrow with fatty obstruction, the victim may experience a shooting pain near the heart, called *angina*. If the plaque lining the vessel walls totally obstructs the passage of blood, then the tissue on the other side of this "roadblock" may die. Such an event is called a *heart attack*, or *myocardial infarction*.

2. *Sticky blood cells (platelet aggregation).* In this situation, the blood cells start adhering to one another and begin forming a clot, as though you had been cut. The clot may cause havoc anywhere in the body and is now called a *thromboembolism*. These clumps of clotting blood cells (thrombus) can find a comfortable spot somewhere in a blood vessel and begin gathering a blanket of fat. The end result may be the blockage of a vessel and death to the tissue on the other side of this roadblock. Or, these sticky blood clumps may instead wander to the brain and lodge themselves somewhere in a delicate artery, choking off nutrient flow to an area of the brain and causing a stroke. A clot that gets caught in a blood vessel of the legs can cause swelling and pain. This is known as *phlebitis*. Internal clotting becomes more likely as humans age.

3. *Hardening of the arteries.* Cholesterol can combine with calcium in the bloodstream to form mineral deposits that begin accumulating along the blood vessel walls. These mineral deposits reduce the elasticity of the vessels and raise the blood pressure. Inflexible and brittle vessels are more likely to burst, causing a stroke or thrombus. Or, the brittle vessels can simply raise blood pressure. High blood pressure, a.k.a. *hypertension*, slowly and perniciously pounds away at the vascular network and eventually may cause organ failure or a heart attack.

4. *High blood pressure.* People can develop elevated blood pressure for reasons besides hardening of the arteries. You have a complex system of hormonelike substances (prostaglandins) and steroids (like aldosterone) that regulate blood pressure. Improper balance of these prostaglandins or steroids can encourage hypertension. Fluid buildup, due to sodium retention or mineral imbalance, can elevate blood pressure. Whatever causes it, when the pressure in your blood vessels goes up dramatically, there is a great

likelihood that one of the vessels may burst, causing stroke or death.

5. *Electrolyte imbalances.* Your heart is a muscle and is operated via remote control through a network of nerves. Both nerves and muscles rely heavily on the "electrolyte soup" of the body. An imbalance in the concentration of any key electrolyte (sodium, potassium, calcium, magnesium or water) can cause spasms, poor heart rhythm, and even sudden death. Also, the heart is one of the few muscles in the body that gets no rest periods. The continuous wear and tear of muscle pumping and a marginal nutrient supply can gradually weaken the heart's pumping ability.

GENERAL RISK FACTORS

Heart disease and hypertension were almost unheard of before the 20th century, and they are still rare in underdeveloped nations. Even though the heart and blood vessels are used continuously, they are not built for failure. For the average American, proper nutrition can keep this delivery system healthy for decades after "normal" deterioration would have set in.

Risk factors for circulatory problems include an excess or deficiency of a wide range of individual nutrients, allergies,[12] overfatness, diabetes, smoking, genetics, hypertension (which is also nutrition-related), serum cholesterol (also nutrition-related), exercise, stress (attitude), and others. See also the chapters on diabetes, eating disorders (obesity), and allergies, since these problems can indirectly provoke circulatory disorders.

This chapter will show you how nutrients can reduce fatty blockages, minimize clotting, dissolve calcified deposits along the vessel walls, maintain the ideal recipe for the "electrolyte soup" of the heart, and keep the whole system working properly. The chapter is divided into sections on the various nutrients that affect circulatory problems.

FATS

Take a bottle of Italian dressing out of your cupboard and notice the distinct separation between the layer of fat and the layer of vinegar and water. Recall the disastrous effect of an oil slick on the ocean. Have you ever tried to wash grease off your hands with just water? Although fats are essential nutrients, life is water-based. Fats are part of the membranes in all cells throughout the body. Fats make up the insulating material that keeps nerve impulses from jumping off the track. Fats are the basis for prostaglandins, a group of potent hormonelike substances that regulate everything from blood pressure to childbirth. Yet, as valuable as fats are to health, they are potential saboteurs from within. Heart disease, the primary cause of death in 20th-century America, is often the end result of fatty deposits clogging the blood vessels near the heart.

The answers seemed so simple a few decades ago. Researchers autopsied heart disease victims and found white fatty substances blocking the blood vessels. The fatty substance was composed mainly of cholesterol. They deduced the obvious: don't eat cholesterol, and you won't get heart disease. Yet the obvious was an overly simplistic conclusion. Your body manufactures more cholesterol than you could obtain from eating eight eggs per day.[13] Many

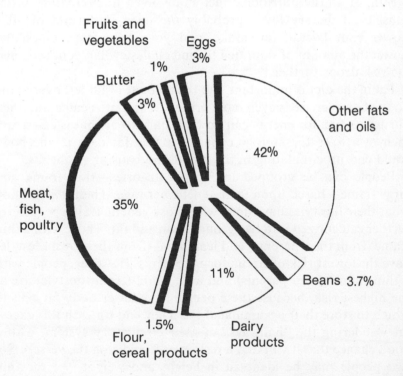

Sources of fat in the American diet.

other nutrients, exercise, and stress were later found to be contributing factors to this fatty accumulation in the blood vessels. The
puzzle became even more complex. Actually, only about one-third
of the population responds to increases in dietary cholesterol with
noticeable increases in their serum cholesterol.[14] Although dietary
fat is an important risk factor in circulatory disorders, equally
important are the nutrients that allow the body to handle fats
properly, such as chromium, selenium, and vitamins C and E.

The "fat as a death squad" theory was dealt a serious blow when
researchers found that Greenland Eskimos consumed a diet with
50 percent more fat than Americans eat, yet the Eskimos had a
near zero incidence of heart disease. To add to the confusion, the
Eskimos were eating very little fresh produce and fiber. Obviously
their low-stress lifestyle and regular activity helped, but something
else was helping them dodge the bullet of heart disease. Scientists
found a fatty acid (eicosapentaenoic acid, or EPA) in the high-fish
diet of the Eskimos that helped to prevent heart disease.

Still, of all the nutritional factors involved in circulatory problems, total dietary fat is probably *the* most important of all.[15]
Lower your overall fat intake, and your risk drops markedly.
Lower the amount of saturated fat and cholesterol in your diet, and
the risk drops further.[16]

Fat in the diet is important, but the amount of fat left over in the
body after exercise is even more critical. Fat that is eaten and then
burned as fuel for energy can do little harm. Fat that is eaten and
then overflows the storage capacity of the fat cells in the body
could end up circulating in the blood and causing problems.

People can be grouped into two categories—thin frame and
large frame—based upon their genetic heritage. Then, based upon
what their lifestyles have done with those genetic traits, people are
further categorized into two groups: lean and fat. Those with a thin
frame (from their parents) and lean build (from their own lifestyle)
have the lowest risk of circulatory problems. However, people with
a thin frame (from parents) and a fat build (from lifestyle) are at
the highest risk, because these people have fewer body fat cells in
which to store their accumulated fat. They end up with this excess
fat wandering the "hallways" of their circulatory system, with a
good chance that it will find a resting spot and clog the vessels. So,
two people may be identical in height and weight, yet the thin
(from parents)/fat (from lifestyle) person is at the greatest risk for

vascular diseases.

How can nutrition influence this fatty accumulation in the blood vessels? In a variety of ways. Merely by losing weight, many people can lower their blood pressure and heart disease risk significantly.[17] A modest reduction in total fat intake with an increase in polyunsaturated fats in the diet will result in a noticeable lowering of blood pressure and serum cholesterol.[18]

HYDROGENATED FATS

Processed fats can also provoke vessel disease. Fats in the food industry are often changed into a different type of saturated fat, called *trans fatty acids*, or *hydrogenated fats*. These hydrogenated fats can have a custom-built texture, shelf life, and viscosity, which benefits the food processor, but they have been shown to raise the levels of fats in the blood.[19] Ironically, hydrogenated vegetable oils are probably even more plaque-forming than the saturated animal fat of butter that they were meant to replace.[20] Hydrogenated fats are similar enough to the fats found in nature that the body will use them, yet they are different enough that they do not have the same abilities once incorporated into the tissue.[21] The liver rearranges the chemical structure of fats to create certain fats that the body needs. Hydrogenated fats reduce the ability of the liver to rearrange and create useful fats.[22] More than 60 percent of all fats consumed in the U.S. are hydrogenated, and the more hydrogenated fat you eat, the more your *bodily* fats will be hydrogenated.[23]

Most fats that are used in restaurants and fast-food places are both hydrogenated and repeatedly exposed to heat, and researchers found that lab animals that ate heat-processed linseed oil had 10 times more unusual fats in their liver than those that ate fresh oil.[24]

POLYUNSATURATED FATS

By increasing your intake of polyunsaturated fats (usually from unprocessed plant foods), you can lower serum cholesterol,[25] lower blood pressure,[26] and prevent the "stickiness" of blood cells.[27]

There may even be a cumulative high blood pressure effect that develops over several generations of bad eating habits. Researchers fed lab animals the polyunsaturated oils from linseed and sunflowers and found that each successive generation experienced lower blood pressure. Normal lab food was reintroduced to the fifth and sixth generations, with the old high blood pressure quickly returning.[28] Perhaps our hypertensive epidemic in this country is due to many decades of marginal nutrition.

The linolenic acid that is found in linseed oil seems to be even more effective at lowering heart disease risk than the more typical polyunsaturated plant oil (linoleic acid) that was used in the above studies. German researchers gave supplements of linseed oil to 41 heart disease patients for three years and found major improvements in serum lipids.[29] Linseed oil even increases the amount of eicosapentaenoic acid (EPA) made in the cells.[30] (EPA has major benefits that will be discussed later.) Linseed oils also increase the amount of alpha linolenic acid and docosahexaenoic acid (DHA) in the body cells.[31] Both of these fats are very valuable, especially for the pregnant woman and developing infant. Unfortunately, the bold flavor and aroma of linseed oil do not lend themselves well to being commonly used in the kitchen. Due to the similarities between linseed and fish oils, cooking with linseed oil smells much like frying fish.

Gamma-linolenic acid (a.k.a *GLA*, or *evening primrose oil*) seems to have some potential in preventing and treating circulatory problems. Eight capsules daily of evening primrose oil (each containing 360 mg of GLA) can lower hypertension that is caused by stress[32] and can also lower serum cholesterol.[33]

OMEGA-3 FATS

Fish oil is no stranger to the healing arts. Cod liver oil has been a remedy for centuries for night blindness and spots on the eyes (corneal xerosis). Both of these conditions are the result of a vitamin A deficiency.[34] Cod liver oil is one of the richest known sources of vitamins A and D. Fishermen from Europe and New England used cod liver oil to ward off rickets (vitamin D deficiency), a disease that left millions of unprotected children with bowed legs and other skeletal deformities. In the late 18th century, a British physician used cod liver oil to treat bone diseases and rheumatism, claiming, ". . . the good effects of it are so well known among the poorer sort that it is particularly requested by them for almost every lameness."[35]

Fish oil has been subjected to a variety of scientific experiments and has passed with honors. It may be the wonder nutrient of the 1980s. The active ingredients of fish oil are EPA and DHA. These omega-3 fatty acids have a unique chemical structure that allows them to do things for the body that other fats, even linoleic acid, cannot do.[36] Your body produces small amounts of EPA. How much and how efficiently varies considerably and could be the reason why some people are more likely than others to get various ailments.

Evidence is mounting that EPA fights heart disease in several ways:

- People who eat at least two ounces of fish per week cut their heart disease risk in half.[37]
- EPA encourages the body to produce prostacyclin,[38] which is a prostaglandin that prevents "sticky" blood cells from forming. EPA in the diet also cuts the production of thromboxane, a prostaglandin that promotes blood cell clumping, by 58 percent.[39] In general, it is quite effective at preventing the blood from clumping, or forming thrombus.[40]
- EPA also helps to regulate blood pressure. Eight human volunteers were given 40 milliliters per day (about 4 tablespoons) of cod liver oil for 25 days. Blood pressure dropped significantly.[41] Researchers also have found that many people with high blood pressure cannot manufacture enough of their own EPA.[42] Another study showed that EPA can lower systolic blood pressure.[43]
- EPA lowers cholesterol and triglyceride levels. Twelve healthy adults were fed diets high in either linoleic acid (the essential fatty acid) or salmon oil. Only the salmon oil diet was able to decrease levels of VLDL (very low density lipoproteins; when present in high levels, heart disease is more likely to occur) and triglycerides, both of which are major risk factors in circulatory disorders.[44] In another study, 20 patients with dangerously high levels of triglycerides in their blood were given various diets, one of them high in EPA. The EPA diet lowered total cholesterol by 45 percent and triglycerides by 79 percent when compared to the control group.[45] In another human experiment, EPA supplements were able to keep se-

rum cholesterol levels low even when the human subjects were fed diets with an additional three egg yolks per day.[46]

● EPA can also significantly decrease angina pain during exercise.[47]

● In animal experiments, EPA was able to improve the chances of surviving a heart attack[48] and increase blood flow so effectively that it minimized damage to the brain during a stroke.[49]

All things totaled, EPA has been judged by experts to be a seriously effective weapon against heart disease.[50] At least two scientists have separately called for a Recommended Daily Allowance to be established for EPA.[51] Other scientists estimate that one-sixth of our fats should come from these magical fish oils.[52] In Britain, fish oil (high in EPA) is used to make margarine, but, alas, the oils are hydrogenated and thus lose their potency as a wonder fat.

Sources of EPA. EPA actually originates in plants and algae. Fish eat enough of these plant sources of EPA to concentrate and store the EPA in their muscle tissue or liver. There are no food sources of EPA in a vegetarian diet that can match the EPA concentration in fish. Yet a lifetime of varied plant food intake will provide measurable levels of EPA, which is certainly better than the very low EPA intake found in the conventional American diet of processed food and high animal fat. Vegetarian sources of EPA include spirulina, an ocean plankton. The best fish sources of EPA are the high-fat fishes, like salmon. Low-fat fishes, like cod, keep their EPA in their liver, which makes cod liver oil valuable, but not necessarily the muscle tissue in cod. Linseed oil (from the flax seed) and purslane (a vegetable common to the European Mediterranean region) are high in alpha linolenic acid, which is similar but not identical to EPA. Alpha linolenic acid may provide some health benefits, but they are not as well documented as EPA.

The dangers of EPA. Can you eat too much of this wonder fat? Yes. As in most areas of nutrition, you can overdo a good thing. EPA both thins the blood (lowers the viscosity) and reduces the stickiness of blood cells (platelet aggregation). These effects help prevent heart disease, yet they also prolong bleeding time, which may be bad for people who have problems with proper blood clotting. One Oxford professor was so impressed with the spate of literature praising EPA that he commenced a diet that was composed almost entirely of fish and included supplements of vitamin E.[53] He developed anemia, dangerously prolonged bleeding time, and plasma vitamin C levels near zero.

Researchers have also noticed that diets that are very high in EPA supplements tend to lower slightly the immune functions in humans.[54] Fish oil also contains cetoleic acid, which may be directly toxic to heart muscle.[55] However, the commercial preparations of EPA have had nearly all of the cetoleic acid, cholesterol, and vitamins A and D removed from the product. But cod liver oil is very high in vitamins A and D, both of which could be toxic if several tablespoons per day were taken for a long period of time. Cod liver oil is also high in cholesterol, which could be detrimental to some people. Finally, fish oils are so polyunsaturated that they can quickly go rancid. Fish oil and EPA need some vitamin C, vitamin E, or another antioxidant to prevent the "rusting" of fat from occurring.

The net result is that 300 to 3000 milligrams daily of EPA or one teaspoon of mint-flavored cod-liver oil may provide noticeable health improvements to a wide range of people. Too much or too little EPA, cod liver oil, or fish could, however, result in some health problems. If a little EPA is good, then more is *not* better.

LECITHIN

Another beneficial fatty substance is lecithin. Lecithin, found in soybeans, is something like a soap in that it can dissolve in both fat-soluble and water-soluble substances at the same time. Therefore, it can prevent the separation of components in food products that have both fat- and water-soluble ingredients and is a popular food additive. This soap-like characteristic of lecithin makes it useful in treating vascular diseases. In one study, over an ounce of lecithin daily was able to drop cholesterol levels by 18 percent in humans.[56] Another study found that lecithin lowered both cholesterol and triglyceride levels in humans.[57]

ZINC AND HDLs

As was mentioned, fat intake is important, but so are the nutrients that help the body to handle fats properly. Too much zinc can deteriorate fat levels in the blood by lowering the beneficial HDLs.

The RDA for zinc is 15 mg per day. Supplements of 150 mg/day lowered these protective HDLs noticeably,[58] at 100 mg/day there was a slight effect,[59] and 28 mg/day of zinc supplements had no effect.[60] Moral of the story: do not take high-dose zinc supplements for long periods of time, lest the benefits of the zinc be outweighed by the potentially elevated risk for heart disease.

FIBER

The whole concept is ridiculous: fiber is indigestible food matter, meaning that it cannot be digested or absorbed by the body. So how can something so useless be so useful? It is.

Fiber is found only in plant foods and is basically categorized into two groups: soluble (can be dissolved in water) and insoluble (cannot dissolve in water). The soluble fibers include pectin (from apples, carrots, grapes, and other fruits), gums, and mucilages (from seaweeds and other plants). Insoluble fibers include lignin (the tough, fibrous part of broccoli stalks, celery, popcorn hulls, and other plants), cellulose (from the bran part of whole grains), and hemicellulose.

Fiber is nature's broom. It cleans out the intestines and keeps toxic substances from being absorbed. It binds fats, cholesterol, harmful metals, and other substances and prevents them from being absorbed.

Unfortunately, Americans consume less than 20 grams per day of fiber. Our food refining often strips the food of fiber. Orange juice, white flour, and potato chips, for example, all have a mere fraction of the fiber that the original foods had. In regions such as Uganda, where the people consume up to five times the amount of fiber that we do,[61] there is near zero incidence of heart disease, overfatness, diabetes, cancer, and gastrointestinal problems.

Fiber has some rather miraculous talents for keeping the circulatory system unobstructed and vital for decades longer than normal. Here are some examples:

• Researchers fed about ⅓ ounce per day of wheat bran to healthy young volunteers. That small supplement increased the subject's normal fiber intake by 35 percent and was able to raise HDLs by 46 percent and decrease LDLs by 25 percent.[62]

- On a very high-fiber diet (100 grams per day, the same as for the Ugandans), patients with dangerously high serum cholesterol levels were able to lower their cholesterol by 13 percent in only 13 days.[63]
- Twelve grams (not quite ½ ounce) of supplemental pectin daily lowered blood cholesterol by 6–15 percent in *healthy* individuals.[64]
- Small amounts of guar gum (5.7 grams daily) added to the diets of six *healthy* human subjects were able to lower serum cholesterol by 16 percent in only two weeks.[65]
- The outer bran layer of grains (especially barley) also contains a substance that has been proven to reduce cholesterol production in the body.[66]
- The oil from rice bran was able to substantially lower various fat levels in both the blood and liver of lab animals.[67]
- Fiber even helps to decrease blood pressure.[68]

There are substances in fiber that are so powerfully beneficial that, if they weren't found naturally in foods, you would need a prescription to buy them. Although all fiber has some beneficial effect, the gelling fibers of pectin, gums, and mucilages are probably the most effective at lowering fats in the blood.[69]

Once again, there is an upper limit on fiber intake. Too much fiber will cause diarrhea, which can be life-threatening if its dehydrating effect continues. Also, fiber binds many metals in the intestines,[70] which is beneficial if the metal is a common toxin like lead but is harmful when the metals are essential minerals that are in short supply in the American diet, such as zinc, iron, and calcium. Increasing the intake of fiber from the average of 20 grams to a more respectable 50 grams daily will provide major health benefits to the circulatory system without seriously lowering the amount of minerals absorbed.

CALCIUM, MAGNESIUM, SODIUM, AND POTASSIUM

Billions of years ago, life evolved in the ocean's primordial soup of water and minerals. Since then, many forms of life throughout the planet earth carry a similar recipe for the ocean within them. All human cells are immersed in a "sea" of salt water of a concentration nearly identical to that of the ocean. Sodium is the main positive ion outside the cells. Potassium became the primary ion inside of living cells. Calcium and magnesium are minor players in this "electrolyte soup" yet are involved greatly in nerve and muscle function. Thus, these four minerals have great importance in the cardiovascular health of humans.

Somewhere between 37 and 50 million Americans suffer from hypertension. There has been no shortage of research on this subject. High-salt diets tend to increase blood pressure because sodium (part of table salt) carries water with it, causing fluid retention in some people.[71] Based upon this simple fact, many experts prematurely stated, "Don't eat salt, and you won't get hypertension." This is only partly true. Cardiovascular diseases are more dependent on the balance of these "electrolyte soup" minerals than on excess sodium.[72] Too little potassium, calcium, and magnesium may be more responsible for high blood pressure in America than too much sodium.

Sodium

Sodium (from salt) is such a useful nutrient in the diet that nature gave humans a specific sensor on the tongue to tell us when a food is salty. In the days before the ubiquitous salt shaker, this tongue sensor was a survival tool. Primitive humans ate considerable amounts of plant foods (high in potassium) and sweated much (losing some sodium) and thus needed to seek high-sodium foods for survival. Today, that salt-seeking instinct may mean our own demise. Food companies know how to get "the hook in the lip" of the consumer. Most processed foods add incredible quantities of salt to increase consumer acceptance. And for decades, many baby food companies added copious quantities of salt to the baby food so that Mom would like the flavor and hence buy it for Junior. And many ready-to-eat breakfast cereals *still* have the same sodium content as potato chips and pretzels.[73]

Americans eat 2 to 5 times the recommended upper limit on sodium intake and 40 times the amount of sodium that is needed for health. Of this massive sodium intake, 30 percent is naturally found in the food supply, 30 percent is added in cooking and at the table, and 40 percent is added by the food processor.[74]

If you shudder at the thought of going without the salt shaker, understand that high-salt diets are an acquired taste, and you can wean yourself of it just as you artificially acquired it. Over a five-week period, researchers gradually cut salt intake until it was at 50 percent of beginning levels for 228 students at a boarding high school in New Hampshire. The students found no difference in taste acceptability of their new low-sodium food.[75] The "norm" can then become a healthier, low-salt program.

For decades, physicians have known that many black people seemed particularly vulnerable to the effects of high blood pressure. A historian may have found the answer to this puzzle. Certain groups of blacks whose ancestors came from West Africa apparently existed on a very low-salt diet for many centuries before being brought to this country. Their low-salt, high-potassium diet encouraged very efficient salt retention. Also, manual labor in the tropics causes considerable sodium loss through sweat. These tribes had no readily available salt source. By consuming the typical high-salt diet that is found in America, these people continued to retain much of that sodium, which then raised blood pressure.[76] At that point, a fabulous evolutionary tool of survival had turned against these people.

Can a low-sodium diet really make a difference? In many people, yes. Ninety hypertensive patients were put on a low-sodium diet for 12 weeks. Eighty percent of the low-sodium group were able to reduce or cease their hypertensive medication, compared to only 33 percent of the control group. As an unexpected bonus, many of these "cured" hypertensive patients reported a significant relief from various pains and depression.[77] Since the brain operates in an "electrolyte soup" of sodium and other elements, it makes sense that an unbalanced formula of electrolytes could instigate both high blood pressure and poor mental health.

Yet sodium excess is not the only answer to hypertension. It may not even be the main answer! Twelve patients, ages 19 to 52, volunteered for a sodium-restricted diet. Blood pressure became lower in seven of these people, but *higher* in the other five people.[78] Apparently, high-salt diets are responsible for high blood pressure in only some people.

Potassium

A critical balance between sodium and potassium exists in the body. A 10-year study involving thousands of men in the Netherlands found that the lower the intake of potassium, the greater the risk for hypertension.[79] By adding 2.5 grams per day of potassium to the diet (which might double the intake for many Americans), blood pressure can be reduced markedly. Since potassium comes primarily from plant foods, Americans would have to eat more plant foods and fewer animal foods. Though supplements would be a viable alternative, they are rigorously restricted by law, despite the fact that taking potassium supplements is risky only for people with poor kidney function. Since there are about 50 million hypertensives in this country and considerably fewer renal dialysis patients, most of whom are well informed on what to avoid, making potassium supplements more readily available would seem to benefit the majority of Americans. Until that happens, however, you can circumvent this strange law by turning to "lite" salt and salt substitutes, which are usually at least half potassium—a cheap and convenient way to bolster your potassium intake. Healthy people can take in up to 10 grams per day of potassium with no side effects. The excess is easily excreted in the urine.

Besides our low consumption of plant food, the way we cook our food robs us of needed potassium. Though steaming is gaining popularity, most Americans still boil vegetables, and in the process lose up to half of the potassium into the cooking water. In contrast, food that is steamed loses only 6 percent of its potassium.[80] If you still insist on boiling your food, you can add potassium chloride (salt substitute) to the boiling water to increase the potassium content of the food.[81]

Low potassium levels can provoke heart problems, some of which may be fatal. Ironically, many diuretic medications given to hypertensive patients cause potassium loss, and less than half of the physicians surveyed in one study recommend a potassium supplement to go with these drugs.[82] Potassium supplements are essential to anyone on diuretic medication, since over three feet of bananas would be required to provide the needed potassium.[83] Because of this, hypotensive drugs could actually make hypertension worse in some cases.

There are several explanations for why potassium is so effective at lowering blood pressure:

1. It competes with sodium in the kidneys for reabsorption, thus leaving less sodium to be reabsorbed in a potassium-saturated system.

2. It dilates blood vessels by relaxing the smooth muscles that surround the vessels.

3. It lowers the output of substances (e.g., angiotensin) that the body produces to preserve the sodium supply.

4. It reduces the flow of stress hormones (catecholamines) that can elevate blood pressure.[84]

Potassium was used effectively 50 years ago to treat high blood pressure, and it still makes sense:

• It has no side effects in people with healthy kidneys.
• It is inexpensive.
• It balances the true optimal state of the body, rather than attempting to temporarily change the natural order of electrolytes with drugs.

Calcium

Calcium is another mineral that can help bring blood pressure back to normal. During a four-year study of 115 women, calcium supplements (1,500 milligrams daily as calcium carbonate) lowered blood pressure in hypertensive patients more effectively than prescription medication.[85] Another study of rural communities in Iowa found that half to three-fourths of the women surveyed consumed less than the RDA for vitamin D. Those women who did consume adequate vitamin D had consistently lower systolic blood pressure.[86] Vitamin D is vital to the absorption and use of calcium in the body.

High calcium intake also reduces the risk of a high blood pressure condition (toxemia) that is common in pregnancy.[87] In rural areas of Guatemala, the diet is low in calories and protein, yet the women have a lower incidence of water retention during pregnancy (preeclampsia) than women in the U.S. The Guatemalans soak their corn tortillas in a calcium solution, which is probably responsible for their amazing pregnancy health amid food shortages and poor medical care.[88]

People drinking hard water (high in calcium and magnesium) have a lower risk for circulatory disorders.[89] One gram of calcium per day even lowered the blood pressure of *healthy* young people.[90] About half of all hypertensive patients seem to respond to this calcium therapy.[91]

Magnesium

Magnesium is another critical mineral involved in blood pressure. Magnesium is important for relaxation of muscles, including those surrounding the blood vessels. It also interacts with the other electrolytes to form the proper "recipe" for the primordial soup of higher life. Lab animals that were fed low-magnesium diets developed higher blood pressure and more constricted arteries than the control animals.[92] And magnesium supplements brought a significant reduction in blood pressure, even in human patients who had been on hypertensive medication for years.[93] Interestingly, victims of sudden heart attack are almost always low in potassium and/or magnesium levels.[94] Magnesium also has been shown to be effective in preventing eclampsia.[95]

Magnesium and potassium are inseparable and interdependent partners in the electrolyte soup of your body. The literature gives us many examples of people whose magnesium levels dropped after they had developed low potassium levels (for whatever reason). The low potassium could be treated only in conjunction with the magnesium.[96]

Magnesium also has been successful in treating certain rhythm problems of the heart (ventricular dysrhythmias).[97] Intravenous magnesium helps prevent potassium depletion that can cause poor heart rhythm in patients taking digitalis medication.[98] And arteries that are even slightly low in magnesium are more likely to have spastic contractions.[99] Perhaps the many sudden-death heart attacks experienced by people who are physically fit are due to the low magnesium levels in their heart. When researchers looked at the magnesium levels in the serum of 100 heart disease victims, only 5 percent showed a deficiency. Yet 53 percent of these people were found to be magnesium deficient when their lymphocytes (blood cells involved in disease resistance) were checked. These scientists concluded that low magnesium levels could instigate a large percentage of heart attacks in America.[100] Since most magnesium is found inside the cells, checking fluid outside the cells (such as serum) can be very misleading. This would be like surveying for poverty incidence in the wealthy bedroom communities that surround our big cities. It just isn't a good representative sampling. Jim Fixx was an exemplary fitness guru who dropped dead of a heart attack at age 52 while running. Low magnesium was likely the problem.

Magnesium intake is very low in America. The Nationwide Food Consumption Survey found that about half of all Americans are consuming less than two-thirds of their recommended intake for magnesium. Another study found that the average magnesium intake for postmenopausal women was less than two-thirds of the RDA.[101] When you consider the proven medicinal values of magnesium, the abysmally low levels of magnesium found in American diets, and the near negligible risk of using magnesium supplements, it's obvious that this mineral could be a major healing nutrient in the war against circulatory disorders.

CHROMIUM

The average adult body contains about $\frac{1}{10,000}$ of an ounce (6 milligrams) of chromium. After more than two decades of research on chromium, it was finally included as an essential nutrient in the 1980 version of the RDAs. Here is a trace element that could single-handedly prevent fat-blocked arteries in up to 25 percent of these patients.

Basically, chromium works in an enzyme system (glucose tolerance factor, or GTF) that helps insulin get glucose through the cell membranes. The favored fuel of many body cells is glucose, and if that fuel cannot go into the cells, many problems develop. The alternative fuels are fat and protein. If glucose metabolism is altered (such as in diabetes or chromium deficiency), then tissue wasting occurs as the body scavenges its own protein stores for fuel. When fat is called upon to be a major source of fuel, the arteries become crowded with fatty substances. The chances of plaque building up then are much greater.

Oral glucose tolerance tests (OGTT) indicate how well the body handles blood glucose. Researchers gave 200 micrograms daily of chromium to 76 *healthy* humans, and all had significant improvements in their OGTT.[102] There was a 1,000 percent difference in the efficiency of chromium absorption among the subjects tested.

Diabetics, with low insulin output, have a much greater risk of heart disease. So do people with a low chromium intake. Chromium deficiencies produced in laboratory animals simulate either diabetes or heart disease or both.[103]

The average daily intake of chromium in the U.S. is 33 micrograms, while the recommended range is 50 to 200. Some scientists recommend that 500 micrograms daily would be a more optimal intake of chromium. Even one-third of all diets designed by registered dietitians have less than 50 micrograms daily of chromium.[104] Scientists at the Human Nutrition Research Center operated by the federal government stated that chromium deficiency is common in the U.S. and is probably a cause of many cases of heart disease.[105] People with severe fatty blockage in their arteries have been found to have chromium levels that were one-third to one-eighth that of normal healthy controls.[106]

As Americans age, our body chromium levels drop off, more as a result of our poor nutrition habits than because of unavoidable deterioration in aging. We can ill afford to lose our stores of this precious mineral, so it is wise to understand the ways our chromium levels can be depleted. First, high sugar intake causes much chromium to be lost. About one out of five calories in America comes from sugar. Second, pregnancy causes a loss of chromium stores to the developing fetus.

As glucose tolerance deteriorates, insulin output increases and heart disease risk skyrockets.[107] But studies with healthy older Americans have found that chromium supplements improve their glucose tolerance measurably.[108] And there are other benefits. Rabbits that were fed high-cholesterol diets and then given chromium injections had the plaque in their arteries dissolved significantly.[109] Human subjects with high levels of fats in their blood (hyperlipidemic) were given 20 grams daily of high-chromium brewer's yeast containing about 48 micrograms of chromium for eight weeks. This is even a lower amount than the lowest acceptable range of intake. Eighty-four percent of the 16 subjects receiving the chromium supplements had major improvements in their blood lipids. Cholesterol levels dropped and HDLs increased.[110] The evidence is becoming almost overwhelming that chromium deficiency probably causes many instances of heart disease.[111]

In the typical American diet, a dependable source of chromium *would* be wheat products, except that refining wheat to white flour removes nearly all of the chromium. Raw cane and beet sugar contain some chromium, while the highly refined end products of these foods contain no chromium. Honey and molasses also contain some chromium.

The ability to take dietary chromium and manufacture GTF within the body varies considerably among humans.[112] GTF is found only in high-chromium yeast. Those people who cannot make dietary chromium into GTF in their body consequently may need to consume GTF from high-chromium yeast.

Supplements of chromium at any level of intake have failed to produce any toxicity symptoms in any laboratory animals tested.[113] With amazing benefits being likely and near zero risk, chromium supplements (especially from high-chromium yeast) seem to be almost mandatory for heart-disease-prone Americans.

CARNITINE

Imagine an old-time steel mill. Workers are shoveling the coal into the furnace to melt down the iron ore. Trucks of coal keep arriving at the furnace site. What if the trucks brought coal faster than the workers could shovel it? Obviously, the pile of coal would build up.

A similar situation occurs in your arteries with fat (the coal) and carnitine (the workers shoveling). Insufficient carnitine leads to a buildup of fats, which then back up into the blood and form plaque. Carnitine is basically a shuttle mechanism to get fat into the mitochondria (the furnace) of the body cells so that energy can be obtained from this foodstuff. Those cells that burn fat abundantly, such as the heart and other muscles, critically depend on carnitine. Carnitine is the "bottleneck" in burning fats effectively. Supplemental carnitine allows most cells to burn fat more efficiently.[114] This not only gives the body more energy but also prevents the fats from building up in the bloodstream.

Preformed carnitine is found only in animal products, hence the Latin root word *carnis*, meaning "meat." Some lower forms of life and possibly certain newborn animals require carnitine in the diet, just as a vitamin.[115] Humans make their own carnitine from lysine, methionine, ascorbic acid, niacin, B_6, and iron. There are two mirror images of carnitine found in nature, the right-handed ("D" for *dextro*) and left-handed ("L" for *levo*). The L form is useful to the body, while the D form either is useless or possibly even dilutes the benefit of L-carnitine.

Most people make enough carnitine to survive until adulthood, yet quite a few humans probably exist at subsaturation levels of carnitine. The world-famous Mayo Clinic has described the symptoms of patients with a carnitine deficiency: elevated fats in the blood and muscular weakness.[116] Unless a substance is essential in the diet, you cannot have a deficiency condition, so some scientists have called for carnitine to be considered an essential vitamin for *some* people.[117] People who develop high fats in the blood may be the ones for whom carnitine should be considered a vitamin.

Numerous studies have linked a lack of carnitine with heart disease:

- Angina pain in heart disease patients was seriously reduced with supplements of 3.5 grams daily of L-carnitine.[118] In another study, carnitine supplements (2 grams daily) reduced angina pain during exercise for human heart disease victims.[119]
- Carnitine supplements in laboratory animals drastically reduced the amount of damage that occurred in heart tissue when the oxygen supply was cut off (ischemic myocardium), which is what occurs in a heart attack.[120]
- Carnitine injections in dogs improved the performance of the heart and caused the blood vessels to dilate.[121]
- In humans, oral carnitine supplements lowered fats in the blood and raised the levels of protective HDLs.[122]
- Carnitine supplements (750–3,000 milligrams daily) reduced cholesterol and triglyceride levels in human patients.[123]
- Heart disease patients were able to exercise more once they were given carnitine supplements.[124]
- Carnitine lessened heart rhythm abnormalities in heart disease patients.[125]
- Carnitine improves overall heart function and its recovery from starvation, abuse, or stress.[126]

Note that lysine, iron, B_6, and vitamin C are involved in the body's ability to manufacture its own carnitine. Deficiencies of these nutrients in the U.S. are quite common and could provoke a carnitine deficiency. L-carnitine (500–3,000 milligrams daily) has the potential of being a true hero in the battle against circulatory disorders.

VITAMIN C AND BIOFLAVONOIDS

There are two very unusual facts about vitamin C: (1) Almost all species of life (except humans and a few other unfortunates) make their own vitamin C. (2) It is the ultimate multitalented vitamin, with more different functions than almost any other vitamin in human nutrition. Humans have lost the ability to make our own vitamin C internally,

Vitamin C (a.k.a. *ascorbic acid*) is very similar in structure to glucose and is made both in life and in vitamin factories from simple sugars. Of the many functions that vitamin C has in the body, several are related to the health of the heart and blood vessels:

- It helps to build tough connective proteins, such as are found in the blood vessel walls of the circulatory system.
- It works as an antioxidant to prevent the destruction of the "good guy" prostaglandin, called prostacyclin.[127]
- It helps to regulate fat levels in the blood in three different pathways.

Disregarding the therapeutic value of high-dose vitamin C, half of all Americans don't even get the RDA, which is 60 mg per day for a 154-pound human. Not only are most Americans low in their intake of vitamin C, but tobacco, certain drugs, stress, pollution, exercise, and other factors can increase the need for vitamin C well beyond the RDA.

Many experts feel that the RDA for vitamin C is actually much too low. Long-term marginal intake of C has been linked to heart disease,[128] and recent studies indicate that our RDA for vitamin C is more of a "survival" guideline than a level which will encourage ideal health. A very new research technique has found that "ideal" levels of C are probably about 10 times the "minimal" intake.[129] That would put the RDA closer to 200 milligrams daily for healthy, nonstressed, younger adults. Many people exposed to tobacco, drugs, stress, pollution, heat, and regular exercise would require more. One thousand milligrams of C (16 times the RDA) promotes better overall health in the elderly. Another study found that elderly men need at least 150 mg of C to maintain decent blood levels of C.[130] And in three out of four university students in Scotland who were found to have substandard levels of C in their blood, researchers were able to triple their plasma levels of C by giving these students only 160 mg, indicating that the body was retaining and using the C, not unlike a dry sponge soaking up moisture.[131]

There probably is also a wide range of vitamin C requirements for humans. Dr. Roger Williams discovered that there was a major difference in the amount of vitamin C that was needed by various guinea pigs.

In a study of Japenese farmers, scientists found that the lower the blood levels of vitamin C, the higher were the risks for hypertension.[132] Vitamin C also has a direct stabilizing effect on blood platelets, helping to prevent them from clumping together into a clot (thrombus).[133] Supplements of 2,000 milligrams daily of C in humans not only prevented blood clumps from occurring, but actually began to break up the clumps that had already formed.[134] In studies of older people with heart disease, 60 percent of the men had unacceptably low levels of C in their blood. After six weeks of supplemental C, these people not only had lower levels of certain fats in the blood, but also had raised levels of the protective HDLs.[135] Rabbits fed diets high in cholesterol get heart disease, but when they receive vitamin C supplements, they do not.[136]

Vitamin C seems to take on these anti–heart disease characteristics only in higher doses. Researchers found that supplements of 1,000 mg daily of C in heart disease patients only slightly increased levels of C in the blood and did not change levels of blood fats or blood clumping tendencies. Yet when they doubled the dose of C to 2,000 mg daily, the breaking up of blood clumps (fibrinolytic activity) increased by 45–62 percent while cholesterol levels dropped by 12 percent.[137]

At lower doses, vitamin C takes longer to act. At 1 gram daily of C, researchers found it took 6–12 months for cholesterol levels to drop significantly.[138] Daily supplements of 1,000 mg were able to reduce the number of clots in leg veins that usually occur after surgery.[139]

Bioflavonoids seem to both help the action of vitamin C and to have their own benefits. Involved in plant photosynthesis, bioflavonoids are found only in plant food. Bioflavonoids were a popular and effective treatment in American health care until about two decades ago, when they were somewhat mysteriously dropped from the list of prescription drugs. Since then, most research on bioflavonoids has been done in Europe and Asia. With about 500 different bioflavonoids, including rutin and hesperidin,[140] and so few chemists who know how to purify these compounds, it's likely that impure mixtures probably led to the "downfall" of bioflavonoids in America. But they are worth pursuing.

Bioflavonoids seem to increase the amount of vitamin C absorbed in the intestines.[141] Rutin, hesperidin, and vitamin C used together were able to increase the blood flow in heart disease patients.[142] Rutin and hesperidin together improved the blood lipid profile while protecting liver tissue in rats with high blood fats.[143] This situation would be similar to the dangerously high blood fat levels commonly found in American men, especially alcohol abusers.

Fragile capillaries can lead to a stroke, heart attack, thrombus, varicose veins, and other problems of the vascular network. Rutin is effective in treating varicose veins [144] and helps to strengthen the tiny capillaries throughout the body.[145] Rutin supplements (200 milligrams daily) also help to clear up the hemorrhoids and gingivitis (swollen, bleeding gums) that plague many pregnant women as the developing fetus sucks vitamin C out of the mother's blood supply. In the days when bioflavonoids were still in the good graces of the FDA, one American physician noted that, over a 10-year period, his hypertensive patients receiving rutin supplements had a much lower death rate than those not getting rutin.[146]

Altogether, it seems that vitamin C and bioflavonoids are quite valuable in preventing and even curing breakdowns in the circulatory system. But can you take too much? Yes, but only if you suddenly *stop* taking it. Taking large (5 grams or more daily) doses of C for a long period and then suddenly ceasing this routine can produce "rebound scurvy."[147]

In addition, some researchers were concerned that high doses of C would trigger kidney stones. But another group of scientists studied 10 people who had been taking 3,000–10,000 mg of C daily for at least two years and found no difference in their oxalate excretion (a by-product of C that is the core of many kidney stones).[148] People with normal kidney functions can tolerate, though probably do not need, up to 15,000 mg daily without any problems,[149] but patients on kidney filtration machines should not consume more than 100 mg of C supplements daily.[150]

How much is "just right"? At least 200 mg of vitamin C per day and up to 5,000 mg daily for those in the maximum-risk category. Two hundred mg daily of the bioflavonoid rutin might also benefit vascular health.

SELENIUM AND VITAMIN E

A more dynamic duo would be hard to find. Both E and selenium work toward making a potent enzyme system (glutathione peroxidase, or GSH) that prevents the destruction of many valuable body substances, including prostacyclin. Vitamin E and selenium also have the ability to help keep the blood flowing smoothly without clumping. Together, they can strongly reduce your risk of getting circulatory disorders. They may even be able to "cure" certain circulatory problems.

Until 1957, selenium was considered to be a toxic trace element. Then, in 1957, researchers found that selenium was essential for health in certain animals. By the late 1960s, selenium had been established as an essential nutrient for human health. Even today, selenium cannot be included in nutritional supplements shipped into Australia, because the Australians still consider it toxic. The need for selenium may have first been noticed in 1935 in a certain part of mainland China, where many people experienced a deterioration of their heart muscle at an early age (Keshan's disease). Scientists then found abnormally low levels of selenium in the soil, Keshan's disease wasn't cured until the late 1960s, when the people were provided with 500–1,000 mcg of selenium daily.[151]

The selenium–heart disease link was strengthened in eastern Finland, which has one of the highest rates of heart disease in the world. Scientists could not explain this, until they found that heart disease patients in Finland had only two-thirds of the selenium blood levels that normal, healthy controls had. The people with the lowest amounts of selenium in their blood had more than a 600 percent greater risk for heart disease than the population at large. The researchers estimated that low selenium intake *alone* was directly responsible for one out of five heart disease victims in Finland.[152]

An American scientist found, in a study of 91 heart disease victims, that the lower the selenium, the greater the heart disease risk and the worse the condition.[153] And death from heart disease and stroke are lowest in the American states where the selenium soil content and hence selenium in the diet are highest.[154] The "stroke belt" along the southeast Atlantic seaboard has the highest frequency of both heart disease and stroke and also has the lowest selenium levels in the soil.

Not only are low selenium levels connected to high heart disease risk, but selenium supplements have been found to have promising curative and preventive properties. For example, supplements of 200 mcg of selenium daily in older patients decreased the clumping activity that often leads to blood clots.[155] Selenium either increases the production or decreases the destruction of prostacyclin, which then lowers the clumping activity of the blood.[156] And by giving rats supplements of selenium, researchers found that GSH activity nearly doubled.[157] This GSH enzyme seems to protect the valuable prostacyclin, which keeps the blood from clumping together. When selenium levels are low, the body has a hard time making enough of the raw materials (arachidonic acid) to produce these healthy blood pressure regulators.[158] By taking 1,000 mcg of selenium along with 200 IU of vitamin E, 22 of 24 patients found significant relief from angina pain.[159] In lab animals, selenium and vitamin E supplements were able to reduce the damage done to tissue when the blood supply was cut off (as occurs in a heart attack).[160]

Vitamin E alone is very protective against heart disease.[161] Six healthy men who took 1,600 IU of vitamin E daily had increased prostacyclin levels and blood that generally was less likely to clump.[162] And in a study of 47 humans, vitamin E (400–1,200 IU daily) was much more effective at thinning the blood than aspirin.[163] Aspirin has been recommended by some scientists as a possible cheap preventive means of reducing the risk of heart disease but has several hazardous side effects, including microscopic bleeding in the intestines that can produce anemia.

One of the symptoms of a long-term subclinical deficiency of vitamin E may be clumping of the blood.[164] Vitamin E may also be responsible for maintaining healthy levels of HDL and LDL factors in the blood to prevent heart disease. Forty-three humans who were given supplements of 800 IU of vitamin E daily for four weeks showed a significant improvement in protective HDL levels.[165] Several physicians have reported using vitamin E on thousands of patients to prevent and possibly cure thromboembolism (clumps in the blood that lodge in dangerous areas of the body).[166] Best of all, they find literally no risks for these levels of vitamin E.

When vitamin E and calcium supplements were given to surgery patients, the risk of fatal pulmonary embolism (blood clot in the lungs) was cut by almost 90 percent.[167] Intermittent claudication (pain in the legs from a clot caught in a blood vessel) has been treated successfully with vitamin E to provide gradual but significant relief.[168] Vitamin E also provided complete or nearly complete relief for 103 out of 105 patients with nighttime leg and foot cramps.[169]

How much vitamin E and selenium would be advisable? Within reasonable limits, vitamin E has no side effects. Doses of 200–600 IU per day would be harmless and possibly beneficial to all.

At the same time as Keshan's disease was cropping up, another area of China was experiencing strange symptoms, including the loss of hair and fingernails, which were found to be caused by a selenium toxicity from selenium-saturated soil. These people had 100 times more selenium in the soil than folks in the Keshan region.[170] Selenium intake should be somewhere between 70 mcg as a bare minimum[171] and 1,000 mcg for high-risk people.

Selenium is found in foods grown on or animals grazed on selenium-rich soil, which doesn't help you pinpoint particular foods that are high in this nutrient. There are no obvious choices here, though Brazil nuts are a very rich source, providing up to 50 mcg per nut.[172] See Chapter 4 for other foods that are *likely* selenium sources. Selenium from natural food sources (e.g., high-selenium yeast) is much less likely to be toxic than inorganic selenium salts, even at very high intake levels. In the Keshan region of China, another group of researchers provided the village people with soybeans, normally a good source of selenium, instead of the selenium supplements. The results showed the same benefits as those that were obtained using the selenium supplements.[173]

GARLIC

Its odor is legendary. So powerful are the fumes of garlic that vampires and plagues were reported to shrink from its presence. I'm not sure about the vampire business, but garlic has a list of well-controlled scientific studies to prove its therapeutic value in promoting a healthy circulatory system:

- Large doses of garlic given to 20 healthy human subjects for six months substantially lowered cholesterol and triglyceride levels in the blood while raising the protective HDLs.[174]

- The same researchers tested 62 patients with heart disease and elevated cholesterol levels. The benefits this time were even more impressive. The amounts of garlic given in this experiment were roughly equivalent to 1 ounce of raw garlic (6–10 cloves) daily. Though few people eat that much and maintain any social life, lower doses would have similar benefits if extended over a longer period of time.
- Garlic also helps to lower blood pressure.[175] Numerous studies with both laboratory animals and humans have left no doubt that garlic has a potent effect in keeping the blood vessels clear and healthy.[176]

I recommend that you use garlic often in cooking. It now comes in a precrushed form in glass jars, for the convenience of chefs in a hurry. If you eat garlic with parsley or other green leafy vegetables, then the chlorophyll will provide a natural breath deodorant. Deodorized garlic tablets are also available, for those who do not like the taste, but whether these pills provide all the same health benefits of natural garlic has not been proven.

HOT PEPPERS

Hot red peppers can be as hostile toward blood clumps in your arteries as they are to some people's taste buds. Red pepper (capsicum family) contains a substance called *capsaicum* that prevents the stickiness of blood cells that lead to blocked vessels. A study in Thailand compared 88 Thais eating the traditional diet full of hot peppers with 55 American whites living in Thailand. The Thais had a 33 percent higher level of breaking up blood clumps (fibrinolytic activity) in their blood.[177]

Though hot red peppers are prohibited from most ulcer diets, researchers found that 3 grams daily of red chili powder (a rather healthy amount) did not affect ulcer healing in 50 patients being treated with antacids for four weeks.[178]

Some claims have been made that capsaicum may create unfavorable changes in cell structures.[179] However, turmeric, another spice commonly used in conjunction with red peppers, contains curcumin, which has been shown to nullify the possible harmful effects of capsaicum.[180] In other words, eat your hot peppers with some turmeric, and you get the benefits without any risks.

Peppers are not only good for you; they are a major improvement over some questionable seasonings. Mexican salsa, Tabasco, many Cajun foods, and recipes from Asia use bountiful amounts of hot peppers. They season food without the typical fat, salt, and sugar that is found in many American recipes.

GINGER, CHICORY, AND YOGURT

There are other "wonder foods" that improve the health of the vessels and heart. One of them is fresh ginger. When high-cholesterol meals were fed to lab animals along with ginger, there was a major reduction in the levels of blood cholesterol.[181] Fresh gingerroot can be found in the fresh produce section of most grocery stores. You can use grated ginger in cooking or make a stimulating tea by adding a small amount of honey and vitamin C powder to 1 teaspoon of grated ginger and steeping the mixture like normal tea. Ginger tea is a healthy, invigorating, and tasty drink. One teaspoon of grated fresh ginger would properly spice up enough food or tea for one or two people.

Chicory is another herb/food that lowers cholesterol levels when eaten regularly.[182] It can be used as a coffee substitute—it has a similar flavor, plus provides some potential health benefits that coffee cannot match.

Yogurt contains a live bacteria culture called *Lactobacillus acidophilus* that appears to have remarkable health benefits, including lowering serum cholesterol.[183]

ALCOHOL

The connection between alcohol and heart disease is a rather complex issue. Early studies found that people who regularly consumed small amounts of alcohol had lower rates of heart disease than nondrinkers.[184] Unfortunately, some people applied the "If a little is good, then more is better" myth to that information. If that were true, then alcoholics would live forever, but we all know that they don't. It *was* later found that small amounts of alcohol encourage the body to produce more of the protective HDLs, yet anything beyond small amounts (two or three drinks per day) began to be counterproductive.[185] Although regular, low alcohol intake raises HDLs, alcoholics have reduced levels of the protective HDLs.[186] "One drink" is considered to be 4 ounces of wine, 12 ounces of beer, or 1 ounce of distilled spirits.

In certain people, alcohol seems to disturb the normal heart rhythm.[187] Excess alcohol intake raises the level of fats in the blood and also blood pressure.[188] One study looked at the blood pressure of hypertensive and normal patients when drinking and not drinking. They found that alcohol raised blood pressure only in the hypertensives.[189] Since alcohol drains the body of certain nutrients involved in proper heart rhythm, the chance of heart palpitations and sudden heart spasms increases with high alcohol intake.[190] Heavy drinkers are often heavy smokers and just plain heavy people. This "heavy" label creates a problem of figuring out which "heavy" is causing the real vascular risk.[191]

Excess alcohol will eventually kill most people in a variety of ways. A study of over 8,000 men living in Hawaii found that drinkers had over twice the stroke rate of nondrinkers. And heavy drinkers had five times the stroke incidence of nondrinkers.[192] Yet small amounts of alcohol are probably a protective factor for most people, say a group of Stanford University scientists.[193]

If you don't drink, then don't start for this reason. There are too many hazards in drinking to consider this mild benefit worth the change in your lifestyle.

SUGAR

A high-sugar diet puts your circulatory system at considerable risk.[194] There are a number of possible explanations for this:

1. High-sugar diets are often associated with high serum cholesterol.

2. High-sugar diets contain no chromium but have abundant glucose to be processed, leaving the body in a chromium deficiency.

3. Simple refined sugar has no fiber and is absorbed quickly into the system, which creates wild swings in blood sugar curves and high insulin output. High insulin output is linked with heart disease.

4. People who eat lots of sugar, which is very concentrated in calories, are often overfat, which is a major risk factor in vascular problems.

5. Even "normal" intake of refined sugars has been found to lower the levels of the protective HDLs.[195]

Twenty percent of the food calories in the average U.S. diet come from sugar. If we could cut that amount at least in half, then sugar probably could be eliminated as a suspect in circulatory diseases.

COPPER AND ZINC

Trace mineral deficiencies or imbalances can play a role in vascular problems.[196] We consume only half of the recommended intake for copper, and low copper intake encourages higher levels of cholesterol. Heart disease victims have about one-fourth the copper levels in their tissue that normal healthy controls have.[197] Copper alone is a factor, but so is the copper-to-zinc ratio.

Zinc deficiencies (both blatant and marginal) are common in America. Zinc is as versatile a nutrient as is ascorbic acid in the number of different body processes that it is involved in. Zinc works in the production of the prostaglandins that help to prevent blood clumping. Lab animals fed zinc-deficient diets have lowered production of these beneficial prostaglandins and are more likely targets for heart disease.[198] Zinc supplements (50 mg daily) given to 23 healthy young men over a six-week period resulted in a significant drop in blood pressure and cholesterol levels.[199] There is ample evidence that the American diet is low in zinc and that zinc supplements would be of value. However, providing zinc supplements without copper could make our current copper problems even worse.[200] Zinc and copper should be in a 10 to 1 ratio in the diet.

OTHER TRACE MINERALS

Silicon is an essential trace element in human nutrition. Silicon deficiency may instigate heart disease.[201] The best dietary sources of silicon would be whole grains. Most silicon is lost in refining the whole grain into white flour. You may recall that the most commonly eaten food in America is white bread.

Although many infants, children, and menstruating women are iron anemic, sedentary adult males are unlikely to be anemic. As a matter of fact, heart disease in some males may be a direct result of *excess* iron in their bodies.[202] High iron stores are directly toxic to the heart. With diets that are rich in iron-ladened red meat, many adult males might find that donating blood several times each year may be an altruistic egotistic way of keeping their circulatory system healthy and helping others while they are at it.

Cadmium is a toxic trace element which is found in small proportions in canned food and industrial pollution. Excess levels of cadmium in the human body are associated with high blood pressure.[203] Diets low in calcium, iron, and other essential minerals encourage the uptake of cadmium since they all compete for sites of absorption in the intestines. High fiber diets tend to bind to cadmium and carry it out of the system. Lead is another toxic trace element that contributes to hypertension and heart disease. Much of our food, water, and air have copious quantities of lead. Lead absorption can be reduced with optimal intake of selenium, fiber, and sulfur-bearing amino acids (like cysteine and methionine).

OTHER VITAMINS

Other vitamins may play a role in heart disease. Of 270 elderly people examined in New Mexico, researchers found those people with higher intakes of thiamine, riboflavin, niacin, B_6, and vitamin D had lower levels of cholesterol and LDL cholesterol in their blood.[204] When niacin was used with a drug clofibrate, the two were able to lower blood cholesterol and reduce the likelihood of recurring heart attacks by 29 percent.[205] A five year follow-up of heart disease patients found that niacin treatment alone lowered illness and death rates.[206] In people who are genetically inclined toward high cholesterol levels, niacin treatment was even effective at *reversing* heart disease.[207] Niacin treatment alone reduced cholesterol levels by 22 percent and triglycerides by 52 percent with an appropriate conclusion by the researchers involved: "To our knowledge, no other single agent has such potential for lowering both cholesterol and triglycerides."[208] Niacin is also a known potent dilator of blood vessels, which may also improve circulation in people with narrowing of vessels.

Vitamin B_6 (40 milligrams daily) is also quite effective at preventing the blood clumping that often leads to heart disease.[209]

QUASI VITAMINS

There is a growing number of nutrients that are not essential for all humans but may be essential for some and useful to others.

Some of these quasi vitamins have potent abilities to keep the vascular network healthy. These quasi vitamins are found in the body yet are not required in the diet since we make a certain amount of them internally. Whether everyone makes enough to ward off heart disease is debatable.

For example, coenzyme Q (a.k.a *ubiquinone* or *CoQ*), a key substance in energy metabolism that works along with vitamin E,[210] has been used by several major hospitals for heart failure patients, and 91 percent of them have shown improvement within 30 days in the pumping ability of the heart, without the usual side effects seen with drugs given to heart failure victims.[211] Also, 10 years of successful experiences in using CoQ to treat heart failure and angina cannot be all wrong.[212] Some early indications are that CoQ (30–60 mg daily) may also help lower blood pressure in some patients.[213]

Another quasi vitamin, lipoic acid, works with thiamine in one of the "bottlenecks" of energy metabolism. Many people may exist at subsaturation levels of lipoic acid. Rabbits fed a high-cholesterol diet along with supplements of lipoic acid had one-fifth the blood cholesterol levels of the controls.[214] Test tube studies show that lipoic acid improves the ability of tissue to use glucose and oxygen.[215] In preliminary findings, lipoic acid lowered cholesterol levels and increased oxygen use by the brain to improve the overall condition of older psychiatric patients. Supplements of 200 mg daily or less may help energy metabolism in some people and hence reduce their circulatory risks.

Pangamic acid (a.k.a *dimethyl glycine* or *DMG*) is a substance found in the body but not required in the diet. Calcium pangamate (a version of pangamic acid) lowered serum cholesterol and raised HDL levels in humans with heart disease.[216] Pangamic acid was able to inhibit cholesterol absorption in the intestines of rabbits that were fed high-cholesterol diets.[217] However, all of this European research is being challenged by other European scientists. Pangamic acid is too new to pass judgment on.

Orotic acid (a.k.a *orotate*) is a building block toward making the nucleic acids RNA and DNA. Orotic acid has been helpful in treating patients who have had heart attacks.[218] In hamster studies, orotic acid improves the strength of heart muscle contractions and shows promise in treating weak hearts.[219] There were no side effects from using 300 mg daily of orotic acid on humans.

Other stepping-stones toward the production of RNA and DNA include inosine and adenosine. Both have been used with some success to lower serum lipids, relieve angina pain, and even improve senility in some cases.[220] Both inosine and adenosine are probably more effective when injected than when taken in oral form.

Forty-six patients with narrowly constricted blood vessels were given chondroiton sulfate, a substance found in the connective tissue of humans and other creatures. The result was lowered blood cholesterol and triglycerides and reduced blood clumping activity.[221]

COFFEE AND TEA

Coffee and tea are among the most ubiquitous beverages in the world. In a study of almost 15,000 healthy adults in Norway, high coffee intake (nine cups daily for men, six cups daily for women) was associated with higher cholesterol levels.[222] In another study, the more coffee they drank, the worse their blood lipid profile became (higher cholesterol/lower HDL levels).[223] Other researchers found that coffee intake provoked higher cholesterol levels *only when* intake was more than two cups per day.[224]

There seems to be a relationship between coffee intake and cholesterol levels, but not between cola or tea intake and cholesterol levels. Therefore, it seems that it is not the caffeine that is doing the harm but perhaps the "typical" coffee drinker's lifestyle.[225] The best scientific guess is that two cups per day is probably safe for most people, while more than five cups per day ups the vessel-plugging risks.[226]

PROTEIN

Protein may play a role in the health of the circulatory system. Studies around the world show that groups who eat diets that are high in plant proteins have a lower risk for heart disease. When animal protein is removed and soy protein substituted, blood cholesterol levels go down.[227] This may result from the higher fat levels that accompany animal proteins, or there may be "something else" in plant protein. Sixty human volunteers underwent changes from vegetarian to normal omnivorous diets and back again. Their vegetarian diets lowered blood pressure, which then was raised when these people went back to their meat-eating ways.[228] Since plant food is an excellent source of potassium, it could be this mineral that has the hypotensive ability in a vegetarian diet. Tyrosine is an essential amino acid and a component of protein. In animal studies, tyrosine lowers blood pressure.[229]

GINSENG

Ginseng is a medicinal root plant native to the cool climes of northeast Asia. It has been used in folk medicine since before the pyramids were built. Modern scientists, by standardizing plant strains and extraction methods, have had considerable success in using ginseng to improve cardiovascular health.

Ginseng is neither useless nor innocuous. It has been shown to decrease (and in some people to increase) blood pressure, improve blood flow and thereby increase mental abilities, improve work capacity and endurance, and improve the elasticity of the blood vessels.[230] It appears that 200 mg daily of Ginsana (standardized ginseng) could prevent or perhaps even reverse some problems of the circulatory system. Excess ginseng (3,000 mg daily), however, may cause anything from mustaches on women to anxiety.

GRAZING VERSUS GORGING

Not only is *what* you eat important, but *when* and *how much* may also be critical. Humans evolved as grazers, not the clock-oriented, meal-eating gorgers that we have become. Eating two or three large meals daily tends to increase the absorption capacity of the intestines as well as the fat-making abilities of certain enzyme systems. Insulin output is higher when large meals are eaten. Spread the same number of calories out over five or six smaller "snacks," and the body is healthier and longer-lived. This concept of periodicity has been shown in reliable studies to lower cholesterol levels and other heart disease risk factors.[231]

NUTRITIONAL RECOMMENDATIONS
DIET BREAKDOWN

To minimize your risk for cardiovascular diseases, these are the percentages of calories that each nutrient factor should contribute to your diet:

25–30 Percent Fat

- Select primarily mono- and polyunsaturated plant fats: soy, corn, safflower, sunflower, olive oils.
- The order of preference for margarine is (1) tub margarine, (2) butter, (3) stick margarine.
- Include a minimum of one 3-ounce serving of high-fat fish in the diet each week, or 1 teaspoon of linseed oil daily, or EPA supplements (up to 3g daily for high-risk people) if the budget allows. One teaspoon daily of mint flavored cod liver oil can be an inexpensive means of providing EPA for those who don't like fish.
- Evening primrose oil (GLA) is expensive but *may* have some value as a healthy fat. If you are at high risk and your budget allows, take 100 to 400 milligrams of GLA.
- Minimize intake of hydrogenated and continuously heated oils.

10 Percent Protein

- At least half of this protein should come from plant sources, including legumes, grains, nuts, seeds, and vegetables. A vegetarian or semi-vegetarian diet can seriously cut heart disease risks.

60–65 Percent Carbohydrates

- Less than 10 percent should be sugar.
- The remaining 50–55 percent of carbohydrate intake should come from complex naturally occurring carbohydrates (grains, legumes, vegetables).

DIETARY GUIDELINES

1. Cut sodium and salt intake to one-half to one-third your normal levels. Use potassium-based salt substitutes in the family salt shakers.

2. At least double your intake of fiber (for the average person). Also, increase your intake of clean water to prevent the fiber from actually constipating the intestinal tract (since fiber binds fluids). Make vegetables, whole grains, fruits, and legumes the main staples in your diet for maximum fiber intake. Slowly add these foods to avoid stomach distress, diarrhea, and flatulence.

3. Eat small and frequent meals, with the larger meals being earlier in the day.

4. Keep alcohol intake at less than three drinks daily (only for those who *can* drink).

5. Keep coffee intake under 3 cups daily.

6. Consume often:
- at least 2 garlic cloves daily
- 1 teaspoon fresh ginger
- red peppers (as much as you can enjoy; remember to use turmeric with them)
- yogurt (1 cup daily)
- chicory (to taste)

DAILY SUPPLEMENTS TO ADD TO YOUR
CORE PROGRAM

Vitamins
E +600 IU
B₃ (niacinamide) +200 mg
B₆ (pyridoxine) +50 mg

Minerals
Calcium +600 mg
Potassium +1,500 mg
Magnesium +300 mg
Zinc +10 mg
Copper +1 mg
Chromium (yeast) +200 mcg
Selenium (yeast) +200 mcg
Silicon +10 mg

Quasi vitamins
Carnitine +1,500 mg
EPA +1,000 mg
Rutin +200 mg
Coenzyme Q +60 mg
Lipoic acid +100 mg
Orotic acid +200 mg
Ginseng (Ginsana) +500 mg
L-tyrosine +2 g

6
THE IMMUNE SYSTEM
Cancer and Other Abnormal Cell Growths

We are losing the war against cancer. In spite of heroic and expensive efforts in medical science, the cancer death rate has increased by 25 percent since 1962. Even after adjusting for changes in age distribution in this country, the cancer death rate has increased by 9 percent over the same period of time.[1] One out of four Americans dies from cancer.[2] Based upon these statistics, a Harvard professor has called the efforts of modern medicine to treat cancer "a qualified failure."

Certain types of cancer are nearly untreatable, including lung, liver, and pancreas cancer. Most conventional cancer therapy leaves the patient weak, lethargic, hairless, nauseous, and low in disease resistance. Many people who do have their cancer medically arrested often experience a new onset of cancer later on. But there is hope. Nutrition is a formidable foe against cancer: as a strong preventive agent, in support of conventional medical care, and perhaps even as a cure for some people.

The whole idea that food could cause or prevent cancer is a relatively new one. In 1950, a group of researchers fed beets or cabbage to different sets of guinea pigs. Next, they exposed the pigs to X-radiation. The cabbage-fed group had a lower rate of hemorrhage and death.[3] The idea that a food could prevent cancer from radiation was totally foreign then. Rather than speculate about some cancer protection role for cabbage, the researchers concluded that something in beets became highly toxic when exposed to radiation. We now know that cabbage can cut the mortality rate in half when animals are exposed to certain levels of radiation.[4] Beets don't cause cancer, but cabbage might prevent it.

Until about 1980, anyone who spoke of a nutrition-cancer link was labeled an eccentric faddist. But the evidence continued to grow. In 1982, the prestigious National Academy of Sciences published its technical book relating many ways in which foods and nutrients can either cause or prevent cancer. We had emerged from the Dark Ages. Since then, the data showing how nutrients can lower your cancer risk by as much as 90 percent have been produced at a lightning pace.

Although heart disease may be the number one cause of death in this country, cancer is the number one fear. Heart disease is pain, debilitation, and death. Cancer, many people think, is worse. It is a strange growth taking over your body. Although cancer is not thought to be communicable, many cancer victims find that their friends and family will not visit them for fear of contracting their illness.

What is cancer? How does it start? Can it be cured? Can it be prevented? What role does nutrition play in cancer?

WHAT IS CANCER?

Basically, cancer is a mistake. It is a group of cells growing out of control that are jeopardizing the normal life processes in that creature. Most of the 60 trillion cells in your body go through regular phases where they grow, split, and form new cells. This "replication" is a fascinating and complex procedure. During replication, the DNA (the cell's "blueprints") must reproduce itself. This process has many steps and possibilities for error. A normal professional typist may make one mistake per page of typing. DNA replication is much more accurate than that. If the information that is encoded on the DNA molecule had to be typed on paper, there would be only one typing mistake per 500 pages! Usually, that mistake is corrected by enzymes or immune factors. Sometimes, however, that mistake is left uncorrected. This new, incorrect DNA may begin making abnormal cells at a very rapid rate. Like an uncontrolled housing project, it begins to take over a region of the body with abnormal growth that interferes with the life processes. Cancer has set in.

The original DNA mistake may have been caused by chemical carcinogens, X-radiation, ultraviolet radiation from the sun, tobacco, certain food components, viruses, free radicals, singlet oxygen, and other possibilities. Free radicals and singlet oxygen are wrecking balls in your body's biochemistry. Dr. Roy Walford of UCLA has called them the "great white sharks" in the chemical sea of life.[5] Free radicals start a chain reaction of cell destruction. This destruction is caused by the unpaired electrons found in free radicals and singlet oxygen that will chemically rearrange substances nearby to placate that unpaired electron. Your body makes a certain amount of free radicals and singlet oxygen in the normal course of living. Your body also makes antioxidant enzyme systems, like GSH, to combat these destructive forces within. By encouraging these antioxidant enzyme systems with optimal nutrition, you can seriously slow down these great white sharks and thereby slow aging (in theory) and lower cancer risk (proven).

Theoretically, all people have regular occurrences of errors in cell division, which are then quickly corrected. If the mistake is not getting any worse, it is considered to be a benign growth, such as fibrocystic breast disease and certain skin growths. When the mistake commandeers all nearby body cells for its own purposes of destroying the body, the growth has become malignant. There are also precancerous growths that are like an inactive volcano about to erupt. Malignant is worse than benign, and benign is worse than normal health. But both benign and malignant tumors are abnormal growths. There is some unknown dividing point at which the benign growth starts interfering with normal life processes and becomes malignant. For that reason, all abnormal body growths (malignant, benign, and precancerous) have been included in this chapter.

HOW DOES CANCER START?

There are many theories, all of which offer some morsel of truth. Chemical carcinogens (like the industrial pollutant PCB and tobacco smoke) can cause mistakes in the DNA replication process.

Chemical pollution in our drinking water, our food, the soil, and even our homes can instigate cancer. Probably, our ever-escalating cancer rate is due to the awesome amounts of pollutants that we are exposed to. People who are psychologically stressed, or sub-clinically malnourished, or genetically vulnerable may be likely to develop cancer from our mushrooming pollution problem.

There is an increasing incidence of known carcinogens in our food supply.[6] Burned proteins, such as from charred or smoked meat, contains benzpyrenes that are known carcinogens.[7] Red dye number 2, cyclamates (artificial sweeteners), and saccharin (artificial sweetener) have each been implicated in causing cancer. Saccharin is still on your grocer's shelves, due to an intense lobbying effort.

Residues of many different pesticides also are found in much of our food supply. EDB (ethylene dibromide) is a pesticide that was sprayed on American grain crops for many decades. In 1983, dangerous amounts of EDB were found on grain crops, and EDB was banned. How many millions of Americans were affected by EDB? We will never be certain.

Other potentially dangerous food ingredients, like nitrates (and nitrites) and coal-tar-based food colorings still remain in our food supply.

DES (diethylstilbestrol), a hormone agent that was used during the 1950s to prevent miscarriages, has also been used as a "morning after" contraception pill, and was used widely in the cattle business to quicken growth. Residues of DES could be found in some of the meat from DES-reared cattle, and DES is now banned for livestock use. (There are undocumented claims that DES is still used in the cattle industry.) DES is a known carcinogen. Researchers found that the daughters of women who took DES during pregnancy were much more likely to develop defects or cancer in their reproductive organs.

Formaldehyde is a common industrial solvent used in everything from particleboard to rugs and plastics. People who live in new mobile homes have a higher rate of cancer of the nasal passage because of the formaldehyde fumes that they are breathing.[8]

People drinking the polluted Mississippi River water in New Orleans have an increased incidence of cancer of the urinary tract, as the body tries to dispose of these deadly chemicals.[9] We are all exposed to a frightening array of cancer-causing agents (more on the subject of chemical carcinogens in Chapter 16).

Sunlight contains ultraviolet radiation, which batters the DNA in the skin cells, creating cross linkages that may become cancerous.

Children living near a nuclear waste site in northern England were found to have a much higher-than-normal incidence of leukemia.

Tobacco is regularly used by 50 million Americans and is a known carcinogen. Even secondhand smoke can elevate your risk for cancer by 50–100 percent.[10]

Other, common factors in American life may have some minor role in cancer incidence: from certain prescription drugs to electromagnetic radiation from TV and FM transmitters, computer screens, color TVs, and photocopiers.

Stress also is a factor. As was mentioned, we all probably experience some abnormal cell growths during our lives. Yet our immune system is constantly patrolling the body for invading bacteria, dead cells, and abnormal cell growths like cancer. The immune factors then destroy these potentially harmful substances. Depression, fear, and other negative emotions reduce the number of "police" immune factors in the body. When the immune system is subdued through negative emotions, abnormal growths are more likely to take over and become a serious problem. In a study of over 2,000 men, depression doubled the risk for cancer.[11] A textbook written by Harvard researchers shows the intimate link between negative emotions and the increased risk for cancer via a crippled immune system.[12] Your thoughts may have a great deal to do with your resistance to cancer. Sometimes the person who seems to be a model of composure can be a boiling cauldron of emotions within. That repression can inhibit normal immune functions, which then allows cancer cells to take over.

Some people have an incredible genetic tenacity against cancer. These people can engulf themselves in tobacco smoke and eat burned meats without any resultant cancer. Yet other people have a genetic vulnerability to cancer,[13] and they must be much more conscious of what their body is exposed to.

CAN CANCER BE PREVENTED?

Yes! In 1980, the National Cancer Institute commissioned a panel of scientists to review the evidence on the nutrition-cancer link. Their report stated that one out of three cancer cells could have been prevented with proper nutrition.[14] That number has since gone up. Away from the normal staid mood that such a cerebral panel normally writes in, these scientists proclaimed: "Spread the message that cancer is not as inevitable as death and taxes." Their technical book, *Diet, Nutrition, and Cancer*, represented a major shift in the acceptance of the nutrition-cancer link. The Japanese government has recently issued its own 12-point program to show its citizens how to prevent cancer, and 8 of these points are nutritionally related, including the recommendation to take reasonable amounts of certain vitamins.[15] Dr. Ames, the chairman of the Biochemistry Department at the University of California at Berkeley and world renowned expert on chemical carcinogens, has listed numerous substances in the diet that can cause or prevent cancer.[16]

As evidence accumulates, the nutrition-cancer connection grows stronger. New estimates say that 90 percent of all cancer is environmentally caused and hence preventable.[17] Environmental factors include foods, pollutants, sunlight, tobacco, etc. Of these environmental factors, nutrition is probably the most important. A conservative estimate states that 30–60 percent of all cancer is nutrition-related.[18] The U.S. has 500 percent more breast and colon cancer than other areas of the world, and much of this dubious distinction is caused by poor nutrition.

Malnutrition may lead to cancer, and cancer may lead to malnutrition. Many cancer victims are malnourished. To compound the issue, conventional medical approaches of chemotherapy, radiation, and surgery often worsen the nutritional status of the patient. The nausea and lethargy induced by these typical cancer treatments can often create clinical malnutrition.[19] The older the cancer patient is and the more progressed the cancer condition, the worse the patient's nutritional status usually becomes.[20]

Nutrition plays a role in the prevention, support, and cure of cancer. Nutrition is probably the single most important factor in *preventing* cancer. Once cancer has started, optimal nutrition is needed for *support* of other therapies. Some nutritional approaches have potential as cures for cancer. It is encouraging that one-third of cancer patients can be treated by conventional medical approaches. But that still leaves two-thirds of the cancer patients with a dim prognosis.

GENERAL RISK FACTORS

Many nutritional factors relate to cancer incidence. Some may prevent it; some may cause it.

- Nutrients that are *likely preventers* of cancer: selenium; vitamins E, A, C; and fiber.
- Nutrients that are *possible preventers* of cancer: manganese, zinc, vitamin B_6, thiamine, vitamin D, niacin, magnesium, and the amino acids L-cysteine and L-methionine.
- Foods that are *likely preventers* of cancer: green and orange vegetables, cruciferous vegetables (cabbage, broccoli, brussels sprouts, cauliflower), seaweed, tomatoes, strawberries, apples, carrots, fish and fish oil, yogurt, garlic.
- Food substances that are *likely instigators* of cancer: excessive fat (saturated and polyunsaturated are both suspect, with the monounsaturated fats from olive oil and dairy products being the most innocuous), psoralens (found in parsnips), burned or smoked protein (like well-done hamburgers), nuts and seeds stored under damp cool conditions, many food dyes, nitrite and nitrate (food preservatives found in most processed meats), sorghum (red and brown variety).
- Food substances that are *possible instigators* of cancer: cholesterol, black pepper, sugar, coffee, alcohol.

VITAMIN E AND SELENIUM

Batman and Robin, the Lone Ranger and Tonto, vitamin E and selenium—all are dynamic duos.

Professors from Cornell University in New York[21] and the University of California[22] have stated that at least 55 different studies show the anticancer effect of selenium. Only three decades after selenium changed categories from "toxic" to "essential," it has become one of the more potent anticancer agents available.

And selenium's effectiveness is further amplified when teamed up with vitamin E. When researchers in Finland examined 51 cancer victims, they found that low selenium levels increased the risk for cancer, but low selenium combined with low vitamin E levels increased the risk even more.[23] Lower blood selenium levels are excellent predictors of who will get breast cancer and fibrocystic breast disease,[24] and so are low vitamin E levels. In a 14-year study of over 5,000 British women, low vitamin E levels in the blood increased the risk for breast cancer by 500 percent.[25] In a Swiss study of over 6,300 adults, people with lower vitamin E levels had much higher risks for bowel cancer.[26]

Prevention

Vitamin E and selenium work together in a potent anticancer, antiaging enzyme system called *glutathione peroxidase (GSH)*. GSH is like a miniature police force that wipes out renegade cells and free radicals within. Fats in the water-based system of life are both essential and potentially lethal. Unsaturated fats can oxidize, or "rust," which sets up a domino effect of cell destruction that can end in DNA damage and cancer. Vitamin E is the only fat-soluble antioxidant in blood plasma,[27] and GSH is unquestionably a critical tool for the body to ward off cancer.[28] The levels of GSH in the body depend greatly on the levels of vitamin E and selenium in the diet.[29] Although vitamin E and selenium each have other functions in the body, their teamwork in this anticancer GSH is well documented.[30]

Vitamin E and selenium are strongly related to cancer incidence. Experts have mapped the selenium levels in the soil across the U.S., then overlaid another map of cancer incidence by states. The correlation is incredible. The lower the selenium level in the soil (and thus the food supply), the higher the cancer incidence of people in that state.[31] South Dakota had the highest levels of selenium in its soil, and Ohio had the lowest. Cancer rates in Ohio are 200 percent greater than those in South Dakota.

Many cancer patients have below-normal selenium levels in their blood.[32] Yet this evidence was criticized because the cancer might have caused the lower selenium levels, rather than low selenium causing cancer. So another study with 10,000 Americans was performed to answer that question. Blood samples were taken at the start of the study and then frozen. Over the next five years, the people in this study who developed cancer had their blood samples unfrozen and checked for selenium levels. Cancer victims were found to have had the lowest levels of selenium in their blood at the start of the study.[33] Low selenium levels in the blood actually *doubled* the risk for cancer.

People in Finland who had plasma selenium levels that ranked in the lowest third had three times the risk for cancer.[34] This means that there is a nearly straight-line relationship between selenium levels and cancer incidence.

Vitamin E also has preventive qualities. Nitrosamines are known carcinogens that result from nitrites (used as a food additive and also found in water from fertilizer runoff) combining with amino acids (from protein foods) in the stomach. Vitamin E (400 IU daily) and C (2,000 mg daily) together were able to cut nitrosamine formation by up to 95 percent in 10 college students.[35] In animal studies, vitamin E inhibited tumor growth in subjects that were exposed to very concentrated levels of DMBA, a carcinogenic portion of tobacco smoke, and completely prevented tumor growth at somewhat weaker levels of DMBA exposure.[36]

When combined with other nutrients, vitamin E and selenium are even more potent against cancer. Lab animals were fed various diets, some of which included nutritional supplements. The animals were then injected with a known chemical carcinogen. The rats that received supplements of riboflavin, niacin, selenium, molybdenum, zinc, and magnesium had marked reductions in the incidence of tumors.[37]

Selenium and beta-carotene (plant version of vitamin A) have been individually shown to have serious cancer prevention abilities. One researcher has proposed that a combination of selenium and beta-carotene would be a most formidable opponent against cancer.[38] This may be more than theoretical chin-stroking. In a study of over 12,000 people in Finland, cancer deaths were highest among people with the lowest intake levels of selenium, vitamin E, and vitamin A.[39]

Support for Conventional Therapy

Not only can vitamin E and selenium prevent cancer; they can also enhance the efficacy of conventional cancer treatment. Selenium helps reduce the toxic effects of the potent anticancer drug adriamycin without reducing the effectiveness of the drug.[40] And vitamin E potentiates the tumor-reducing ability of chemotherapy agents.[41] Selenium supplements even helped to prevent the recurrence of tumors in lab mice after they had been treated with more conventional therapy.[42] This is important, since many cancer patients often experience recurring tumors. Both vitamin E and selenium can prevent these "aftershock" tumors.

Curative Powers

Selenium and E are definitely effective at preventing abnormal growths, and they seem to help support conventional therapy once a tumor begins, but can they treat cancer? In precancerous and benign growths, perhaps.

Selenium has been shown to improve the efficiency with which DNA can repair itself after being exposed to damaging substances.[43] At high intake levels, selenium is directly toxic to cancer cells.[44] Selenium supplements not only retarded the growth of tumors in human breast tissue (test tube study) but also slowed breast tumor growth in mice by 80–93 percent.[45] The amounts of selenium used on these mice, if converted to human terms, would be equal to roughly 25 mg daily, which is 125 times the upper limit that is stated by the RDA. This therapeutic range should only be used by qualified health care professionals, however. It could be dangerous. Selenium is also a potent stimulant to the immune system, which is important since many cancer patients fall prey to other infectious diseases.[46]

Vitamin E may also have curative powers. Supplements of vitamin E were able to soften hardened breasts and shrink cysts in 16 women with premenstrual syndrome. In 20 other women, supplements of vitamin E relieved breast tenderness and caused cyst regression.[47] Another researcher reported that 70 percent of the women treated with vitamin E supplements (895 IU daily) experienced relief of their breast cysts.[48] Vitamin E may be able to reverse other precancerous growths in the body.[49]

Recommended Amounts

What level of these wonder nutrients would be considered minimal, optimal for normal people, therapeutic for sick people, and toxic? The National Academy of Sciences has recommended 50–200 mcg daily as the safe range for selenium intake. However, this estimate is based on animal studies and may need to be adjusted upward somewhat for humans, who are typically exposed to myriad carcinogens. There is very good evidence that the upper limit (200 mcg) established by the National Academy of Sciences is too low.[50]

The average American diet contains about 33 mcg of selenium daily. For healthy, nonstressed, nongrowing adults, 70 mcg daily would be necessary to replace the selenium that is excreted.[51] A follow-up study found that 80 mcg daily was necessary to replace the selenium that was being lost in the stools and urine of 27 human subjects.[52] Yet some people may be able to adapt to a low intake of selenium over many generations. New Zealanders live in a land of minimal population and low stress which has helped them adapt to an average intake of 24 mcg daily of selenium. Perhaps New Zealanders can get along with less selenium than we can. Our cancer incidence says that we are doing a plethora of things wrong. Our low selenium intake could be one of the factors that encourages cancer.

Selenium intake beyond the RDA would probably decrease cancer risks for many people, say some professors at Cornell University in New York. They suggest 600 mcg daily as a safe and "pharmacological" dose to stem the rising tide of cancer.[53]

Based on the data from animal studies, one part per million provides excellent cancer prevention along with other benefits. For humans, this converts into 400–1,000 mcg daily. Given our selenium intake from food, this would require daily pill supplements of 200–800 mcg for adults. Children would be best protected with a daily supplement of 100 mcg.

Depending on the source of selenium and the person taking it, toxicity may start at anywhere from 2,000 to 5,000 mcg of selenium daily. There are regions of China where the average adult male consumes 700 mcg daily without any apparent side effects.[54] The National Research Council has estimated that 2,400–3,000 mcg daily would be required to produce symptoms of selenium toxicity.[55] The Chinese who experienced selenium toxicity were eating about 5,000 mcg daily.[56]

The form of selenium is important, too. Organic selenium is better tolerated, better absorbed, and less likely to cause toxicity than inorganic sodium selenite. Supplements of either organic or inorganic selenium were given to lactating mothers in Finland. Although both forms of selenium supplements increased the mother's circulating levels of blood selenium (the organic form was slightly more effective at this), only the mothers who were taking organic selenium from yeast had extra amounts of selenium present in their milk.[57] Most selenium naturally found in food is bound to the amino acid methionine. This seleno-methionine complex improves bioavailability and circulating levels of selenium in the blood.[58]

Food sources of selenium are greatly dependent on the selenium content of the soil that they were grown on. Selenium in the soil is generally more concentrated in the western U.S. than the eastern part of this country. Although soybeans are not a particularly rich source of selenium, the selenium in soybeans is very well absorbed.[59] Brazil nuts are an unusually rich source of selenium, containing as much as 50 mcg of organic selenium per nut.[60]

FIBER

Early in this century, food scientists were busy making new and different food products. They found that removing the fiber from grains and other foods made these products easier to work with. They promoted these products as "purified," as though something was wrong with the fiber that nature put into our food supply. You may recall that the most commonly eaten food in America is white bread, which has negligible fiber when compared to whole wheat bread. As our dietary fiber intake declined, the incidence of a new set of "diseases of civilization" increased dramatically. Cancer, heart disease, overfatness, diabetes, appendicitis, hemorrhoids, and other problems descended upon the American people with a vengeance.

Fiber is useless, since it cannot be digested or absorbed, but its value *lies* in its uselessness. *Because* it is not absorbed, fiber can bind toxins and hurry them out of the intestinal tract before they can cause problems.

In 1969, Dr. Burkitt, an English physician, returned from a stay in Africa and reported the incredibly low incidence of cancer among Africans, who consume three to four times the fiber levels of civilized Western nations.[61] Dr. Burkitt proposed that fiber intake might have something to do with this major difference in disease incidence. Dr. Burkitt was probably right.

Grain fibers contain phytates, which were once thought to be useless or even harmful since they bind essential minerals and carry them out of the system. Yet new evidence indicates that, by attaching to iron, phytates lower the danger of cancer-causing microorganisms in the intestines by grabbing their much needed iron supply.[62] This would explain why diets that are high in fat and meat while being low in fiber are often at the top of the list for cancer risk.

In a study of 871 men in the Netherlands, researchers found that people in the lowest 20 percent of fiber intake had a 300 percent increase in their risk of death from cancer and other diseases.[63] A slight increase in fiber intake to 37 g daily (25–50 percent higher than normal levels) would drop cancer risks greatly.

Fiber also speeds up the trip that food takes through the intestines, thus reducing the exposure of the intestinal walls to whatever carcinogenic substances are found in the food supply.[64] Cruciferous vegetables, like broccoli, cabbage, brussels sprouts, and cauliflower, are quite effective at preventing intestinal cancer, says the National Research Council.[65]

Fiber absorbs fats, cholesterol, heavy metals, drugs, and other problem-causing substances. Fiber also prevents bacteria in the intestines from degrading cholesterol into a known carcinogen (deoxycholic acid). And it greatly reduces the toxicity of many substances. Lab animals were fed a low-fiber diet and then exposed to a variety of toxins, including drugs and certain questionable food additives. Many of the animals got sick, developed cancer, or died. Another set of similar animals were fed a high-fiber diet and then exposed to the same variety of chemical pollutants. They were unharmed.[66]

In comparing carnivorous versus vegetarian diets, researchers found that high-meat/low-fiber diets encourage higher circulating levels of certain hormones that raise the risk for prostate cancer.[67]

While fiber is a serious weapon in the war against cancer, you shouldn't try to switch from a low-fiber diet to a high-fiber diet overnight. Too much fiber can lead to diarrhea, which can cause dangerous fluid loss. Excess fiber can also bind essential minerals to create deficiencies. And some fibers are metabolized by bacteria in the intestines and hence give off gas (flatulence). By slowly increasing your fiber intake and also consuming some live cultured yogurt, you can minimize flatulence (see Chapter 17 for more information on how to control flatulence). None of these limitations are a problem when fiber is consumed in normal healthy quantities of 50–100 g daily. Slowly build up to this level by adding a little fiber each week.

VITAMIN A

Vitamin A is one of the more mysterious substances in human nutrition. It has a variety of different forms and participates in many different chemical reactions in the body. Vitamin A is found in the human body as retinol, retinaldehyde, and retinoic acid, and it is involved in at least three completely different functions: in cell growth and differentiation, reproduction, and vision.[68] Vitamin A is considered by experts to be "the most efficient quencher of singlet oxygen thus far discovered,"[69] which is significant because singlet oxygen is something of a "wrecking ball" in the biochemistry of the body, causing aging and cancer. And low vitamin A consumption has been linked to cancers at many different sites:

- Vitamin A may be one of the most formidable anticancer weapons that a smoker can use. In a 19-year study of over 2,000 healthy men, researchers found that smoking men who were in the lowest one-fourth for beta-carotene (plant version of vitamin A) consumption had an 800 percent increase in their risk of lung cancer.[70]

  When scientists compared the nutrient intake of 447 lung cancer patients with 759 healthy control subjects in New Mexico, they found a substantially lower intake of beta-carotene in the cancer patients.[71] When 763 lung cancer patients in New Jersey were examined, low carotene levels increased cancer risks by 130 percent above those with high carotene levels.[72]

- Of 191 Italian women studied, those who averaged less than 3,300 IU of beta-carotene daily had eight times the risk of developing cervical cancer when compared to healthy controls, consuming at least 5,000 IU daily.[73] In 78 women admitted to a hospital for treatment of cervical cancer, 2 out of 3 were low in at least one of the nutrients tested for: beta-carotene, folate, and vitamin C.[74]

- When researchers looked at all stomach cancer victims in a four county region of Pennsylvania, they found that low intake of vitamin A doubled the risk for stomach cancer.[75] (Vitamin A plays an important role in maintaining the lining of the stomach.)

- Of over 5,000 British women studied, those with the lowest intake levels of beta-carotene had higher risks for breast cancer.

- Over 450 million people (mostly adult males) in Africa, Asia, and the south Pacific regularly chew betel nuts, which substantially increase the risk for mouth cancer. When a group of betel nut chewers were given supplements of vitamin A (15,000 IU) and beta-carotene (45,000 IU) daily, the degenerative changes in mouth cells that precede cancer decreased by two-thirds.[76]

Low levels of *serum* vitamin A also were linked to the incidence of cancer at various sites, including the lung, bladder, breast, and endometrium (the lining of a woman's uterus).[77] In Georgia, 3,100 volunteers were followed for cancer incidence over the next 12 years. Regardless of race, sex, or age, there was a major connection between low serum retinol levels and the incidence of cancer.[78] Egyptian patients with bladder cancer had markedly lower serum carotene and serum retinol levels.[79] In a Swiss study of over 6,300 adults, low beta-carotene levels elevated lung cancer risk, and low vitamin A levels increased stomach cancer risk.[80] And the evidence goes on, relating vitamin A or, more often, beta-carotene to cancer risk in the colon,[81] prostate,[82] and other parts of the body. Taking in all the data, an Oxford physician estimates that optimal intake of beta-carotene *alone* could reduce cancer incidence by a third.[83]

Not only is vitamin A a potent defender against cancer attacks, but its ability to stimulate the immune system makes it quite valuable when treating cancer patients with traditional methods.[84] Large doses of vitamin A blunt the toxic side effects of chemotherapy and radiation therapy. When cancerous animals were given large doses of beta-carotene, researchers were able to increase the chemo- and radiation therapy levels and hence achieve a "cure" in 92 percent of the animals tested.

Can vitamin A cure cancer? Probably not. There are no guaranteed cures for cancer today. Topical applications of retinoic acid (a version of vitamin A) have been found to be quite effective at treating precancerous skin changes on the body resulting from too much sun exposure.[85]

Beta-carotene is a thirsty sponge in the body for soaking up free radicals that can create deviant cells. Beta-carotene is also incredibly effective at stimulating the immune system to protect the body. But there is a big difference between prevention and cure. In cells that are at optimal doses of beta-carotene it is almost impossible to produce a cancerous growth. Yet that information has been misinterpreted to mean that beta-carotene can cure cancer.[86] It is much easier to repel foreign invaders at your own shores than to purge them from the country once they have established themselves throughout the land.

So vitamin A and beta-carotene are proven bodyguards against cancer. But many foods are full of A. How could any Americans be deficient in this potent anticancer nutrient? After protein-calorie malnutrition, vitamin A deficiency is the most widespread malnutritive condition in the world.[87] In southeast Asia, amid the tropical splendor of fresh green foliage that is full of beta-carotene, it is not considered "macho" for men and young boys to eat green plants. About 250,000 children each year go permanently blind from vitamin A deficiency in southeast Asia alone because these foods are not part of their cultural diet. Vitamin A is quite available but often ignored in the diet throughout the world. In order to prevent the widespread diseases that result from low A intake, some Central American countries have fortified commercial white sugar with vitamin A. Several regions of southeast Asia add vitamin A to flour and MSG.[88]

Americans have not been spared in the widespread deficiency of vitamin A. About one out of three Americans is low in vitamin A intake. Even more common than blatant deficiencies are the borderline deficiencies. Researchers find that a large percentage of people in America and Canada have serum levels of A that are indicative of a marginal deficiency.[89] Many postmortem studies of Americans have found reduced liver reserves of vitamin A. In other words, though we have a minimal problem with raging deficiencies of vitamin A, we may have many people who are marginally low in A, which increases their risk for cancer.

How much vitamin A is enough, too little, too much? The RDA is 5,000 IU for vitamin A, which will probably prevent any symptoms of deficiency in most healthy people. There is plenty of evidence to indicate that 25,000 IU of beta-carotene could both stimulate the immune system and lower cancer incidence without bringing any risk whatsoever. Vitamin A as retinol is definitely toxic at certain levels of intake, while beta-carotene is very nontoxic. One case was reported of a 32-year-old nurse consuming over 4 pounds of carrots daily along with other food sources of beta-carotene. She developed stomach pains, nausea, vomiting, headaches, and loss of menstrual cycle.[90] The symptoms quickly abated once she ceased her unusual weight loss program. So you *can* overdose on beta-carotene, but it does take some effort.

Vitamin A in retinol form (animal version) is another story. Adults consuming 50,000 IU of vitamin A daily for long periods of time will probably develop symptoms of vitamin A toxicity, which include weakness, bone pain, hair loss, skin problems, orange hue in the skin and eyes, headache often similar to that of brain tumors, elevated calcium levels in the blood, and even psychosis.[91] Pregnant women should be diligent about avoiding excessive amounts of preformed vitamin A, since either an excess or a deficiency of A during pregnancy can lead to birth defects.

We've seen that there are many benefits from having higher serum levels of vitamin A and beta-carotene. Will supplements increase these levels? Yes. In one study, 376 healthy adult volunteers were given either placebo or any of six different intake levels of vitamin A supplements. The more A they took, the higher were their serum retinol levels.[92] Five percent of the subjects taking 22,500 IU daily of retinol showed mild symptoms of vitamin A excess: dry, itchy eyes.

Since there are nearly a thousand different versions of vitamin A, known as *retinoids*, it has been difficult for scientists to standardize measurements of vitamin A. Different versions of A have different levels of effectiveness in the body. One retinol equivalent (RE) equals about 5 IU. One IU equals 0.3 mcg of retinol.[93] If you find that confusing, you are not alone. Most health care professionals still don't understand the various units of vitamin A.

VITAMIN C

Only a few species in nature need to eat vitamin C, and humans are one of them. Vitamin C has many different functions in the human body, and it works against cancer in a variety of ways:

- It stimulates the immune system to attack the newly sprouted abnormal cells.
- It is a free radical scavenger, mopping up free radicals to prevent destruction of the DNA.
- It stimulates the production of interferon, a potent anticancer agent in the body.[94]

- It blocks the formation of carcinogenic nitrosamines in the stomach.[95]

The presence of vitamin C in the body inhibits cancer and the absence of vitamin C increases cancer risk. The incidence of cervical dysplasia (a precancerous condition of the cervix) was seven times greater in women who consumed less than 60 mg of vitamin C daily than in the better-nourished and healthier controls.[96] When 78 women with cervical cancer were compared to 240 healthy controls, the cancer victims had significantly lower levels of folate, beta-carotene, and ascorbic acid.[97] These vitamin levels dropped even further in the cancer patients after they underwent surgery.

Smokers bind up large amounts of vitamin C through tobacco use, as much as 500 milligrams of ascorbic acid per pack of cigarettes. Smokers also have much lower levels of circulating ascorbic acid. People who are well nourished with vitamin C are less likely to get cancer of the esophagus, stomach, bladder, and other areas of the body.[98] In a study of over 6,300 Swiss adults, low levels of vitamin E, vitamin A, and beta-carotene predicted *certain types* of cancer, but low levels of vitamin C increased the risk for *all types* of cancer.[99]

Vitamin C does not cure cancer.[100] But in many cancer patients, high doses of C (10,000 mg daily) are able to extend the quality and quantity of life by an average of 300 days.[101] Other studies have not shown the same results. Perhaps using chemotherapy and radiation deadens the immune system, so that vitamin C supplements are of little value when applied with conventional medical approaches.[102] Of 139 patients with lung cancer, most had blood levels of vitamin C indicating a deficiency, with some people testing in the scurvy range.[103] These cancer patients were then given supplements of 1,000 mg of C daily for three days, then 200 mg daily for the next two weeks. Their blood levels of C rose closer to normal. Tumors hoard vitamin C. Merely through binding up much vitamin C, tumors could bring sickness and weakness to the cancer patient.

There was a 400 percent difference in the amount of vitamin C absorbed by four human subjects,[104] indicating that a wide range of absorption efficiency may create health risks for some people. Fresh fruits and vegetables are the richest source of vitamin C and bioflavonoids. Bioflavonoids may work by themselves or in conjunction with vitamin C to increase cancer resistance. Test tube (in vitro) studies have shown bioflavonoids to be directly toxic to cancer cells.[105]

Everyone should consume at least 250 mg of ascorbic acid each day from food or supplements. A more optimal level for most people would be about 1,000 mg daily. Smokers and those exposed to pollutants should get 1,000–5,000 mg. Cancer patients, AIDS victims, and other critically ill people can show marked improvement (though no cure) by using 5,000–10,000 mg daily.

Time-release pills are of no advantage, they cost extra, and they may actually be less absorbable than other forms of vitamin C supplements. Powdered crystals of ascorbic acid are quite inexpensive and can be purchased from numerous mail order vitamin supply houses. Using this vitamin C powder as both a food preservative (making your own salsa or tomato preserves) and a tartness agent in foods will provide you with cheap nutritional protection against a variety of common ailments, including cancer.

FAT

When saturated fats were implicated in heart disease, scientists began recommending diets high in polyunsaturated fats. Some cardiac recovery programs were even spoon-feeding their patients corn, soy, and safflower oil. However, scientists soon learned that diets high in polyunsaturated fats increase the risk for cancer, [106] which makes sense. Polyunsaturated fats have vulnerable double bonds that can easily be attacked by free radicals to create a domino effect of cell destruction. This fat "rusting" (a.k.a *lipid peroxidation*) could probably be prevented by vitamins E, A, and C and selenium. Yet many people are low in their intake of these fat-processing nutrients. The best source of vitamin E would normally be the same plant oils that bring polyunsaturated fats, yet the heat processing that is used to extract plant oils is quite destructive to the vitamin E. Cold-processed oils are a better source of vitamin E.

Vulnerable polyunsaturated fats are not the only link between fat and cancer. Americans have a 500 percent greater incidence of cancer of the breast and colon than the rest of the world,[107] and we eat more fat than most other countries. There is probably a connection there. When 50 bowel cancer patients were compared to healthy controls, the cancer victims consumed 16 percent more kilocalories, 14 percent more fat, and 21 percent more carbohydrates (primarily from sugar).[108] Cancer of the ovaries also is related to fat intake. When 16,000 California women were examined, researchers found that eating three eggs per week tripled the risk of getting cancer of the ovaries over women who ate one egg per week or less. Eating fried foods five times per week tripled the risk of getting cancer of the ovaries when compared to eating fried foods three times each week or less.[109] In a study of 26 countries, researchers found that animal fat was the main predictor for ovarian cancer.[110] A high-fat diet also increases the risk of developing fibrocystic breast disease (a condition that sometimes develops into cancer).[111]

Fats that are exposed to intense heat combine with protein to form benzpyrenes, which are known carcinogens. Animal tissue that is burned, as in well-done meat and smoked meat, has been shown to be a major cancer risk to the stomach.[112] Even smelling the fumes of burned fat has been shown to raise the risk of cancer in the nasal passages.[113]

Is it the fat in the diet or fat stored in the body that causes the problem? Either or both are possibilities. Stored body fat is probably a risk factor by itself. Overfatness is a major risk factor of cancer in general[114] and breast cancer in particular.[115]

Fat not only encourages cancer by itself, but it heightens the carcinogenic properties of toxic substances. Researchers fed various groups of animals high- or low-fat diets and then exposed them to different chemical carcinogens. The animals who were fed a high-fat diet had much more cancer than the low-fat group.[116]

Not all fats are "bad guys," however. Although excess fat in the diet or body may increase cancer risks, there are a few "wonder" fats that may actually protect against cancer. Prostacyclin is one of the prostaglandins that seem to work toward cleaning up cancerous growth in the body.[117] It is known that fish oils of eicosapentaenoic acid (EPA) and docosahexaenoic acid (DHA) stimulate prostacyclin production while inhibiting its opposing force in the body, arachidonic acid byproducts.

These special omega-3 fats may be cancer preventers and conditional cancer "cures." The omega-3 fatty acids found in fish oil (EPA and DHA) were used in animal studies to drastically reduce the size and weight of breast tumors,[118] Gamma-linolenic acid (often called *evening primrose oil* from the plant that yields much of this "wonder" fat) also has potential as a therapeutic agent against cancer. Research in cancer wards in South Africa has shown that GLA and vitamin C were able to reduce the pain and abdominal swelling (ascites) of cancer victims.[119]

Essentially, Americans eat too much fat in the diet, store too much fat in the body, and generally eat the wrong kinds of fat. All of this contributes to our cancer woes.

MINERALS

A number of minerals may play a role in cancer incidence.

Calcium

Calcium attaches itself to fats in the intestines and carries them out with the feces. This action could account for calcium's cancer prevention abilities. In a 19-year study of 1,954 men at Western Electric in Chicago, researchers found that lower vitamin D and calcium levels were coupled with higher risks for cancer of the colon and rectum.[120] The men with the highest calcium intake had one-third the colon cancer rate of the men consuming the least calcium. Vitamin D serves to increase calcium absorption, its transport through the blood, its deposition in the bones, and its general use in the body. Vitamin D can be produced in the body when the skin is exposed to sunlight. Places of the world where sunlight is more abundant have lower rates of colon cancer than the cloudy climes. Thus, calcium supplements, even if not absorbed, may still be quite useful by preventing cancer in the intestines.

To test this theory, researchers used 10 healthy adults who were all at high genetic risk of developing cancer of the colon. They found abnormal cell growths (colonic crypts) in the lower intestines that are common in people with cancer of the colon. They then gave the 10 subjects 1,250 mg daily of calcium (as calcium carbonate) and later retested the cells in the bowels. The cells were now more normal and less likely to erupt into colon cancer.[121] Supplemental calcium may serve the purpose of mopping up excess fat in the intestines to prevent the destructive effects of fat. This should be encouraging news, since only lung cancer kills more Americans than colon cancer.

Zinc

Zinc is a multitalented mineral that works in many systems in the body, including disease resistance and new cell production. Serum zinc levels are markedly lower in patients with cancer of the esophagus,[122] lungs,[123] and prostate gland.[124] Rats that are given zinc supplements and then exposed to carcinogens have fewer tumors.[125]

Societies that have corn and wheat as dietary staples have 80–90 times the risk for cancer of the esophagus when compared to societies where sorghum, millet, cassava, and yams are staple items.[126] Scientists propose that magnesium, zinc, and niacin are the nutrients that are found in lower levels in the corn- or wheat-based societies.

So, it would seem that zinc might be a potent cancer preventer. But wait. Other studies have shown that low zinc levels in the diet slow down tumor growths[127] and that high zinc intake can be associated with a higher risk for certain types of cancer.[128] How does one rationalize that? Zinc competes with other minerals for absorption and use by the body. Perhaps when zinc competes with toxic minerals, like cadmium, the net result is a lower risk for cancer. Yet, when zinc competes with selenium for absorption, the net result is a higher risk for cancer.

Also, zinc is used by all rapidly dividing cells, even cancer cells. So a zinc deficiency could slow the growth of some tumors. It is likely that optimal zinc intake is a valuable anticancer force, while too much and too little are both cancer-inducing situations. High-dose supplements of zinc without selenium to compensate for the competitive absorption factor could increase the risk for cancer. This is just another illustration that nutrition is truly a question of balance. Since the average American consumes roughly half of the RDA for zinc, daily supplements of 15–30 mg of zinc (as zinc gluconate) would be a healthy idea for most adults.

Molybdenum

Molybdenum is a trace mineral that played a key role in the esophageal cancer that plagued a certain region of China for nearly 2,000 years. Researchers found that the soil in that region was very low in molybdenum. By fortifying the soil with molybdenum and providing supplements of vitamin C to the people, scientists have seen a marked drop in the incidence of cancer in that region.[129]

Low molybdenum levels in the soil of the African Bantus is probably related to their high rate of esophageal cancer, too.

Molybdenum is also a powerful scavenger of free radicals.[130] Molybdenum supplements in rats have provided excellent protection against chemical carcinogens.[131]

The molybdenum content in soil varies considerably from region to region, so plants are an unpredictable source of molybdenum. Also, much molybdenum is removed in food refining. So supplements of molybdenum (150–500 mcg as sodium molybdate) might be a valuable cancer prevention measure.

Vanadium

Vanadium is an obscure but essential trace element in human nutrition. Researchers at the University of New Hampshire inflicted chemical carcinogens in the breast region of laboratory mice, some of which had been given vanadium supplements. The mice given vanadium supplements remained cancer-free longer with no side effects from the supplements.[132] Vanadium is lost in most food-refining procedures, so the highly refined diets of Americans may be low in vanadium. This may be one piece in the big puzzle of cancer in this country. The best food sources of vanadium are plant oils, such as soy, corn, and safflower.

Copper

Copper is another essential metal that could play a role in protecting you against cancer. The average intake of copper in the U.S. is roughly half of the RDA. Also, the higher the intake of sugar, the lower the absorption of copper.[133]

Copper is bound within the blood in the form of ceruloplasmin, which is one of the more important antioxidants in the bloodstream. Ceruloplasmin acts to keep hemoglobin iron from rusting. Hemoglobin oxidation could create free radicals that could instigate abnormal growth, such as cancer. Both copper and zinc are involved in a crucial anticancer enzyme called *superoxide dismutase (SOD)*. There are several different types of SOD enzymes containing different trace minerals. SOD and ceruloplasmin both act as "fire extinguishers" throughout the body to squelch free radicals that could be the beginning of strange growths. Also, copper salts provided measurable protection against cancer when added to the diets of lab rats that were exposed to chemical carcinogens.[134]

Manganese

Manganese is another essential trace mineral in human nutrition. One version of SOD contains manganese. SOD manganese is important in fighting free radicals that constantly arise in the body and may produce abnormal cell growth. *All* tumors that have been studied to date have markedly lower-than-normal levels of manganese-containing SOD.[135]

Cadmium

Cadmium is a toxic trace mineral that is found in tobacco smoke, industrial pollutants, and in small amounts in canned foods. Cadmium and zinc compete to install themselves in the prostate gland. If cadmium is available in large quantities and is deposited in the prostate, cancer is more likely.[136]

PROTEIN AND AMINO ACIDS

Proteins and their building blocks of amino acids may play some role in cancer incidence and prevention. Burned proteins become benzpyrenes, which are known cancer-causing agents. Excess protein in the diet may also bring on cancer. In a study involving 50,000 households in Germany, scientists found a link between high protein intake and the risk of pancreatic cancer.[137] Cancer of the pancreas is one of the least treatable of all cancers. The same study found that high alcohol and sugar intake were related to stomach cancer incidence. The average American consumes about 50 percent more protein than recommended levels. High-meat diets are known to elevate the risk for colon cancer,[138] possibly due to the intestinal bacteria that thrive on meat and create DNA-altering materials as a result.

Yet on the flip side, some amino acids seem to provide a certain amount of cancer protection. A variety of studies have shown that methionine protects DNA from free radical and other destruction.[139] When lab animals were fed diets deficient in methionine and cysteine (both are sulfur-containing amino acids), they had lower levels of enzymes that protect against cancer.[140] Cysteine also protects against pollutants and may be a potent life extender. Lab animals who were injected with cysteine lived much longer than the control group.[141]

Aging usually results in lower circulating levels of sulfur-containing compounds (like cysteine and methionine) that protect against cancer and cell destruction.[142] These sulfur-containing amino acids of cysteine and methionine may provide the body with the raw materials to slow down aging and bizarre cell growths like cancer. Arginine is another amino acid that has been used experimentally to slow the growth of transplanted tumors in lab animals.[143]

So, excess or burned protein may invite cancer cells. Yet certain amino acids may prevent cancer or even slow it down once it has started. Some other amino acids may provide crucial support for cancer patients who are being treated with conventional medicine. Researchers at Harvard University found that tube feedings that contained a 250 percent increase in the amount of branched-chain amino acids (leucine, isoleucine, valine) promoted major improvements in the patients' health.[144] Many cancer patients develop cachexia, a condition of tissue wasting, loss of organ function, apathy, weakness, and other metabolic problems. Since they cannot eat, they are often tube-fed. The richer solution of branched-chain amino acids stimulated the growth of tissue protein and albumin, which is a major improvement for these people.

COFFEE AND ALCOHOL

In a study of over 8,000 men living in Hawaii, those who consumed more than 16 ounces of beer daily had an increased risk of rectal cancer. Wine and whisky consumption were related to an increased risk of lung cancer.[145]

Fibrocystic breast disease involves lumps in the breast that sometimes lead to cancer. Coffee drinking increases the likelihood of women having fibrocystic breast disease. A physician at Ohio State University studied 47 women with fibrocystic breast disease who consumed at least four cups of coffee daily. He was able to convince 20 of them to abstain from their caffeine (coffee, tea, chocolate, colas) habit. Of these 20 women who abstained, 16 had complete remission of their breast lumps. Only 1 of the 27 nonabstainers had her fibrocystic lumps disappear. The remaining 26 women had to be treated medically.[146]

Yet, another study looked at 2,651 women with newly diagnosed breast cancer. They found little or no correlation between coffee intake and breast cancer.[147] Researchers often have a difficult time eliminating the other influences in coffee and alcohol consumption. People who drink lots of coffee and alcohol may also be involved in tobacco use, high sugar intake, sedentary lifestyle, and other risk factors that may be more harmful than the coffee itself. Heavy alcohol drinkers usually eat less, leaving open the possibility of numerous vitamin and mineral deficiency states. Which of these risk factors is the real culprit? It seems that most healthy adults can consume one or two cups of coffee daily and one or two alcoholic beverages without any elevated risk for cancer, *if* their diet and other lifestyle factors are ideal.

B VITAMINS

Folacin is a B vitamin that is involved in directing new cell growth in the body. Rapidly dividing cells need adequate folacin; otherwise growth will be stunted or mistake-prone. Abnormal folacin metabolism is commonly found in cancer patients.[148] Oral contraceptives increase the need for folacin. Forty-seven young women with cervical dysplasia who had been using oral contraceptives were recruited for a study. Some were given 10 mg daily of folacin (25 times the RDA), and others were given vitamin C as a placebo. Four women in the folacin group were completely cured. No one in the placebo group was cured, while 4 women in the placebo group had now developed cancer.[149] Folacin plays a key role in cells that must multiply often. When cell division goes awry, cancer may result.

Eighty percent of all cancer patients, regardless of the site of the tumor, excrete virtually no riboflavin in their urine. Most healthy people excrete measurable amounts of riboflavin daily.[150] Low riboflavin intake may be a cancer risk factor, or cancer growths may create unusual riboflavin metabolism.

Vitamin B_6 has been shown to inhibit cancer cell growth in culture dishes and even lends greater cancer resistance to mice that are given injections of skin cancer cells.[151] About 40 percent of Americans are low in their intake of B_6.

ANTICANCER FOODS

Yogurt is a salubrious milk product that has been fermented with a special type of bacteria, *Lactobacillus acidophilus*. In test tube studies, yogurt was able to stimulate human cells to produce more interferon, one of our body's most effective anticancer substances.[152] In lab animals, researchers found that yogurt colonies were able to substantially reduce the amount of cancerous products being produced by other intestinal bacteria.[153] Yogurt with live bacteria cultures is a very valuable food for many health reasons. It may even help to defend the body against cancer.

Cruciferous vegetables are composed of the cabbage family of broccoli, brussels sprouts, cauliflower, and cabbage. These special vegetables seem to be elite members of this anticancer food group. Cruciferous vegetables contain noteworthy amounts of sulfur, which may be responsible for their cancer protection. Recall the cancer protection imparted by the sulfur-bearing amino acids cysteine and methionine.

Guinea pigs fed a high-cabbage diet before being exposed to X-radiation had a lower incidence of mortality and hemorrhaging.[154] Another group of animals fed cabbage before being exposed to lethal doses of X-radiation had less than half the mortality rate when compared to animals fed oat and wheat bran.[155] The vice president of research for the American Cancer Society, Dr. Frank Rauscher, told his annual gathering in 1983 that *something* in brussels sprouts inhibits cancer in lab animals. Indoles may be the "magic" compound in cruciferous vegetables that wards off cancer.[156]

Chlorophyll is the green pigment in plants that captures the sun's energy in photosynthesis. Chlorophyll may also prevent cancer.[157]

Extracts from the roots and leaves of wheat sprouts have also shown some cancer prevention abilities.[158]

In a five-year study of 1,271 Massachusetts residents over 65 years of age, investigators found that high vegetable intake only mildly lowered cancer risks. Yet people who ate strawberries or tomatoes on a weekly basis had the lowest cancer rate of all.[159]

Different groups of lab animals were fed various diets, including a variety of seaweeds, and then exposed to a known chemical carcinogen. The seaweed-fed rats had markedly lower rates of tumors than those not fed seaweed.[160] Garlic has also been found to have antitumor properties in lab animals.[161]

Dr. Max Gerson was a renegade physician who created a rigorous raw food vegetarian program for cancer patients. Though there are no controlled studies to "amen" his work, he did report as-tounding anecdotal claims of success. There are theories about why such a diet might be effective against cancer, including the high potassium-to-sodium ratio that is found in vegetarian diets.[162]

POTENTIAL CANCER FIGHTERS

DMSO (dimethyl sulfoxide) has potential in the war against cancer. A 3 percent solution of DMSO in the drinking water of mice resulted in nearly a 50 percent reduction in fatal cancer cases.[163] Unfortunately, most DMSO preparations sold over the counter are of very low purity compared to the research quality DMSO used in the above studies. This is an experimental substance.

Ginseng is a root herb whose first prescription was written before the pyramids were built. Most American researchers have given up on this substance due to impure preparations, mixed results from studies, and frustration in trying to get standardized plants. Too bad. European and Asian scientists have been finding impressive results with purified ginseng. It has been shown to reduce the incidence of mammary tumors and leukemia in mice.[164] With literally hundreds of studies supporting the idea that ginseng is a "rejuvenator" par excellence, it merits further attention in American health care circles. More information on ginseng is found in the chapters on the Circulatory System, Muscular System, and Aging.

Laetrile (amygdalin) is a cyanide-containing substance that was promoted as a cancer cure. No decent scientific studies have been able to endorse this product. One hundred seventy-eight patients in good condition were given laetrile with no noticeable improvement in their condition.[165]

RNA and DNA are the crucial nucleic acids which carry the "blueprints" of new cell growth and the ability to execute those building plans. Some crude research indicated that supplements of various nucleic acids and their precursors could lower the incidence of mammary tumors in mice.[166] Later studies found that rats injected with RNA and DNA preparations lived twice as long as those not given nucleic acids.[167] Another group of rats with chemically induced tumors lived much longer when given injections of RNA.[168]

The real hope of nucleic acids working against cancer seems to be centered in a synthetic nucleic acid preparation called Poly A/ Poly U. Thirty milligrams daily of intravenous Poly A/Poly U was given to 155 women who had been treated for breast cancer. A 4-year follow-up showed that those women receiving the Poly A/ Poly U lived longer than the placebo group.[169] It is unlikely that oral supplements of RNA or DNA would survive the acid bath of the intestines and have any benefit to humans.

SOD (superoxide dismutase) is an enzyme found in the human body with various minerals at its center, including zinc, copper, and manganese. SOD is a valuable scavenger of free radicals and therefore is responsible for checking the destruction of DNA which could result in cancerous growth. Injections of SOD increased the lifespan and survival rate of hamsters with induced tumors.[170] Yet, once again, this is a substance that is worthless in oral supplement form, since it would be destroyed in the intestines and absorbed as indistinguishable fragments.

A very unusual but possibly useful agent against cancer is the oil from green coffee beans. When green coffee bean oil was added to the diets of mice they had measurable increases in their glutathione peroxidase (GSH) levels.[171] GSH is an important cancer fighter in the human body.

FOODS THAT INCREASE CANCER RISK

Pancreatic cancer is the fourth leading cause of fatal cancer in this country. Twenty-three thousand of the 25,000 new cases diagnosed this year will not survive the disease, since only 2 percent of the victims live beyond 5 years. With such poor success at treating the condition, researchers at Johns Hopkins University sought lifestyle factors that might predict the disease. The risk was high with white bread intake and smoking, and lower with raw fruits, vegetables, wine, and diet soda.[172] With the numerous nutrients removed from white bread, it is hard to guess which vitamins, minerals, protein, or fiber are responsible for this increased risk for pancreatic cancer.

Sugar may play a role in cancer incidence. In 50 patients with bowel cancer, investigators found that the cancer patients consumed 21 percent more sugar than the healthy controls.[173]

In lab mice, black pepper appears to have some ability to change cells and may induce cancer when consumed in large amounts.[174]

Sorghum is a grain that is commonly grown in the tropical regions of the world. Certain strains of red and brown sorghum seeds contain so much tannin (a bitter component found in teas and other plants) that not even birds will eat them. Cultures that use these high-tannin sorghums as food staples have much higher rates of cancer of the esophagus than those that don't eat sorghum.[175] Therefore, high-tannin foods are suspect for cancer provocation.

Parsnips contain psoralens, which readily cause cancer in laboratory animals.[176]

Storing nuts or seeds in damp conditions can promote a deadly mold that produces the carcinogen called *aflatoxins*. You cannot taste or smell aflatoxin infestation. Monkeys fed small amounts of aflatoxins eventually develop liver cancer, which is one of the more incurable types of cancer.[177]

The fatty marbling in beef and pork often concentrates the carcinogens, pesticides, and other pollutants that the animal has been exposed to. Do not eat marbling. (More on pollution and cancer will be discussed in Chapter 16.)

NUTRITIONAL RECOMMENDATIONS

DIET BREAKDOWN

To minimize your risk for cancer, these are the percentages of calories that each nutrient factor should contribute to your diet:

25–30 Percent Fat
Balance polyunsaturated, monounsaturated, and saturated fats in roughly equal proportions. Omega-3 fats (e.g. from fish oil) should contribute at least 10% of your polyunsaturated fat intake.

10 Percent Protein
At least half of this should be from plant food.

60–65 Percent Carbohydrates
These should be primarily complex naturally occurring carbohydrates from vegetables, grains, and legumes.

DIETARY GUIDELINES

1. *Consume often:* green and orange vegetables, cruciferous vegetables, seaweed, tomatoes, strawberries, apples, carrots, low-fat plant food, fish, cod liver oil (1 teaspoon daily), yogurt (live culture), garlic.

2. *Minimize consumption of* fatty meats, black pepper, sugar, fat, cholesterol, canned food, coffee, alcohol.

3. *Avoid* burned protein, parsnips, food dyes, sorghum (red and brown varieties), nuts and seeds stored in damp conditions, fatty marbling on meats.

4. *Increase fiber* intake until it is two to three times your current level. Bowel movements should be at least daily, and stools should float.

DAILY SUPPLEMENTS TO ADD TO YOUR CORE PROGRAM

Vitamins
Selenium   +400 mcg
   (from yeast)
A   +1,5000 IU
   (beta-carotene)
Riboflavin   +10 mg
   Rutin   +200 mg
   Folacin   +400 mcg

Minerals
   Calcium   +800 mg
   Zinc   +10 mg
   Molybdenum   +150 mcg
   Vanadium   Although 30 mcg daily of supplemental vanadium
                  may be valuable, very few supplements contain
                  vanadium
   Copper   +1 mg
   Manganese   +8 mg

Quasi vitamins
   Ginseng   +200 mg
   L-cysteine   +2 g
   L-methionine   +2 g

7
THE IMMUNE SYSTEM
Disease Resistance and Wound Healing

The classic novel *Moby Dick* showed what can happen when wounded people are poorly nourished. Sailors in those days spent months eating little more than dried white bread and salted meat, and several of Melville's sailors experienced the reopening of wounds that had allegedly healed long ago. This can happen. Poor nutrition during wound healing provides subpar tissue rebuilding, which can come back to haunt you for a long time to come.

For centuries, people have thought that "fickle fate" pointed out who would get sick and who wouldn't. That just isn't true. People usually get sick for very predictable reasons. There is plenty of evidence to show that both nutrition and emotions play key roles in determining who will get an infection.

People who are overly stressed, depressed, or lonely are more likely to contract all sorts of infectious diseases and even cancer. The thymus gland is responsible for making many of the immune soldiers that destroy invading microbes. Stress causes the thymus gland to shrink. This field of mind-immune interplay, called *psychoneuroimmunology*, is a major factor in people's health.[1]

Did you ever notice how people often get sick just before that critical job interview or that long awaited vacation? Stress (both

153

good and bad) lowers the body's ability to fight off infections. Happy and expressive people get sick less often. For thousands of years, priests, shamans, mystics, and healers have recognized the power of the mind in health. Now 20th-century science also recognizes that power. In 1918, a Japanese researcher noticed that "mental excitation" (stress) worsened tuberculosis.[2] More recently, a variety of studies have shown that your attitude directly affects your disease resistance:

- Medical and dental students had lowered immune abilities during exam time.
- People who lose their spouse have markedly diminished immune capacities.
- Military cadets under great stress were more likely to get mononucleosis.[3]

A major factor in staying healthy is staying happy.

Diet also plays an important role in disease resistance and wound healing. Numerous times throughout history, a plague has been preceded by a famine.[4] The famine created a food shortage, which brought on malnutrition, and shortly thereafter came the devastating plague. In 1347 A.D., the bubonic plague (a.k.a. the Black Death) killed about 75 million people, or about half of the known world at the time. As recently as 1918, a flu epidemic killed about 21 million people. Interestingly, each of these pandemic plagues followed a major war. Wars are remarkably effective at starting a plague. Burn the crops and draft the farmers. Bring in foreigners with exotic pathogens unknown to the visiting region. Add immense stress, which is unavoidable in wartime, and you have the makings of a major famine/plague.

But beyond these blatant cases of malnutrition, the normal American diet with its marginal supply of nutrients also affects our disease resistance. There is a direct relationship between the quality of diet and the efficiency of the immune system in warding off infections.[5] Lung infections, for example, are more common in people who are malnourished.[6] In the underdeveloped regions of the world, malnourished children are 18 times more likely to die from infections than their better nourished peers, and when they eat tainted food their gastrointestinal infections last two to three times longer.

Most people can accept the fact that severe malnutrition can impair the body's ability to fight off infections and heal wounds. Yet new evidence shows that above-RDA levels of certain nutrients can provide above-normal healing rates. Remember, the RDAs are intended for "normal" people who are in good health and not under any stress. Wound healing and infection fighting would definitely be considered stress situations. Nutrition also enhances the effectiveness of vaccines. A controlled study of 100 elderly men showed that improved nutritional status enhanced the value of vaccinations against the flu virus.[7]

Subclinical (less obvious) malnutrition is common in the U.S., and clinical malnutrition is quite common in American hospitals, as revealed by eminent scientists during the early 1970s.[8] Amazingly enough, patients were literally starving to death amid the high-tech wizardry of 20th-century medicine. This hospital malnutrition causes much disease and many complications while it also slows the healing process. Currently, about 25–50 percent of all patients who are in the hospital longer than two weeks show signs of clinical protein-calorie malnutrition.

Ten years after hospital malnutrition was exposed, the trend continues unabated. In a modern Houston hospital in 1982, physicians found that *all* of the 129 surgery patients examined had at least one indication of significant nutritional depletion, with 42 percent being clinically malnourished.[9] A 1985 British study found that one-third of the assessed patients had measurable protein-calorie malnutrition and nearly all were in negative nitrogen balance, which causes tissue wasting.[10] And 61 percent of the 152 men examined in a Veteran's Administration hospital in Virginia were considered to be malnourished.[11] But nutritional assessment of hospital patients is still not a standard practice. If all patients were screened for their nutritional status, the average hospital stay could be cut by at least one or two days, and billions of dollars could be saved in annual health care costs.

The ability of your body to heal from wounds, broken bones, surgery, infections, and burns depends greatly on your nutrient intake because the healing process is fueled *entirely* by nutrients from the diet. Patients recovering from a bone fracture require 25 percent more calories than normal. In patients with major trauma or infection or both, the calorie need goes up by 30–55 percent. And some seriously injured people need 200–300 percent more calories and protein, requiring up to 200 g of protein and 5,000 kilocalories per day. The need for most vitamins and minerals also increases proportionately. Ironically, sick people are less likely to eat even "normally," much less consume these new super-proportions of foods. For that reason, supplemental nutrition is a vital link in the recovery process for the infected or wounded person. Malnourished people are much more likely to contract infections, complications, stay longer in the hospital, and die during recuperation.

Nutritionists who specialize in tube feedings (parenteral nutrition) usually recommend, "If the stomach works, then use it." Yet many sick people can't or won't eat. In that case, tube feedings are better than starving the patient. When patients were tube-fed for six days prior to surgery, the overall risk of morbidity and mortality dropped by 50 percent, and the risk of death and infection fell to one-third that of the unsupplemented patients.[12]

If hospital staffs took five minutes to conduct serum albumin and percent-body-fat measurements, they could quickly find patients who are undernourished and therefore at high risk for complications. Serum albumin relates to protein intake, and protein intake strongly correlates to the overall quality of the diet.[13] These two measurements are fairly accurate at assessing bulk nutrient intake, such as calories and protein. But they do not do justice to the need for various vitamins and minerals that are also crucial to proper healing.

WHAT HAPPENS IN THE WOUNDED PERSON?

Whether you have a broken bone, a bruise (contusion), a large cut (laceration), a burn, or other offenses to the body, wound healing involves four separate phases:

1. *Inflammation*: includes arresting the bleeding and beginning the clot formation.
2. *Migration*: special cells (fibroblasts) move toward the wound site to initiate the repair of the connective protein collagen.
3. *Proliferation*: a gathering of specialized wound repair cells (fibroblasts and others) begin the collagen repair process.

4. *Maturation*: rebuilding of skin tissue (reepithelialization) and formation of scar tissue.

The clotting procedure is a cascading effect of enzymes and proteins that results in a scab formation over the wound to seal off the area. Clotting caps the leaking blood vessels and blocks the entrance of outside invading organisms. In a clot, fibrin forms "threads" over the damaged area.

A variety of nutrient factors can affect the clotting process. The bulk materials that form a clot are made of protein. Vitamin K is a critical ingredient that works in the liver to make these clotting proteins. EPA (from fish oil), vitamin E, capsaicum (from hot red peppers), aspirin and related compounds, and Coumadin (a drug prescribed for patients with vascular disease) all thin the blood. These agents all slow clotting and prolong bleeding time. This effect can be valuable in reducing the stickiness of blood cells that can plug up the blood vessels, but it can be bad in people who are undergoing surgery. Dentists, physicians, nurses, and other health care professionals should question their patients about the use of these agents, because they can markedly slow down clotting and increase the chance for major blood loss.

Nutrients provide the raw materials to rebuild damaged tissue and the fuel for this reconstruction. Bulk nutrients, like protein and calories, are critical to the wounded person. Nutrients involved in new cell growth, like zinc, vitamin C, vitamin A, folacin, B_6, and B_{12}, are also in great demand in the sick person. Nutrients to bolster the immune system, like B_6, selenium, zinc, and vitamin C, help to prevent an infection while the body is temporarily vulnerable. Usually blood has been lost and new blood must be created. This process requires copper, iron, protein, B_6, folacin, zinc, and B_{12}. All of these phases need energy and the vitamins that allow energy metabolism to proceed, like thiamine, niacin, riboflavin, biotin, pantothenic acid, and chromium. All totalled, nutritional status is a major factor in how quickly a person will heal, how strong the mended tissue will be, and the risks for complications and infections during recovery.

A number of individual nutrients have been well documented as enhancing wound healing and disease resistance, including zinc, selenium, vitamin A, vitamin C, protein, and certain individual amino acids.

ZINC

Among its many other functions in the body, zinc is involved in all new cell growth. Wound recovery requires considerable protein building and the replication of DNA and RNA, all of which need copious quantities of zinc. Infections call for a stepped-up production of immune "soldiers" to battle invading organisms, which also requires lots of zinc.

The American diet provides about one half to two-thirds of the RDA for zinc. Zinc-deficient animals have a reduced ability to heal. Surgeons have given zinc supplements (usually about 150 mg daily) to their surgery patients with marked improvements in the speed and strength of wound healing.[14] Zinc supplementation restores proper immunity in a wide variety of conditions.[15]

Are zinc supplements effective because so many people are zinc-deficient or because high doses of zinc bring the immune system beyond "normal" abilities? Wounded humans are known to have measurably lower serum zinc levels and also to excrete more zinc in their urine than normal.[16] But once again, it's a matter of balance: long-term excessive zinc intake (over 300 mg daily for several months) will actually lower the immune response.[17]

Older adults are at particular risk for a zinc deficiency. In one study, *healthy* older adults were given 220 mg of zinc sulfate twice daily for one month. There was a measurable increase in their blood levels of disease resistance factors (T-lymphocytes).[18]

Zinc supplements can reduce surgery recovery time by up to 43 percent. In the 10 surgery patients who were given 150 mg of zinc sulfate daily, recuperation time averaged 46 days. The patients receiving the placebo took an average of 80 days for recovery.[19] When zinc supplements were given to patients with stomach ulcers, healing time dropped to one-third that of the control group.[20] Not all follow-up studies have had the same success, however, so it seems that zinc is only one of the nutrients involved in the wound healing procedure.

Not only does zinc help build immune bodies to fight infections, but zinc itself may be directly toxic to invading bacteria and viruses. A young girl with leukemia was being given various drugs and nutrition supplements for her condition. Just to try something different, she kept a zinc tablet in her mouth and let it dissolve completely. She noticed that her cold and sore throat went away almost immediately. She told her father, who told a researcher friend, who corroborated the claim with a double-blind experiment. Sucking on zinc tablets (three 50 mg tablets of zinc sulfate per day) can reduce the duration and severity of colds and sore throats.[21]

Down's syndrome is an incurable genetic defect that leaves its victims with intellectual retardation and often a lowered disease resistance. When Down's syndrome children were given 135 mg of zinc supplements daily for two months, they showed remarkable improvements in their immune functions.[22]

Zinc supplements also have proven to be more effective than the drug of choice (penicillamine) for treating patients with Wilson's disease, an inherited disorder causing toxic levels of copper storage in the body.[23] Zinc probably works in Wilson's disease because it competes with copper for absorption sites in the intestines.

AIDS (acquired immune deficiency syndrome) is creating a near panic situation in various parts of the world, including America. This disease is unusual for many reasons. It may lie dormant for 5–10 years before surfacing to destroy the immune system. In only a few years, AIDS has sprung from near obscurity into the disease limelight. So far, 40,000 Americans have died from it. Yet that number could increase dramatically in the near future. Blood-to-blood or blood-to-sperm contact must be made in order to get it, which means that those who engage in polygamous sexual contact, drug abusers who share dirty needles, and recipients of donated blood are at the greatest risk for contracting AIDS. There is no cure, no vaccine to prevent it, and most AIDS patients die within a year from a multitude of infections, since their immune systems have been crippled.

Yet, curiously enough, only about one-third of the people who have been exposed to the virus have contracted AIDS or even the milder version, *called AIDS-related complex.* What happened to the other two thirds? Several scientists have noticed that nearly all AIDS victims show very low serum zinc levels. Zinc status in the U.S. is generally deplorable, and it may be even worse among men who have frequent intercourse, since sperm-making requires large amounts of zinc. Promiscuous sexual behavior could create an impressive zinc loss through the semen and prostate fluid that is spent.[24] The remaining low body zinc levels could depress immune abilities and make AIDS infection more likely in those who are exposed to the virus. A well-nourished immune system, especially with respect to vitamins A and E and zinc, could be a major factor in protecting people who are exposed to the AIDS virus.[25]

There is ample evidence that well-nourished people would be less likely to contract the AIDS virus.[26] AIDS may have its greatest impact on poverty regions of the developing nations. In Africa, AIDS is also known as the "slim disease," since its victims are primarily very thin undernourished people. The highest incidence of AIDS in America is in Belle Glade, Florida, a region of poor people, not addicts and homosexuals. John Beldekas, Ph.D., found that AIDS victims had markedly reduced symptoms when fed a vegetarian diet. AIDS was first found in the 1970s among people in central Africa who were eating monkey meat. One theory states that the AIDS virus started off as a reasonably innocuous virus found in green monkeys in Africa. When people ate this monkey meat, the virus mutated into its current deadly immune-crippling form. There is reason to believe that a well-balanced vegetarian diet may offer a certain edge of extra protection against AIDS.

SELENIUM

Why selenium is so effective at encouraging proper disease resistance is somewhat of a mystery. Perhaps selenium helps to protect a potent hormonelike substance (prostacyclin) that promotes immune factors, while limiting the antagonistic force (leukotrienes) that might lower disease resistance. Possibly selenium provides a shield for the body's "warriors" as they douse the invading organisms with lethal free radicals. Thus, the bacteria and viruses die, but not the body's immune factors, which are left to combat more invaders. Whatever the reason, selenium is critical to healthy immune functions and is commonly in short supply in the American diet. Tobacco and alcohol reduce the amounts of selenium available in the body.[27]

In animal studies, selenium supplementation has produced up to a 30-fold increase in the activity of the immune system.[28] High doses of selenium supplements even slow cancer growth in various animal experiments, indicating that the immune system is helping to destroy the invading cell growth.[29]

When intake of selenium is ideal, animals are able to produce more antibodies in response to invading foreign proteins. This means that selenium can improve the value of vaccinations. Indeed, selenium supplements in lab animals were able to increase the effectiveness of malarial vaccines,[30] and supplements in calves doubled the immune response to a vaccine for leptospirosis (infections obtained from other animals, rodents, or disease-infested swamps).

VITAMIN A

Vitamin A has a couple of known roles in the body that relate to wound healing and disease resistance: (1) It is involved in cell division, which occurs at an increased pace during wound healing. (2) It is crucial to the health of the mucous membranes and their mucous production, which are the first-line defense against invading microbes.

People and animals who are low in vitamin A have reduced immune functions and are more likely to get infections.[31] Above-normal doses of vitamin A may be able to elevate the immune system beyond "normal" abilities. When supplements of vitamin A are given in high doses, the immune system shows increased effectiveness.[32] Wounds heal faster with supplemental vitamin A.[33] Burn victims almost always have lower vitamin A levels in the blood, which can then be returned to normal with high dose supplements of vitamin A.[34]

A variety of studies have found that precariously high doses of vitamin A (500,000–1.5 million IU daily) are able to prevent the immune-suppressive effects of chemotherapy, radiation therapy, and surgical anesthetics. Yet these doses of vitamin A could be toxic. Some new evidence indicates that the nontoxic version of vitamin A (beta-carotene) may have the same benefits without the same risks.

Diabetics are notoriously vulnerable to infections and poor wound healing. Vitamin A supplements have been able to encourage markedly the disease resistance and wound healing processes in surgical diabetic patients.[35] Vitamin A also helps to prevent ulcers in traumatized patients[36] and to accelerate the healing of stomach ulcers (150,000 IU daily).[37]

Vitamin A is crucial to people who are sick, wounded, infected, or recovering from surgery. Although vitamin A (as beta-carotene) is easily obtained in the American diet from green and orange fruits and vegetables, many Americans are still low in this immune-bolstering vitamin. For those who don't get enough vitamin A in their diet, supplements provide a viable alternative. In some cases, intake of vitamin A beyond levels that could be obtained from food can have amazing healing effects.

VITAMIN C

Collagen is the tough connective protein that is referred to as "the glue" that keeps all tissue in the body together. It is a primary ingredient in skin, muscles, cartilage, bones, and blood vessels. Vitamin C is vital for collagen synthesis and thus for wound healing. Vitamin C is also important to the production of immune bodies to ward off infections, and it accumulates in burn sites.[38]

Supplements of vitamin C (500–3,000 mg daily) have been quite effective at speeding up wound healing in humans.[39] In a double-blind study involving 94 older patients, 1,000 mg of vitamin C daily helped their bruise healing.[40] High-dose supplements of vitamin C improved the healing of pressure sores[41] and leg ulcers in thalassemia (an inherited blood disorder) patients.[42] All of these patients were considered to be "normally" nourished and not vitamin C–deficient. One gram of vitamin C supplements daily also helped to prevent the blood clotting that often occurs in the legs of post-operative surgery patients.[43]

Vitamin C also does an amazing job of mobilizing the body's immune system against infections. Supplements of 2–5 g of vitamin C daily increase the activity of lymphocytes[44] and improve the migration and mobility of leukocytes, all of which makes for a more effective immune system.[45]

Vitamin C is deadly against many viral infections. One gram of vitamin C daily was able to reduce the duration and severity of colds by an average of 37 percent.[46] Although various studies have found mixed results using vitamin C against the common cold, one study attempted to quell the controversy by using matched pairs of identical human twins. The vitamin C group got 19 percent fewer colds, duration of colds was 38 percent shorter, severity was 22 percent less, and intensity was 20 percent less than in the placebo group.[47]

The herpes virus plagues as many as 20 million Americans. In a double-blind study, vitamin C (600 mg daily) and bioflavonoids (600 mg) cut healing rate time in half for oral herpes sores.[48] Some physicians also claim excellent results when giving very high doses of C (20,000–100,000 mg daily) for severe viral infections, such as hepatitis and mononucleosis.[49] Up to 10 percent of all blood transfusion patients get hepatitis, which is a severely disabling viral infection of the liver. Large *oral* doses (3,200 mg daily) of vitamin C could not lower the incidence of hepatitis in patients receiving blood transfusions.[50] But large *intravenous* amounts (7,000 mg daily) nearly eliminated the hepatitis scourge in human transfusion recipients.[51] Guinea pigs given injections of vitamin C showed increased survival time when infected with the rabies virus.[52]

Many scientists consider the loss of immune functions to be a progressive and nonnegotiable result of aging. Yet in a placebo-controlled experiment, healthy normal older adults receiving injections of 500 mg of ascorbic acid daily had measurable improvements in their immune systems.[53]

Sick people are able to tolerate more vitamin C. In healthy people, daily oral doses of more than 10,000 mg may produce diarrhea. AIDS victims can tolerate up to 40,000 mg of oral vitamin C before the diarrhea sets in.[54] Some physicians report extended quality and quantity of life for AIDS victims when given high-dose vitamin C, though no one claims this is a cure.

Bioflavonoids may help the function of vitamin C. One American study showed that bioflavonoids improved the efficiency of absorbing vitamin C.[55] In European studies, bioflavonoids were found to be effective in slowing bacterial, fungal,[56] and viral infections.[57]

Are large doses of vitamin C necessary for everyone to reap these benefits? Maybe not. Even though Americans have plenty of available food sources for vitamin C, many people don't get even RDA levels. In a study of over 4,000 people in Florida, from different strata of life, researchers found that 17–72 percent of these people were at suboptimal levels of vitamin C. Half of the institutionalized elderly in this study exhibited clear signs of scurvy![58] Just getting ourselves up to RDA levels (60 mg) of vitamin C would improve disease resistance and wound recovery in many people.

Recent studies show that about 200 mg of ascorbic acid daily provides tissue saturation in most normal healthy humans. People under stress, surgery and burn patients, the elderly, and those using drugs, alcohol, or tobacco could all likely benefit from using up to 3,000 mg of ascorbic acid daily. The risks are near zero, the potential benefits are significant, and the cost is very low.

PROTEIN AND AMINO ACIDS

Protein is probably *the* most important of all nutrients in the disease resistance and wound healing business. Although it seems ludicrous amid our food abundance, many Americans (especially the elderly and poor) are low in protein intake. Protein-calorie malnutrition was found in 21 of the 51 (41 percent) elderly Canadian people studied.[59] Their immune systems had a very marginal ability to resist infections.

Not only is bulk protein intake crucial, but there are certain amino acids that can stimulate the disease resistance and wound healing capacity of the human body. Lysine (about 1,000 mg daily) helped 84 percent of the herpes victims tested.[60] Lysine is a limiting essential amino acid, meaning that it is essential in the human diet and is often the amino acid in a food that limits the value of the protein because so little lysine is available. Lysine is low in grain foods and is lost during the refining, baking, and even toasting of bread.[61]

Methionine, a sulfur-bearing amino acid that is found in high levels in beans and eggs, is another limiting essential amino acid. When lab animals exposed to toxins were given supplements of methionine, they had improved weight gain and reduced mercury concentrations in their tissue.[62]

Arginine is a nonessential amino acid, meaning that you can make *some* internally when your body is provided the nine essential amino acids. You do need arginine, but you can make some from other amino acids. Hence, most normal healthy people probably do not need it in the diet. But supplements of arginine have been very effective at stimulating disease resistance and wound recovery. Large doses (up to 30 g daily) of arginine were shown to stimulate the immune system of humans.[63] Lower doses of arginine also help to promote wound healing.[64] The thymus gland resides in the abdomen cavity and is very important to disease resistance.

During stress, the thymus gland often shrinks, and people get sick, regardless of whether that stress was good or bad. Arginine supplements stimulate the thymus gland to maintain its proper size and lymphocyte output.[65] Ornithine is another nonessential amino acid that stimulates the thymus gland for enhanced immune function.[66]

Taurine is a nonessential amino acid that does not fit many of the standardized rules for amino acids. People who are ill have a reduced ability to make their own taurine. Consequently, taurine may be a conditionally essential nutrient for the sick person and the premature infant.[67]

OTHER MINERALS

Iron deficiency, which is quite common in America, often lowers the immune response in people.[68]

Copper deficiency in laboratory animals lowers the antibodies that are available to fight infections.[69] When animals are infected with dangerous bacteria, the death rate is much higher in the copper-deficient animals.[70] Copper deficiency in animals can produce emphysema.[71] The average copper intake in America is roughly half of the RDA.

OTHER VITAMINS

Vitamin E

Vitamin E also plays an important part in disease resistance. In animal studies, supplements of vitamin E bolstered the production of antibodies and helped to protect against bacterial and fungal infections.[72] However, a human study did not have the same promising results, so this issue needs more investigation.[73] Yet supplements of both vitamin E and selenium were able to reduce the swelling in various areas of the body.[74]

Plastic surgeons find that about one third of all breast implant patients develop "puckering" around the wound site. With vitamin E supplements taken internally (2,000 IU daily), the rate of "puckering" dropped to 19 percent of the patients.[75] Vitamin E supplements (1,000 IU daily) were also able to lower the incidence of postoperative problems in surgery patients.[76]

Topical vitamin E from gelatin capsules is used by some people to help heal skin burns and wounds. Many people report good results with this treatment, but some people are sensitive to topi-cally applied vitamin E and will develop a rash.[77]

Vitamin E (200–600 IU daily) and calcium (500 mg daily) have been used in tandem in six different experiments on postoperative humans to reduce the incidence of complications. Postoperative patients who did not receive the vitamin E and calcium supple-ments had 200 percent more blood clots in the legs (peripheral venous thrombosis), 600 percent more cases of blood clots stuck in the vessels of the lungs (pulmonary embolism), and 900 percent more fatalities from pulmonary embolism.[78]

B Vitamins

Of all the B vitamins, B_6 is probably the most crucial to the healthy functioning of the immune system. B_6 deficiencies in hu-mans leave the immune system woefully depressed in a variety of ways,[79] and supplements can aid the immune system. For example, vitamin B_6 supplements 50mg/day have been shown to help the immune function of both normal older adults and renal dialysis patients.[80] Unfortunately, 40 percent of Americans have been found to be deficient in B_6, and it could be a prime limiting nutrient in American health care.

Pantothenic acid is a B vitamin that is involved in energy pro-duction and antibody formation. It has measurable bacteria-killing abilities.[81] Supplemental pantothenic acid accelerated the healing process in lab animals following surgery.[82] In intestinal surgery patients, pantothenic acid supplements helped to bring back nor-mal intestinal motility sooner.[83] Pantothenic acid also is used up more quickly during physical and mental stress. Lab animals who were supplemented with pantothenic acid were able to survive twice as long in cold water as unsupplemented animals.[84]

The name *pantothenic acid* is derived from the Greek word *pantos*, meaning "found everywhere." Although pantothenic acid is widely distributed in most plant and animal foods, it is also lost in food refining. Americans do not get even RDA levels of panto-thenic acid. In one study, the average intake of pantothenic acid for teenagers was 5.5 mg, or about half of the RDA.[85] For nursing home residents, the average intake was one third of the RDA.[86] The researcher who discovered pantothenic acid, Dr. Roger Wil-liams of the University of Texas, believes that the RDA for pantothenic acid (10 mg) is too low, which means that most Americans aren't getting even marginal amounts of this nutrient, much less the higher optimal amounts that would encourage better wound healing.

Folacin is a B vitamin that is intimately involved in new cell growth, such as occurs in wound healing and the making of immune soldiers for disease resistance. Burn victims show an increased loss of folacin by-products by as much as 10 times the normal level.[87] With many Americans marginally nourished in folacin, supplements of folacin during wound recovery would probably speed healing. Topically applied folacin was able to improve gum tissue healing dramatically in human patients.[88]

Riboflavin supplements have been used in eye surgery patients to prevent infiltration of blood vessels in the cornea (corneal vascularization).[89] Although most forms of malnutrition increase the vulnerability of humans to infections, a riboflavin deficiency seems to *lower* the growth of malaria microbes in various hosts.[90] However, starving the host in order to discourage the parasite is a questionable approach to disease prevention.

Vitamin D

Vitamin D deficiency can be common in the elderly, among those who don't drink milk (since milk is fortified with vitamin D), and in people living in cloudy climates. Vitamin D supplements were able to speed up the bone reformation process in human subjects who were low in vitamin D levels.[91]

OTHER HELPFUL NUTRITION FACTORS

In addition to the vitamins, minerals, and amino acids discussed above, other substances, which are not essential in the diet of normal healthy people, show promise in promoting wound healing and/or disease resistance.

Coenzyme Q

Coenzyme Q is a substance that works at a key juncture in energy metabolism. Supplements of CoQ (30–60 mg daily) stimulate the human immune system.[92] Oral supplements of CoQ have also been effective at speeding up recovery in certain gum diseases.[93]

Isoprinosine

Inosine is a precursor (raw material) that eventually ends up as DNA, RNA, or ATP in the body. A derivative of inosine (isoprinosine) has been found to have impressive antiviral activities.[94]

Carnitine

Carnitine is a shuttle system for fat burning in the furnaces of body cells. The more efficient the fat-burning process, the less protein the body will use for fuel. Only protein can build tissue, yet protein, carbohydrate, or fat can provide the fuel for life's metabolic processes. This fact can be quite critical when a patient is recovering from a wound and is showing nitrogen loss or lean tissue wasting as the body burns its precious protein reserves. When L-carnitine was added to the parenteral nutrition (tube feedings) for lab animals, the nitrogen balance improved measurably.[95] This means that more protein is left for the wound repair process.

DMSO

DMSO (dimethyl sulfoxide) is a liniment that is used commonly on the sore muscles of athletes and race horses. Its uses have now spread into other areas of health care. Although the purity of DMSO sold on the shelves is questionable, pure DMSO (topically applied, of course) may help heal skin infections.[96]

Yogurt

Yogurt is a dairy product that has been fermented with the bacteria culture *Lactobacillus acidophilus*. This bacteria is quite effective in protecting the body from outside pathogens. Yogurt helps to cure stomach and intestinal upsets from the flu or food poisoning.[97] Yogurt douches have long been a common folk cure for vaginal tract infections. Now there is scientific proof to support these claims. Physicians were able to cure 93 percent of vaginal tract infections by giving the women injections of *Lactobacillus* vaccine (made from the yogurt bacteria).[98] Women who were vegetarians and consuming garlic, ginger, chili peppers, and moderate amounts of alcohol were less likely to get urinary tract infections.[99]

Essentially, there are many nutrition factors that prevent infections, cure them quicker once you get them, speed healing to wounds and burns, and generally make the recovery process a quicker, less dreadful experience. More information becomes available every day:

- Garlic is an ancient wonder herb/spice/food. It is quite effective in strengthening the immune system and is directly toxic to certain strains of viruses, bacteria, and fungi.[100]
- Ginseng is another ancient but effective substance used against infections.[101]
- Brewer's yeast is the richest source of GTF chromium, which is important for proper glucose metabolism. Glucose is the favored fuel for tissue rebuilding, which helps to explain why diabetics have such a problem with disease resistance and wound repair. Brewer's yeast has improved the immune abilities in a variety of animal studies.[102]
- Eicosapentaenoic acid (EPA) is a special fatty acid found in fish oil that can markedly enhance the body's immune functions.[103]

Healing nutrients in combination with the wonders of modern medicine could markedly reduce hospitalization time for Americans. In reviewing 90 years worth of records in a Scottish hospital, one scientist found that the improved survival statistics for modern surgery are due more to improved diet and hygiene than to specific medical procedures.[104] Healing nutrients can be an incredibly effective method to help avoid illness or to recover more quickly after infections, burns, wounds, and surgery.

NUTRITIONAL RECOMMENDATIONS

For maximal recuperative powers, start this program at least a week prior to surgery and continue with it throughout the healing period.

FOLLOW THE CORE DIETARY PROGRAM, PLUS

DIETARY GUIDELINES

1. Add three to six protein exchanges to the Core Program.
2. Consume often: garlic and live cultured yogurt.

DAILY SUPPLEMENTS TO ADD TO YOUR CORE PROGRAM

Vitamins
  Vitamin A   +20,000 IU
   (beta-carotene)
  Vitamin D   +400 IU (for bone healing)
  Vitamin E   +200 IU
  Riboflavin   +20 mg (for eye surgery)
  Vitamin B$_6$ +50 mg
  Folacin   +400 mcg
  Vitamin C   +2,000 mg
  Pantothenic acid   +100 mg

Minerals
  Calcium   +500 mg
  Zinc   +50 mg
  Iron   10–50 mg (depending on blood loss)
  Copper   5 mg
  Chromium   +200 mcg
   (from yeast)
  Selenium (from yeast)   +200 mcg

Quasi vitamins
  L-carnitine   +1,000 mg
  EPA   +1,000 mg
  Coenzyme Q   +60 mg (especially for gum problems)
  Ginseng   +200 mg
  Bioflavonoids   +500 mg
  L-lysine   +1,000 mg
  L-methionine   +2,000 mg
  L-arginine   +2,000–30,000 mg
  L-ornithine   +2,000 mg
  L-taurine   +3,000 mg

8
THE IMMUNE SYSTEM
Food Allergies and Sensitivities

If you want to stir up some controversy among an eclectic blend of health care professionals, bring up the subject of food allergies. It's guaranteed to stimulate at least a brisk discussion, if not an argument. Probably no other field of health care has more unfounded claims, peripheral practitioners, and placebo effects. Physicians who specialize in allergy treatment are the highest-paid specialty group with the least number of procedures that have been proven in double-blind experiments. There are three basic categories of allergies: (1) inhalant (like ragweed and pollen), (2) ingestant (from foods consumed), and (3) contact (like poison oak and ivy). Proper nutrition can almost totally eliminate food allergies. The link between nutrition and inhalant or contact allergies is vague. The rest of this chapter deals exclusively with food allergies. In spite of all the confusion and the limited quantity of reliable information, one thing is certain: food allergies do exist, and they often express themselves in the most unusual physical and mental symptoms.

Food allergies are more than just a bothersome problem. They have been proven to be a possible cause in heart disease,[1] diabetes,[2] irritable bowel syndrome and diarrhea,[3] arthritis,[4] marked changes in behavior and emotions,[5] migraines,[6] and many other symptoms. When 28 patients with irritable bowel syndrome and diarrhea were given a diet specially formulated to avoid common offending foods, *all* of them improved, and half of them were found to be biochemically allergic to various foods.[7] After six weeks on a special diet that avoided common allergenic foods, 75 percent of the 46 arthritics tested had major objective improvements in their arthritis condition.[8]

The confusion in the field of allergies is understandable. The average American is exposed each day to about 63,000 different chemicals in our food supply and environment.[9] Millions of other substances are made in our body. The chance that one or more of these substances will not get along with others is quite good. And the chance that someone will be able to detect just which interaction is doing the harm is quite poor.

Many of you are familiar with the runny nose and swollen itchy eyes of a hay fever sufferer, or the itchy skin sores from poison oak and poison ivy, or the severe reaction some people have to bee stings. Each of these is an allergic reaction. Scientists are now finding that food allergies are also quite common and can affect any part of the mind or body.

Allergies may exist in some people only when certain food combinations are consumed or only when the individual is under stress. Since our personal biochemistry can change somewhat as we age, some people grow out of allergies, and others grow into them. Some people can react to almost undetectable levels of offending substances. In other people, reactions occur only after repeated exposure. In many people, an allergic reaction happens when their exposure to various allergens (substances that induce an allergy) reaches a cumulative crescendo. So, the fact that you ate something that you are allergic to does not mean that allergic symptoms will occur immediately. Allergic reactions probably surface when your level of allergen exposure reaches a certain critical mass. That turning point is something like the point at which a container of liquids overflows. A teaspoon here, a cup there of fluid, and eventually the container overflows. It is the *overflowing* that produces the overt allergic symptoms. This is just one of the many reasons why allergies are so difficult to pinpoint.

Also, the common overt symptoms of inhalant allergies (e.g., the swollen eyes and runny nose) are just the tip of the iceberg. Ninety percent of the allergy problem lies beneath the surface as internal ailments.

For the purposes of this chapter, a food *allergy* is a reaction to a food protein, while a food *sensitivity* is a reaction to some other component of food (e.g., additives or salicylates).

Conservative estimates indicate that 8 percent of the U.S. population suffers from some type of allergy.[10] More realistic estimates put the incidence at two to three times that number.[11] This means that somewhere between 19 and 57 million Americans are allergy victims and could benefit considerably from this chapter.

WHAT CAUSES AN ALLERGY?

Basically, an allergy is caused by an overzealous immune system that attacks the body itself. The immune system is designed to seek out foreign substances in the body and destroy them, which protects us from infections. In allergic people, the immune system not only destroys the invading food protein that has been mistakenly absorbed into the bloodstream; it also begins to wreak havoc on the body.

The healthy digestive tract renders food in the diet into smaller molecules for absorption into the bloodstream. In 90 percent of healthy people, small amounts of undigested food proteins are able to pass through the intestinal wall intact and enter the bloodstream.[12] In most people, this situation does not create any problem. In food allergy victims, the immune system swarms all over the food proteins in the bloodstream and then begins attacking the body itself.

When you cut yourself, some bacteria probably enter the wound, where they are greeted by your circulating immune bodies. The immune system recognizes these invading bacteria as foreign proteins and destroys them. The large protein molecules from the food that made it into the blood supply are also recognized as foreign invaders. The immune bodies destroy the food protein. When the antigens (food proteins) build up in the bloodstream, the immune bodies can become overwhelming in number and initiate a "feeding frenzy." By now, the numbers of circulating immune bodies are so high that they begin to attack the body's own tissue. This is called an *autoimmune* (*auto* as in "self") response because the immune system is attacking the host.

If this autoimmune attack occurs in the upper respiratory tract, then wheezing, sniffling, and sneezing often develop. We have all seen this in hay fever sufferers. When this autoimmune response occurs in the skin region, hives, welts, itching, and swelling can occur. Most of us have experienced this from poison oak or poison ivy, which are allergens that are absorbed through the skin to do their mischief. Both hay fever and poison oak are considered environmental allergens since they are inhaled or rubbed on.

The same autoimmune response can occur with food allergies. If the autoimmune response is in the pancreas region, then diabetes can be the result as the pancreas is destroyed. If the gastrointestinal tract is attacked, then diarrhea, cramps, Crohn's disease (a dangerous intestinal inflammation), and other forms of distress can ensue. If the bone joints are the site of the autoimmune response, then arthritis may be the result. If the brain is the site of the autoimmune attack, then behavioral changes may develop. Asthma, eczema, hives (urticaria), and other symptoms often are the result of an allergic reaction to food. Up to 12 percent of all preschool children suffer from eczema, which involves itchy lesions on the skin surface.[13] Many of these difficult-to-treat and seemingly unrelated conditions may be caused by food allergies.

Food allergies can also influence your mood. Allergies can affect any part of the body, including the brain. Possibly the autoimmune attack causes swelling of the brain, or perhaps it changes the blood-brain barrier (a special filtration sieve that is unique to the blood vessels in the brain) to allow substances into the brain that normally are excluded.[14] The net effect could be mood changes, lethargy, poor attention span, reduced intellect, or any other possible variation in mental abilities. Depressed patients have twice the normal incidence of allergies.[15]

Nursing infants can even have allergic reactions to substances that are in mother's milk as a result of mother's diet. Onions, garlic, caffeine, and other "loud"-flavored foods can pass into the breast milk to offend the infant. Or mother's allergies may be manifested in her breastfeeding infant. One-third of all infants with colic were cured when their mothers stopped drinking cow's milk.[16]

HOW TO DETECT ALLERGIES

A number of diagnostic tests are used in the field of allergies, but none of them are satisfactory. Other areas of health care have such neat and tidy means for detection—X-rays show broken bones quite dramatically; angiograms can peer into the blood vessels to detect blockages—but there are no such dramatic and definitive detection devices for allergies.

Allergy diagnosis can come from any of the following tests:

Skin testing involves making a series of scratches on the skin surface and placing various substances inside the wound. If a red spot develops, an allergy is suspected. This test is expensive, painful, and not very reliable.

Radioallergosorbent test (RAST) involves sending a sample of the patient's blood through a complicated device that allegedly can detect allergies by bombarding certain blood components with radiation. This too is expensive and of dubious reliability.

Basophil histamine release is a complex laboratory technique that is accurate but is also expensive and time-consuming. Currently, this method is suited only for research work.

Cytotoxic testing draws the patient's blood and places various likely offenders in the blood to see if blood cells are destroyed. The test can be done in front of the patient in the doctor's office. This method is very controversial.

Provocative sublingual testing places a sample of suspected allergens under the tongue of the patient. Then the clinician tests the patient's arm strength by pushing against the arm. The theory is that an allergic reaction will reduce arm strength and the patient's resistance to the therapist's push. This method is also very controversial.

Patient response is probably the most useful, although the least scientific, of all the methods. Essentially, it means "If the food offends you, don't eat it." Although most scientists would like to have double-blind reproducible results to placate their curiosity, such is not always possible in the complex chemical milieu of the human body. In the study mentioned in the beginning of this chapter, all of the patients with various gastrointestinal problems were helped via the special diet, but in only half of the patients was the food allergy corroborated by clinical tests.

The patient response method is based on common sense that has significant merit. If wheat makes you ill, don't eat it. Looking for laboratory proof can be costly and sometimes misleading. What if the laboratory tests indicate that you are not allergic to wheat, yet every time you eat it you get sick? Which should you believe, a fallible series of people and test tubes or your own body?

WHY ARE ALLERGIES BECOMING SO COMMON TODAY?

Perhaps allergies have always been with us but were undiagnosed. Perhaps more health care professionals are willing to take unconventional approaches, like allergy treatment, to solve unusual patient problems. If this is true, then allergies *have* always been around. Most experts agree, however, that allergies are becoming more common today, and several theories have been proposed to explain this trend:

LOW INCIDENCE OF BREASTFEEDING

Only 10–20 percent of American babies are nursed until six months of age. This is truly a tragedy. Human milk is made *by* humans *for* humans and is very unlikely to cause an allergic reaction. Infants who are breastfed are not only less likely to get an allergy as infants but also less likely to develop allergies later in life.[17] Cow's milk and soy formula are more likely to cause an allergic reaction.

EARLY INTRODUCTION OF SOLID FOODS[18]

Nature has provided humans with an unusual feature that allows a breastfeeding mother to share her extensive disease resistance abilities with her newborn babe. In the normal adult intestines, the immune factors provided by mother's milk would be destroyed. Yet the infant has a unique intestinal tract, with large "windows" that are suited specifically to allow these immune proteins to pass into the infant's blood.[19] As the infant ages, these "windows" close up. Thus, a young infant is very vulnerable to food allergies with these "windows" that allow large protein complexes to pass into the bloodstream. Mother's milk does not create a problem. Other foods might.

When food other than mother's milk is fed to the infant before six months of age, the large proteins from the food can slip through these special "windows" and provoke an allergic reaction that may sensitize the infant's immune system for the rest of his or her life. Early introduction of food other than mother's milk increases the chances of that person's developing allergies now and throughout life.

THE RESTRICTIVE DIETARY SELECTION IN AMERICA

There are many thousands of different types of fruits, vegetables, legumes, grains, nuts, eggs, dairy, poultry, fish, and other edible items. There are over 20,000 edible varieties of plants alone. Yet the average American restricts his or her grocery store selections to no more than 20 regular items. With small amounts of these food proteins regularly slipping into the bloodstream, a progressive accumulation may cause an allergic reaction. People who eat a wide variety of foods are less likely to encounter food allergies.

MANY AMERICANS ARE DEFICIENT
IN A VARIETY OF NUTRIENTS

A healthy body is less likely to go awry and attack itself with an autoimmune reaction. Scientists have found, for instance, that a marginal deficiency of vitamin E can provoke the autoimmune response that occurs in allergies, and supplements of vitamin E seem to stabilize certain autoimmune conditions.[20] Any one or all of these vitamin and mineral deficiencies present in Americans could create an abnormal immune system that surfaces through allergic reactions.

POLLUTANTS

Pollutants can change the normal workings of the digestive and immune systems. Any substance that contaminates the body could be considered a pollutant. Alcohol can alter the permeability of the intestinal wall and allow substances into the system that normally would be kept out. Drugs, tobacco, pesticides, and industrial toxins can all make a healthy system unhealthy. Pollution can create an abnormally permissive intestinal tract that absorbs substances it normally would keep out. Pollution can create an abnormal immune system that is more likely to attack the body, so a body infested with pollution is more likely to develop an allergic reaction.

STRESS

Here is a fascinating issue. The new field of psychoneuroimmunology has established a definite link between the mind and the immune system. Depressed and stressed people are more likely to get infections and cancer and to die younger than their happier peers. Stress can change the absorption efficiency of the intestinal tract to allow more food proteins to enter and excite the immune system into an autoimmune attack. This brawl between food proteins and immune bodies may spread to the brain and produce behavioral disturbances.[21] In other words, the mind started it, and the mind gets it back. As the stress of 20th-century living seems to build, we must learn to control our emotions better, lest the mind (stress) ends up creating new ailments for us to contend with.

HOW TO TREAT FOOD ALLERGIES

Two main food programs exist: (1) the elimination diet and (2) the rotation diet. These programs are almost self-explanatory, yet we shall delve into them in detail. In addition to varying the food intake, a variety of nutrients can help provide relief to the food allergy patient. The intent of the supplements is twofold: (1) to reduce the swelling and inflammation that are so common in allergy victims and (2) to nourish the person to prevent an abnormal immune reaction caused by a malnourished system.

THE ELIMINATION DIET

This method assumes that you are so sensitive to a food that you cannot have any of it. How small an amount can provoke an allergic reaction? Quite small, unfortunately. In a recent incident reported in the national press, a 12-year old boy who knew he was allergic to peanuts bit into a piece of chocolate birthday cake at a friend's party and instantly spit it out. He did not chew or swallow any of the cake, since he immediately detected a peanut flavor—a small amount of peanut butter had been used to make the chocolate frosting. The boy was immediately taken to the hospital, where he died. The skin under the tongue can absorb substances (like allergens) and bring them into the body, as users of nitroglycerin for heart conditions will attest. Some people can be very sensitive to even the smallest amount of an allergenic substance.

People who are allergic to corn may be so sensitive that they also react to corn syrup, which is basically pure sugar with tiny traces of corn protein left over. They may even react to synthetic vitamin C supplements, which are often made from the corn syrup sugar, which would then have infinitesimal amounts of corn protein left over in the vitamin C.

THE ROTATION DIET

This program is designed for people who are not quite as sensitive to their allergens. They may get sick if they drink milk every day, but not if they have it once a week. Thus, the offending foods are rotated weekly or monthly to avoid buildup of these allergen by-products in the blood. The sensitivity of the individual will dictate how severe his or her dietary restrictions must be. Ultrasensitive people cannot go on the rotation program.

DETECTING THE ALLERGENS

Both the elimination program and the rotation program are based upon detecting the offending food(s). Two phases are involved:

1. *Cleansing period.* During this four-day phase, the patient is allowed no food. This cleanses the system of residual allergens. The patient is provided with electrolytes, hypoallergenic vitamin and mineral supplements, and specially filtered water. This fasting period is not recommended for diabetics and other people with brittle health problems. These people should avoid fasting and go straight into the hypoallergenic diet.

2. *Organized food introduction.* After the initial four-day cleansing period, a hypoallergenic diet is introduced. This consists of foods that rarely instigate allergy trouble, including rice, apples, carrots, pears, turkey, olive oil, black tea, and lamb. Infants are given commercially prepared hypoallergenic formulas containing casein hydrolysates, which are partially digested proteins. If no allergic reaction to this hypoallergenic diet is seen, then every four-

day period one more food is introduced, usually selecting first from among the suspect hyperallergenic foods listed below. If the person reacts to the hypoallergenic diet, the process is started over, and these hypoallergenic foods are introduced one at a time. Notes are kept on any effect (either physical or mental) from the foods introduced.

The foods that are most likely to cause allergic reactions (hyperallergenic) include eggs, milk, wheat, beef, corn, peanuts, soybeans, chicken, fish, nuts, mollusks (like clams, oysters, mussels), and shellfish (like shrimp and lobster). Note that most of these foods are quite commonly found on the American shopping list.

Once all offending food substances have been identified, the patient is sent home with a list of foods to avoid or rotate in and out of the diet and information on how to shop for and cook these foods. With proper compliance, that may be the end of the patient's problems.

HELPFUL SUPPLEMENTS

Certain nutritional supplements can help lessen the allergic reaction. Histamine, a substance produced by your body's immune factors, is a major contributor of various symptoms in allergic reactions. Antihistamines block the effect of histamines and are a major drug category used against allergies. Bioflavonoids have been effective as antihistamines in lowering allergic reactions.[22]

Other nutrients have also proven helpful: Fish oil (EPA) helps to lower the production of leukotrienes, which are inflammatory agents that encourage tissue swelling.[23] Preliminary evidence indicates that fish oil may be quite effective in reducing the allergic response.[24] Vitamin E and selenium have lowered the inflammation process of arthritis in test animals and veterinarian practice.[25] This anti-inflammatory principle may help to provide relief for human allergy sufferers.

FOOD SENSITIVITY

While food allergies are controversial and confusing, food sensitivities provide controversy and confusion to the 10th power. The Food and Drug Administration (FDA) is charged with ensuring the immediate safety of food additives. In the American food supply, there are 2,800 FDA-approved additives and another 10,000 additives that are incidental to the agriculture and food-processing business.[26] Although it is unlikely that anyone will die immediately upon ingestion of approved additives, no one can predict what will happen if the sensitive consumer eats large amounts of these "safe" additives. Nor can anyone predict the possible interactions of food additives. No one eats just one additive. When additives are mixed, they may have deleterious effects that do not occur when consumed one at a time. The net effect is that a number of food additives are becoming a source of health woes for many people. Skin problems (angioderma, hives, eczema,), sinus conditions (rhinitis), asthma, hyperactivity, and migraine all are possible symptoms of intolerance to food additives.[27]

COMBINED EFFECTS OF FOOD ADDITIVES

Food additives are tested individually for safety in laboratory animals. Yet most Americans eat hundreds of different food additives together each day. What are the synergistic reactions from these additives?

A researcher asked the same question. He gave one group of laboratory animals a small amount (2 percent of their diet) of red dye number 2 (once approved, now banned), another group cyclamate (artificial sweetener once used, now banned), and another group a food emulsifier (polyoxyethylene sorbitan monostearate). None of these animals showed any adverse reactions from these additives. Next, the researcher gave both red dye number 2 *and* cyclamate to another group of animals. This group suffered diarrhea, balding and scruffy fur, and retarded weight gain. Another group of animals were given all three additives at once. The members of this group all died within two weeks.[28]

The moral of this story is that no one eats just one additive, that testing additives in various combinations with other additives would be astronomically expensive, and that combinations of certain additives may cause poor health in certain sensitive individuals.

POTENTIALLY HARMFUL ADDITIVES
AND INGREDIENTS IN FOODS

There are some FDA-approved food additives that can still be quite harmful to certain humans.

Metabisulfite

Metabisulfite is an antioxidant used widely in the food industry that could kill any of the 500,000 asthmatics in this country.[29] Metabisulfite and other sulfur agents are used in preparing fresh produce, potatoes, and wine and in restaurant salad bars. Although various consumer groups have attempted to get this additive banned or at least a caution label listed on the foods that contain it, nothing has been done to protect these half million vulnerable asthmatics. Federal legislation is currently pending to make sulfite warnings mandatory on all products that contain this questionable additive.

MSG

Monosodium glutamate (MSG) is a flavor enhancer that was developed as a synthetic and inexpensive alternative to the original Oriental flavor enhancer, glutamic acid, that was made from seaweed. Excessive MSG intake can cause chest pains, labored breathing, and a flushing sensation within 20 minutes after ingestion. MSG may cause tumors in the brains of developing animals. For that reason, MSG should be particularly avoided by pregnant and lactating women and young children. Since Oriental foods use copious quantities of MSG, the "Chinese restaurant" syndrome has surfaced as the name for MSG poisoning. Vitamin B_6 (50 mg daily) almost totally prevents MSG toxicity.[30]

Aspartame (NutraSweet)

Aspartame is an FDA-approved artificial sweetener that is now encountering some problems. Perhaps none of the researchers who studied aspartame's safety had any idea of how much aspartame some people would consume. Some people are drinking up to 2 gallons of aspartame-sweetened beverages daily. Many of these aspartame fans have been experiencing seizures, twitching, and other nerve problems.[31] In most people, small amounts of aspartame are probably safe, but not huge quantities. Once again, pregnant and lactating women and young children should avoid aspartame.

Molds, Antibiotics, and Tartrazine

The mold that is found in fermented foods, like cheese, yeast, bread, wine, and yogurt, may cause food sensitivity problems for some people.

Most dairy cattle are given regular amounts of antibiotics in their food supply to reduce the possibility of infection and hence the rejection of that batch of milk by federal inspectors. Cow's milk contains varying levels of antibiotics, which can create a reaction in some people.

Yellow dye (tartrazine) can invoke a reaction in people who are sensitive to aspirin and other salicylates.

Candida

Candida albicans is a yeast mold that is found in the bodies of most humans and also lives on many carbohydrate foods. *Candida* is the organism that produces vaginal tract infections in women. In normal healthy people, *Candida* causes no problems. But in others—those with poor nutrient intake, those who are taking long-term antibiotics, those who are under stress, and those who have other health problems—*Candida* can create symptoms ranging from arthritis to migraine headaches. *Candida* infections may be more of a symptom of an underlying problem than the problem itself. The *Candida* organism is considered to be an opportunistic organism, meaning that it is able to prey only on people with a lowered immune response.[32] It is quite possible that pollution exposure blunts the normally healthy immune system in some people and opens the door for a *Candida* infection. People with *Candida* infections should have a complete physical and mental review by a qualified health care practitioner. Something, beyond the *Candida* infection, is wrong with people who have this problem.

The superficial treatment for *Candida* infections includes Nystatin (an antiyeast medication), a diet low in carbohydrates, and a staunch abstinence from sugar. Sugar is a favorite food for yeast. The more in-depth approach would be a comprehensive physical examination.

THE FEINGOLD DIET

Dr. Ben Feingold was a nationally respected allergist with 30 years of clinical and teaching experience and departmental director in a large San Francisco hospital. For a woman with hives (urticaria), he provided a basic diet that avoided likely food allergens. Two weeks later, he was called by the woman's psychiatrist, who was anxious to hear what Dr. Feingold had done. This woman had undergone years of intense psychotherapy and drugs for her emotional problems—all to no avail. Then, suddenly, within two weeks after beginning Feingold's diet, this woman's emotional problems dissipated. Her skin and mental problems cleared up simultaneously.

After further testing of this strange phenomenon, Feingold became convinced that many people suffer from emotional disorders as reactions to certain food substances. The Feingold Diet was born, amid a maelstrom of criticism. After more than a decade of strident attack, research now proves that Feingold's basic concept improved behavior in 62 of 76 hyperactive children, with 21 being completely cured.[33] Even the National Institute of Health has admitted that dietary modification improves the behavior of some hyperactive children.[34]

Feingold's first success was to cure a woman who had both hives and emotional disorders. In a recent study, 75 percent of the 86 children tested in double-blind fashion had marked relief from their hives when many food additives were omitted from their diet.[35] More recently, scientists have discovered that Feingold's Diet had mixed results when tested by other researchers because it was not a salicylate-free diet, as he thought he was recommending.[36] His principle was right, but his food restriction list wasn't.

The new revised Feingold Diet (a.k.a. the oligoantigenic diet) involves omission of high-sugar snack foods, most processed and refined foods, and food additives. Additionally, foods with salicylates, amines, or MSG must also be avoided.

The following foods contain one or more of those suspect food ingredients: chocolate, grapes, oranges, cheese, peanuts, corn, fish, melons, tomatoes, ham, bacon, pineapple, apples, pork, pears, tea, coffee, caffeine, nuts, cucumber, bananas, carrots, yeast, apricots, and onions.

The basic oligoantigenic diet is high in vitamins, minerals, fiber, and complex carbohydrates. It adheres to the Senate Dietary Goals. It is also relatively easy to comply with. The more intense Feingold Diet (which restricts salicylates, amines, and MSG as mentioned above) requires more diligence by its participants. Yet, for millions of children, the effort would be most worthwhile.

Why does Feingold's Diet work? Is it because of what the child is getting (vitamins, minerals, protein, fiber) from the new high-nutrient diet or because of what the child is no longer getting in the form of questionable additives and excessive sugar? No one really knows. For whatever reason, about one-third of all hyperactive children improve when placed on this nutrient-dense, additive-free diet.

Most hyperactive children are given potent prescription drugs that have side effects such as headaches, drowsiness, and stunted growth. No hyperactive child has a deficiency of amphetamines, any more than a person with a headache has an aspirin deficiency. The drugs merely treat the symptoms, not the cause. Dietary modification costs nothing, has no side effects, and at the very worst will improve the child's health. At best, this diet will cure the hyperactive child. With 10–20 percent of all American children now classified as hyperactive,[37] the nutritional approach deserves more use in the health community.

TREATMENT OF FOOD SENSITIVITIES

The take-home lesson here is that some people react to some food additives. Rather than spend a great deal of time sorting through the questionable versus the safe additives, it is best just to avoid additives whenever possible. A general rule would then be: Don't eat processed foods. If the food item has a label, it probably contains some food additives. Shop the perimeter of the grocery store, where fresh produce, fresh meats, dairy, and breads are found. Venturing into the deep, dark interior of the store increases the intake of food additives, reduces the nutrient intake, and adds measurably to the food budget.

You could spend many thousands of dollars in a hospital unit attempting to isolate the food items that may be causing your health dilemmas. Or you could try the diagnostic procedure outlined in this chapter. Identifying food allergies requires a certain persistence and Sherlock Holmes mentality, but it can be well worth it for people who have suffered too much for too long.

Once you find out what dietary components are offensive to you, either avoid them completely (elimination diet) or allow them in small regulated quantities (rotation diet). Food allergies and sensitivities are probably at the root of many vague and untreated conditions in America.

9
AGING

"You just can't win. I know a guy who took out a million dollar's worth of life insurance policies, and he died anyway."
Robert Orben

Death is nonnegotiable. However, *when* you die and in *what condition* seems to depend very much on how you live. Nine out of 10 Americans die from conditions that are caused by lifestyle and hence under the control of the individual.

A few decades ago, there was a flurry of important medical discoveries, including inoculations to prevent plagues like polio. The public was so relieved and impressed that we all sat back and expected medical science to discover cures for all disease—even death. It hasn't happened yet, and it probably won't happen in our lifetime. Scientists are now telling us that the best hope for having a long and resplendent life is to take charge of your lifestyle, including nutrition, exercise, attitude, and pollution avoidance. Hence, *you*, not some distant researcher, hold the keys to a longer life.

What is aging? What is the condition of the average older adult in America? What physical and mental changes occur in aging? What does lifestyle have to do with aging? How well nourished is the older adult in America? Does the older adult have unique nutrient needs? Can nutrition influence mental vigor, disease resistance, and wound healing and possibly extend life? All of these

186

questions will be answered in this chapter. Optimal nutrition throughout life can help make the "golden years" longer-lasting and more brilliant.

WHAT IS AGING?

His bald head, wrinkled skin, and deteriorated health were the classical picture of an old man dying from old age. Yet, this "old man" was actually a six-year-old boy who was dying of progeria, a rare disease in which the aging process is accelerated 10-fold. This disease provides limitless tantalizing hope for scientists to be able to "crack" the code of aging. If the rate of aging can be sped up markedly, as in progeria, can it also be slowed down? In the 20th century, it is unlikely. In the 21st century, perhaps.

In 1979, Dr. Leonard Hayflick, a researcher who made some of the more important discoveries in the field of aging, found that nearly all human cells are able to divide and rejuvenate themselves only 50–55 times.[1] Whenever wear and tear, abuse, or just plain time takes it toll on the tissues, the cells divide and bring new vigor to the body. This rejuvenating cell division would be kind of like fixing your house when a part of it wears out. This theory is sometimes spoken of as "organ reserve," meaning that each of us has a certain ability to bounce back from abuses that are heaped upon our bodies. Once that "savings account" reserve of 50–55 cellular divisions has been used up, however, that person begins to age quickly.

Alcoholics, drug addicts, and people who are exposed to great physical or emotional stress use up their "organ reserve" much more quickly than the rest of us. These people probably age sooner and die younger. Old age basically sets in when you have exhausted your "organ reserve" of cellular divisions. Challenges (like exhaustion, stress, and sickness) that young people recover from easily can derail the health of an older person for a much longer period of time.

A basic tenet of slowing the aging process is to use these precious 50–55 cellular divisions sparingly. Some people have a genetic tenacity that is enviable. For whatever reason, they age more slowly and are more vigorous when they are older. Regardless of your genetic background, optimal nutrition can probably help you to improve on whatever normal life span your ancestors have experienced.

The lesson here is that your cellular genes may be likened to denim jeans. When first new, these jeans seemed indestructible, and some people treat their jeans (and genes?) accordingly. Yet they do wear out, and toward the final wearings of the jeans many people are remorseful that they had not taken better care of them. Are you prematurely aging your jeans (genes) through a destructive lifestyle?

There are several theories about what causes cells to wear out and force us to use up our 50–55 cell divisions:

- The *Clinker Theory* attributes the physical decay of aging to the accumulation of debris. This "sludge" of oxidized lipids and partially completed proteins compose the pigments known as "age spots."[2]
- The *Lipid Peroxidation Theory* proposes that cell membrane oxidation leads to the destruction of this outer coating of body cells and begins the accumulation of waste matter within.
- The *Autoimmune Theory* claims that normally protective antibodies change allegiance and begin attacking the body from whence they came.
- The *Somatic Mutation Theory* states that growing and dividing cells are eventually inactivated with age.
- The *Wear and Tear Theory* relates aging to the mechanical and chemical exhaustion of the body.
- The *Free Radical Theory* is one of the more popular explanations for aging. Free radicals are substances (like hydrogen peroxide) that have an unpaired electron that can hungrily attack and destroy most living tissue. These free radicals have been called the "great white sharks" in the biochemical sea of life. Free radicals attack protein and fatty tissue, thus setting up a domino reaction of destruction. The slowing of these free radicals could likely extend the quality and quantity of life.

THE AVERAGE OLDER ADULT IN AMERICA

Many young people have a distorted vision of aging. They consider the older adult to be synonymous with a withered, feeble-minded, limping figure with diminished sensory equipment and bladder control. Actually, this semifunctional person is in the minority among older adults in America. Two out of three people in America over age 65 are in decent health. Only 5 percent live in nursing homes.[3] Retired from work and free of the responsibility of child rearing, some older adults are having the time of their lives.

With improved health care, America has experienced a "graying." In 1900, only 4 percent of our population were over age 65. Today, that percentage has tripled to 12 percent. The average life span for men and women in America is now 71 and 78 years respectively.[4] Yet all is not well for today's elderly.

Once past the gauntlet of youth and middle age, the average life span for an older adult male has not increased in this century. It is wonderful to see vigorous people today living well into their 80s, yet 200 years ago Thomas Jefferson and Benjamin Franklin were also old and productive people in their 80s, and 400 years ago, so was Michelangelo. As far back as 2,400 years ago, Hippocrates was considered an old but productive person who lived well into his 80s. In other words, though the *average* life span has increased dramatically through improved hygiene and neonatal care, people who are 80 years of age are now and have always been considered old for humans.

Ninety-eight percent of all older adults in America are using some type of prescription medication, with the average person taking six different types of drugs.[5] Yet there are no disease conditions today (including heart disease, diabetes, and cancer) for which current medical treatment has a better chance of success than the best medical care of 1951.[6] The incidences of heart disease, hypertension, cancer, diabetes, osteoporosis, arthritis, mental ailments, hemorrhoids, diverticulosis, and other common ailments have risen continuously and unabated since the early part of this century. Our high-tech "Star Wars" era of medical science has been mostly impotent against the rising tide of "diseases of civilization." All of these degenerative diseases are most prevalent in the elderly. None of these statistics boast of good health for the older American, nor of modern medicine's ability to improve the quality of life.

The talented people and impressive accoutrements of 20th-century medicine have taken an impractical route toward improving the health of Americans. All the effort and expense that has gone into emphasizing emergency care for people who are ill rather than providing preventive and supportive care for people who are still in decent health. This approach has had an insignificant or even negative impact on the quality of life for the older adult. I say "negative" impact, because the availability of high-tech wizardry has made nutrition seem like a primitive and unexciting tool to the physician. Too bad. Again, nutrition, along with other preventive measures, could take care of health problems—at the source and before they blossom into serious illness.

THE PHYSICAL AND MENTAL CHANGES OF AGING

Most bodily functions diminish somewhat with age. Yet there is no need for the drastic deterioration of mind and body that often occurs in America's elderly. Many people think of older adults as being less mentally agile. Yet the Baltimore Study found that healthy elderly people have memories that are as accurate as those of younger people.[7] Blood flow in the brain of *healthy* older adults was comparable to people 50 years younger. Although there is an undeniable 10 percent loss in brain volume in older adults, this shrinkage is probably due to a compacting that occurs as the spaces between brain cells lessens.

In addition, even though an octogenarian may not have the same stamina and enthusiasm for sex as a 20-year-old newlywed, sexual activity need not cease as people age. People who were sexually active when younger usually continue their sexual vigor into old age. "Use it or lose it" takes on renewed meaning for mental, sexual, and physical abilities in older adults.

Yet there *are* some common losses that occur with age:

- The pumping efficiency of the heart decreases by about 30 percent.
- The ability of oxygen to pass through the lungs and permeate the body tissue decreases by 50–70 percent.
- The velocity of nerve transmissions diminishes by 15 percent, which means that reflexes are slowed.
- Basal metabolism declines by about 20 percent, which seriously reduces the calorie needs of the older adult.
- The filtering capacity of the kidneys is about half that of younger adults.

- Minerals begin leaving the bones, with an average loss in height of two inches for men and eight inches for women by the time they are in their 70s.[8]
- Digestion and absorption are less efficient.
- Glucose tolerance is lowered, which reduces mental and physical energy levels.
- Serum lipids (fats in the blood) are elevated.
- Eighty percent of the elderly have no teeth.[9]

Remember, these figures are averages, as in "normal." Although "normal" is often thought of as being "unavoidable, typical, to be expected," "normal" health statistics in America actually can be more a consequence of the semisuicidal lifestyle that is so "normal." You can probably improve on these figures, if you are willing to take responsibility for your nutrient intake and other lifestyle factors.

There are many examples of people who live vigorously into their 90s with full use of their faculties. A number of well-respected researchers estimate that we should be able to live vigorously for 100–140 years, if we take care of ourselves.[10] It is our own self-imposed limitation of a risky lifestyle that reduces the quality and quantity of life for so many people.

The typical American experiences a gradual deterioration of body and mind that begins around age 50. Healing nutrients can show you how to slow down the aging process. The younger you are and the closer you adhere to these guidelines, the better are your chances of vastly improving on the statistics of "normal" health and life span for the older American.

WHAT DOES LIFESTYLE HAVE TO DO WITH AGING?

Plenty. Nothing can stop the aging process. But optimal nutrition can slow it down.[11] Through proper foods and supplements, you can dramatically improve your chances of having an exuberant and lengthy life. Nutrition is related directly to heart disease, hypertension, cancer, and diabetes, which are the leading causes of death in America. (See the chapters on each of these conditions for more information.) Nutrition is related to mental vigor, immune functions, and other processes that seem to deteriorate as people age.

Exercise also relates intimately to life span. As mentioned earlier, scientists have found that many health problems of aging may result from disuse of the body (i.e., sedentary lifestyle).[12] Also, the skin problems that are so common in the elderly are nearly identical to the skin problems found in malnourished people.[13] Although aging is unavoidable, it appears that "normal" lifestyle in America probably accelerates the aging process.

HOW WELL NOURISHED IS THE OLDER ADULT IN AMERICA?

Malnutrition is rampant among older adults in this country.[14] Older adults, as a group, are even more malnourished than the average younger adult. One study found that affluent and well-educated elderly people were deficient in vitamins B_{12}, E, B_6, and folacin and the minerals calcium and zinc.[15] Another study found that Americans age 80 and older were deficient in an average of 10 different nutrients.[16] In a third study, half of the older adults were consuming deficient amounts of vitamins A and C and the minerals calcium and iron.[17]

I mentioned earlier that older males living alone are even worse off nutritionally,[18] with many being at great risk for contracting scurvy![19] Half of the institutionalized elderly in Florida were found to have clear signs of scurvy![20] Although requirements for vitamin C probably increase with age, about two-thirds of elderly women don't even get the RDA levels of intake for vitamin C.[21] Among the elderly, rampant deficiencies have been found:

- The elderly consume roughly one-third of their RDA for pantothenic acid.[22]
- They consume about half of the RDA for zinc.[23]
- Postmenopausal women consume about 60 percent of their RDA for magnesium.[24]
- Of 135 elderly women admitted to a hospital in Scotland, two out of three had a deficiency in one or more of the four vitamins studied (ascorbic acid, thiamine, riboflavin, pyridoxine).[25]

In order to be considered deficient in these studies, the person had to be consuming less than 70 percent of the RDA. Any who were consuming between 70 and 99 percent of the RDA for a nutrient were not categorized as deficient.

Scientists have found that body levels of vitamin C progressively decline with age, indicating either an increased need or a reduced efficiency for absorbing and using vitamin C as people get older. Due to a reduction in the efficiency of nutrient use, the elderly probably need greater-than-RDA levels for certain nutrients. Also, 98 percent of the elderly use some type of medication, and many drugs increase the need for various nutrients, which worsens an already bad nutrition situation.

Older adults are also beginning to feel the cumulative effects of decades of seemingly insignificant unhealthy lifestyle practices. By age 65, the average American has consumed 100,000 pounds of food, plus or minus a few tons.[26] A marginal diet consumed over the course of many decades gradually brings about subclinical malnutrition that fades ever so subtly into raging overt malnutrition. Some people do not even notice the effects of their poor food selection until later in life. We know this to be true in many of the common degenerative diseases in America: heart disease, cancer, hypertension, obesity, osteoporosis, diabetes, liver and kidney problems. It takes a while to arrive at such poor health. For many people, this transition from decent to bad health is so gradual that they do not connect their poor dietary habits to the erosion of their health.

Many factors may lead to reduced food intake or poor food choices. Older adults often live alone, cook for themselves, have lower incomes, have lower appetites, suffer the emotional loss of friends, are without cars, lack teeth or properly fitting dentures, and have poor sensory perception of food. That is, their ability to taste foods is reduced. As we age, we lose up to 80 percent of our taste buds. Zinc is important to taste bud maintenance. Since most older adults are low in their zinc intake and since poor taste acuity is a classical symptom of the zinc deficiency many older adults suffer, it should not be surprising that supplements of zinc were able to improve taste awareness in a group of older adults.[27]

Much of what the elderly eat is highly refined convenience foods. White bread and crackers are the most commonly eaten foods by older adults in America.[28] Altogether, a large percentage of older adults in this country are seriously malnourished, and that malnutrition almost certainly contributes to the many health maladies facing these people.

DO OLDER ADULTS HAVE
UNIQUE NUTRIENT NEEDS?

Yes. They probably need greater-than-RDA levels of certain vitamins, minerals, and protein. Older adults are not identical to 20-year-olds, in looks, performance, biochemistry, or nutrient needs. The RDAs that are used today were published in 1980 and compiled years before then. A great deal of newer data says that older adults should have their own set of RDAs.[29]

As we age, various changes take place in our metabolism. Digestion and absorption are less efficient. The efficiency of the body to scavenge nutrients and keep them in circulation diminishes.[30] Various diseases that are rare in younger people are quite common in the elderly, thus emphasizing the need for certain protective nutrients against these diseases. For a variety of reasons, older adults need greater-than-RDA levels of nutrients.

In spite of the fact that older people need more than the RDA of vitamin B_6,[31] 92 percent of older women and 90 percent of older men don't even get two-thirds of the RDA for vitamin B_6.[32] In order for the large and complex molecule of vitamin B_{12} to be absorbed in the intestines, a series of steps must take place. B_{12} absorption is hindered in many elderly people.[33] Folacin requires digestion and activation for its proper use. Some people, especially those with a B_{12} deficiency, do not activate folacin well.[34]

Pernicious anemia, the B_{12} deficiency condition, used to be quite common among the elderly. No doubt it has not disappeared today but has just been misdiagnosed as various other conditions, including fatigue and mental problems. In a group of patients with pernicious anemia, injections of B_{12} provided a noticeable improvement in red blood cell count in only 24 hours![35] It usually takes weeks or months to bolster red blood cell count. Researchers have found that by depriving a microorganism (Euglena) of its vitamin B_{12}, they can duplicate the effects of aging in human cells.[36] Many ailments of the body and mind that are commonly thought to be synonymous with aging could be due to a B_{12} deficiency.

Among the nutrients involved in maintaining healthy energy metabolism are thiamine, niacin, riboflavin, biotin, pantothenic acid, and chromium. As lab animals age, their efficiency in absorbing thiamine is reduced.[37] Although *most* Americans are low in chromium (which reduces glucose tolerance), the average older adult has a glucose tolerance that would put him or her in the category of "diabetic" if compared to healthy younger people. One study took 76 *healthy* older Americans and gave them 200 mcg daily of chromium. *All* 76 people showed improved glucose tolerance.[38] Some of the symptoms of aging are due to long-term subclinical malnutrition.

Biotin status largely depends on bacteria producing this vitamin in the encouraging environment of a healthy gut. Drugs (especially antibiotics and alcohol) can reduce the already limited capacity of a poorly functioning gastrointestinal tract to make biotin. Riboflavin deficiency is common among older adults throughout the world. Essentially, a variety of nutritional reasons are responsible for low energy levels in older adults.

Osteoporosis (hollowing of the bones) and osteomalacia (softening of the bones) are common ailments found in the elderly. Both can be caused by a low intake of vitamin D, which is common among older adults.[39] Older adults who were eating the same food and exposed to the same amount of sunlight as younger adults had lower vitamin D levels.[40] After being consumed in the diet or manufactured in the skin, vitamin D must then be activated by the kidneys and liver before it is ready for use by the body. Older adults have a diminished ability to activate vitamin D.

Both disease resistance and serum vitamin C levels decrease with age. Low levels of vitamin C could be partly responsible for this drop in immunity. The muscular contractions of the intestines slow down as we age. For many older adults, this slowed motility results in constipation. Of 43 elderly patients studied, 79 percent were receiving some type of medication for constipation. For 10 weeks, their diet was changed to high-fiber foods. In all people tested, high fiber helped or "cured" elimination problems.[41] Perhaps aging increases the need for fiber beyond that of younger people.

The National Academy of Science established the protein RDA with a margin of safety to protect almost everyone. That is, everyone except the elderly, say researchers at the Massachusetts Institute of Technology. They examined 15 healthy elderly people and found that the RDA of protein was not adequate for these people.[42]

Basal metabolism (the rate at which your body burns its fuel) slows dramatically as we age. Older adults need less than the RDA for calories in order to avoid overfatness.[43] This creates a truly complicated issue. Older adults need fewer calories (i.e., overall food intake) yet more nutrients than younger adults. This makes the *quality* of foods that are consumed ever so critical for older adults. It makes a rational supplement program almost mandatory for the health of the older adult.[44] Unfortunately, only 3 percent of physicians in America consider a multiple vitamin and mineral supplement to be important.[45]

Few health care professionals investigate why the body of the older adult is not working right. They usually offer temporary "bandages" of medication to sedate the symptoms rather than trying to make the body work right by giving it the nutrients that it is lacking. Hence, much money and effort is wasted.

MENTAL VIGOR

The cumulative effects of many violations of nutritional rules come home to roost in the senior years and often become most apparent in the loss of mental acuity. In many cases, the first symptom of malnutrition in the older adult is mental problems.[46] About 15 percent of people over age 65 suffer from Alzheimer's disease, some due to poor nutrition.

Nutritionists once thought that the mind was relatively unaffected by diet. They thought that the brain would take what it needed and avoid substances that it didn't need. Not so. Actually, the brain is even more vulnerable to malnutrition than other bodily organs. The brain takes more oxygen than any other organ on a per-weight basis, which makes nutrients build the red blood cells that deliver the oxygen very important. The brain is very selective about using blood glucose for fuel, while other parts of the body are more flexible in which fuel (carbohydrate, fat, protein, alcohol) they will use. Being at the pinnacle of nature's accomplishments, the brain is also at the pinnacle for specific nutrient needs and problems.

Of 182 elderly women admitted to a mental hospital in England, one-third had unacceptably low levels of either the B vitamins or vitamin C.[47] In each of these patients, the degree of malnutrition was related directly to the severity of mental symptoms.

VITAMIN C

Older dementia patients (usually Alzheimer's disease victims) were found to have very low levels of vitamin C in their blood plasma and white cells. With supplements of only 50 mg of vitamin C daily (83 percent of the RDA), blood levels of vitamin C rose by 500 percent in these patients.[48] The vitamin C did not improve the Alzheimer's condition, but the elevated blood level of vitamin C after supplementation shows that these people were very low in body vitamin C levels. In another study, researchers created situations in which lab animals had high levels of iron and low levels of vitamin C in their brains. This imbalance is similar to what happens in many American men who eat much red meat (high iron) and little fresh produce (low vitamin C). Iron is an oxidizing metal, and vitamin C is an antioxidant that can slow down the destructive effects of iron. The lab animals experienced very high levels of fat "rusting" in their brains, which was slowed down when they were given supplements of vitamin C.[49] Continuously low levels of vitamin C intake may be related to the onset of Alzheimer's disease in some instances.

ALUMINUM VS. FLUORIDE

High levels of aluminum also are found in the brains of Alzheimer's patients. Aluminum cookware can contribute small amounts of aluminum to the diet, which increases as the acid content of the food increases. Cooking pineapple and tomato-based foods in aluminum cookware would be considered a risk factor here. More significant aluminum sources include silicoaluminate (an anticaking ingredient added to all commercial packaged goods, including salt), aluminum-based antacids, and even aluminum-based antiperspirants that are absorbed through the skin.

The more fluoride that is in the diet, the lower the absorption of aluminum, since the two minerals compete for absorption sites in the intestines.[50] Regular decent intake of fluoride hardens teeth to prevent cavities, hardens the bones to prevent osteoporosis, and lowers the risk for Alzheimer's disease. Still, many cities resist putting fluoride in the drinking water.

ANTIOXIDANTS

The brain is composed primarily of fatty tissue. Antioxidants, like vitamins A, E, and C and the mineral selenium, slow down the deterioration of those fats, which may be responsible for a considerable portion of mental problems in the elderly. Sixty percent of Alzheimer's victims have abnormally low levels of vitamin E in their blood.[51] In lab animals, vitamin E and selenium supplements have been able to reduce significantly the rate of fats "rusting" in the brain.[52] A primary source of vitamin E in the American diet should be the wheat germ found in whole wheat bread, yet *the* favorite food of older adults in America is white bread, which has almost zero vitamin E.

Also, vitamin E is a fat-soluble vitamin whose absorption depends greatly on the ability of the intestines to absorb fats in general. Older adults often have lower levels of vitamin E due to fat malabsorption problems. In one case study, a man with severely hindered fat absorption eventually developed nerve and muscle disorders until he could no longer walk. Researchers found very low levels of vitamin E in this man and began giving him intramuscular injections of E. Within six months he was much better.[53]

With American food staples including refined grains and heat-treated hydrogenated fats, marginal vitamin E deficiencies are common. Over the course of decades, these mild deficiencies could become a major problem.

VITAMIN B$_{12}$

Both vitamin B$_{12}$ and folacin also play key roles in maintaining a healthy brain, yet deficiencies are not uncommon. B$_{12}$ deficiency is common in people over 40 years of age who are of northern European descent.[54] Scientists do not know why people of northern European extraction have a more difficult time absorbing B$_{12}$, yet this description applies to about 45 million Americans. Forty-six percent of 200 elderly psychiatric patients had blatantly low levels of either B$_{12}$ or folacin.[55] Another researcher estimates that at least one out of five elderly psychiatric patients suffers from masked B$_{12}$ or folacin deficiency as the primary cause of their ailment.[56] The first symptoms of B_{12} deficiency usually surface in the central nervous system as irritability, impatience, and forgetfulness. Some elderly manic patients have been found to have nothing more than a serious B_{12} deficiency.[57]

THIAMINE

A British study found that many elderly patients developed severe confusion after their surgery. Of the 64 patients studied, most had unacceptably low thiamine levels.[58] Many elderly people lie precariously close to a thiamine deficiency. The stress of surgery dips these low levels well under the acceptable range, and dementia and confusion are often the result.

These are just a few of the areas where nutrition relates to mental functions. Mental problems for the older adult can often stem from poor circulation to the brain or from accumulated pollutants like lead in the brain. Allergies can create symptoms of confusion or mood swings. (See Chapters 4, 8, 10, and 16 for more information on how nutrition can influence mental acumen.) If an older adult develops bizarre behavior and has no history of psychiatric illness, then malnutrition should be a primary suspect.

DISEASE RESISTANCE
AND WOUND RECOVERY

Many health care professionals consider waning immunity to be an inescapable fact of aging. But is the aging more responsible for poor immune function, or is poor nutrition at fault? There is an impressive volume of data indicating that poor disease resistance of the elderly could be closely related to their poor dietary habits.

A group of Canadian researchers examined 51 people over age 60 and found protein-calorie malnutrition in 21 of these people. These blatantly malnourished elderly were given protein, calorie, vitamin, and mineral supplements for eight weeks and then examined again. All subjects showed major improvement in various factors that relate to immune competence.[59] These people will now be able to thwart infectious ailments more effectively. In another study, 100 elderly men were examined, with 30 of these found to be malnourished in at least two different indices. All 30 were given flu vaccinations. Researchers then took half (15) of these men and provided them with dietary supplements, while the other 15 served as controls. After four weeks, the 15 who received supplements and nutritional advice showed major improvements in their antibody levels against the flu virus.[60] Not only does nutrition improve disease resistance, but it heightens the effectiveness of vaccination programs.

The elderly, like most other people, do not eat enough zinc. Of 99 elderly patients examined, two-thirds had low serum zinc, while more than half had low dietary intake of zinc.[61] Although 58 of these people were taking nutritional supplements, only 1 of them was getting any zinc in their pills. Another experiment found that high doses of zinc enhanced the immune function of even healthy older adults.[62]

Many older adults are easily bruised, and their bruises heal very slowly. Low zinc levels may be partly responsible for the "purple spot" bruising (purpura) that seems indigenous among older adults. Forty geriatric patients, ages 65 to 99, were examined. Half of them had major cases of purpura, and those with the lowest plasma zinc levels had the worst cases of bruising.[63] In another study on bruising, 94 institutionalized elderly were given 1 g (1,000 mg) of vitamin C supplements daily in blind fashion. The vitamin C raised plasma and leukocyte levels of C, reduced bruising (purpura), and stimulated a small weight gain.[64] The same amount of vitamin C was also able to improve overall clinical health and weight gain in older hospital patients.[65] In a blind study, researchers found that injections of 500 mg of vitamin C daily provided major improvements in the immune abilities of healthy older adults.[66]

Pantothenic acid is involved in disease resistance, wound healing, and arthritis. In separate studies, supplements of pantothenic acid accelerated wound healing in animals and reduced the pain and stiffness of rheumatoid arthritis in humans.[67] In a typical nursing home that was assessed for pantothenic acid in the patients' diet, the average amount offered on the meal plates was about one-third of recommended levels.[68] Researchers also pointed out that, due to plate waste, the elderly may have been consuming even less.

Cataracts are common in the elderly. A riboflavin deficiency, common in the elderly, can lead to cataracts. Most older cataract patients have lower-than-normal levels of riboflavin.[69] Riboflavin supplements have been used after eye surgery to improve oxygen flow to the cornea and prevent blood vessels from growing in the area.[70]

Some of the eye problems experienced by older adults may come from cumulative exposure to the sun's ultraviolet radiation. When researchers saturated eye lenses with vitamin E and then exposed the lenses to sunlight, the lenses experienced only one-fifth the damage compared to the unprotected lenses.[71] Given the dissolving ozone layer that used to protect us from excessive ultraviolet radiation, there will probably be a sharp increase in the incidence of cataracts in the coming decades. Vitamin E might help prevent these.

Malnutrition in the elderly can be caused by drug-nutrient interactions, poor taste buds, and poor budgets or by reduced efficiency of digestion, absorption, and metabolism. So it seems that both aging and malnutrition are responsible for the progressive deterioration that occurs in America's elderly. Since the aging is "incurable," why not work on the quite curable malnutrition? The end result can be older adults whose joys often outweigh their problems.

POSSIBLE NUTRITIONAL LIFE EXTENDERS

One of the better documented ways to live longer is through "undernutrition without malnutrition." Essentially, this means living in a constant state of semistarvation and eating only high-quality foods. This concept seems to work for both laboratory animals[72] and humans.[73] But considering the penchant that the average American has for food, perhaps it is unrealistic to expect anyone to take this suggestion. It means never eating until full, especially during developmental years. It means meals should be only of nutrient-dense foods, such as fresh produce, grains, beans, nonfat dairy, and organ meats. Any takers?

ANTIOXIDANTS . . . PLUS

On a more realistic note, researchers at the National Institute of Aging have reviewed the many proposed theories on nutritional supplements to stem the tide of aging.[74] They found that the nutritional antioxidants vitamins A, C, and E and the mineral selenium "deserved further investigation." Going beyond this speculation, researchers in Europe divided 100 healthy older women into three groups, giving them supplements of vitamin E, vitamin C, or both. After one year, the group receiving both vitamins E and C had decreased lipid peroxidation (internal "rusting" of fats) levels throughout the body by 25 percent.[75]

You might recall that one of the biggest drops in efficiency during aging is the ability of the body to bring oxygen to the cells through the lungs. Tissue destruction in the lungs via oxidation is the problem, and antioxidants may be the solution. There is suggestive evidence that vitamin E, basically an antioxidant, might retard the aging process.[76] And vitamin E, vitamin C, and selenium used together have shown an ability to slow the oxidation of the lungs.[77] Another author has proposed the supplemental use of vitamin E along with selenium and coenzyme Q to retard aging and make old age more vital.[78]

Vitamin E and BHT are potent antioxidants that are used almost interchangeably as preservatives in fatty foods. Supplements of both E and BHT used together slowed the accumulation of age pigments in lab animals.[79] However, BHT is both poorly tested and difficult to find. BHT should not be considered a longevity agent.

SULFUR

A sulfur-bearing amino acid named cysteine shows great potential as a life extender.[80] Researchers have also found that animals have a shorter life span when raised on a low-sulfur diet. Though sulfur is considered an essential nutrient, very little is known about deficiency states.

APRICOTS

The Hunzas of Pakistan eat copious quantities of apricots and have been credited with longer-than-normal life spans.[81] Dr. Whipple, a Nobel laureate, stated in 1934 that the rejuvenative powers of apricots are comparable to the value of liver. Though apricots are a decent source of fiber and vitamins A and C, no one really knows what the alleged life extension agent may be in apricots.

BIOFLAVONOIDS

Bioflavonoids are a group of vitamin-like substances which assist in plant photosynthesis. An elite medical journal in 1955 sang the praises of bioflavonoids, "Taking everything together, there can be little doubt that flavonoids are not only useful therapeutic agents in conditions of capillary fragility, but have many diverse actions in the body."[82] For some elusive reasons, bioflavonoids suddenly fell into great disfavor with the medical community and were "blacklisted" by the Food and Drug Administration in 1968. Yet the honored *Dorland's Medical Dictionary* (25th ed., p. 1371) still describes one variety of bioflavonoid (rutin) as "used to reduce capillary fragility." Bioflavonoids have been shown to be effective at improving blood flow, improving blood lipid profiles, antibacterial and anti-viral capacity, detoxifier of pollutants, and overall stimulant.[83] Bioflavonoids are lost in food refining, such as rendering oranges into orange drink. Best sources of bioflavonoids include the outer pulp of citrus fruits, buckwheat, other plant foods, and even honey (since it is gathered from plants). Bioflavonoids even enhance the value of vitamin C by increasing absorption efficiency.[84]

ALCOHOL

Alcohol has been the demise of millions of humans. Yet low, regular intake of alcohol seems to improve the overall physical and mental well-being of older adults in rest homes.[85] Not only does alcohol do us the favor of raising "good cholesterol" (as was discussed in Chapter 5), but wines contribute a substance called *GABA*, which helps to promote sleep. The problem is that many older people drink excessively out of boredom or loneliness. The net result, especially for males living alone, is less food consumed, yet more nutrients are needed due to the drug-nutrient interactions of alcohol.[86] Judicious use of wine with evening meals seems to help the heart, appetite, moods, and sleep. Most long-lived people and cultures around the world have boasted of low but regular intake of their own "home brew" alcohol. These people fermented their own beer and wine, and thus the supply was limited. Nothing stronger than wine can be made without elaborate distillation equipment. Hard liquor should be avoided.

GINSENG

Ginseng is another possible life extender that has been either ignored or scorned in this country. It has been used since before the pyramids were built. It is still chewed by Russian cosmonauts in space to prevent infections. Henry Kissinger and Chairman Mao used it. It is standard issue in the backpacks of Chinese and Vietnamese soldiers. Five thousand years of use among millions of adherents can't be all due to the "placebo" effect. The problem with ginseng arose when researchers were unable to find standardized concentrations of ginseng in the plant roots. Methods of extraction and concentration varied. Results were mixed. Ginseng became unofficially "blacklisted" and lampooned by many U.S. scientists. Yet, in Europe and Asia, scientists found ways to standardize plant yields and the method of extraction. From that point, their experiments became much more fruitful and reproducible.

Ginseng (200 mg of standardized Ginsana daily) has been shown to stimulate the central nervous system and the immune system, increase stamina and vigor, improve blood flow and mental abilities in older adults, improve coordination and reflexes, and enhance sex hormone production.[87] Do not overdo a good thing: use less than 500 mg daily. Again, people taking up to 3,000 mg of ginseng daily have experienced everything from mustaches on women to nervousness, insomnia, and diarrhea. As a tea, ginseng is probably nothing more than a social beverage. In concentrated tablet form, Ginsana can enhance vitality and perhaps even longevity for some people.

TAURINE

Taurine is a renegade amino acid. Among its other uses, taurine has been found effective in protecting membranes from destruction[88] (such as occurs in aging) and in lowering blood pressure while improving heart muscle tone for patients with congestive heart failure.[89] We can make some taurine ourselves, but it is probably a dietary essential for both young and sick humans because in these unique stages of life we cannot make enough taurine.[90] Our ability to make taurine is also probably reduced as we age.

NUTRITIONAL RECOMMENDATIONS

1. Core diet with the following changes.
   A. Older adults are at greater risk for fatty deposition along the vessel walls, therefore reduce fat and cholesterol intake even further.
   B. Older adults often have a diminished glucose tolerance, therefore reduce sugar intake even further.
   C. Older adults have lowered intestinal motility, therefore increase fiber and fluid intake for healthy bowel functions.
   D. Older adults have a lowered efficiency in protein use, therefore add about 20 grams per day of protein.

DAILY SUPPLEMENTS TO ADD TO YOUR CORE PROGRAM

Vitamins
Vitamin D   +200 IU
Vitamin E   +200 IU
Thiamine   +15 mg
Riboflavin   +15 mg
Niacinamide   +60 mg
Vitamin B_6 +50 mg
Vitamin B_{12} +100 mcg
Folacin   +400 mcg
Biotin   +300 mcg
Vitamin C   +1,500 mg
Pantothenic acid   +50 mg

Minerals
Calcium   +600 mg
Potassium   +1,000 mg
Magnesium   +300 mg
Zinc   +30 mg
Iron   +10 mg
Copper   +3 mg
Manganese   +5 mg
Chromium   +200 mcg
Molybdenum   +150 mcg
Selenium   +200 mcg

Quasi vitamins
Choline   +1,000 mg
L-carnitine   +500 mg
EPA   +1,000 mg
Coenzyme Q   +60 mg
Taurine   +2,000 mg
L-cysteine   +6,000 mg
Bioflavonoids   +500 mg
Ginseng   +200 mg

10
THE NERVOUS SYSTEM
Emotions, Behavior, Intellect, Pain, Sleep, Tremors

"Everyone seems crazy but you and me. And I'm beginning to wonder about you."

Anonymous

NUTRITION AND BEHAVIOR

Nutrition has a potent influence on the mind. There is not only plenty of scientific evidence to support that, there is also a swelling stack of newspaper clippings:

A man in San Francisco shot the mayor and mayoral assistant but received a sentence of only five years in prison. He pleaded temporary insanity due to hypoglycemia from eating too much sugar-laden food. The "Twinkies defense" was born.

A Missouri man sucked on throat lozenges throughout the drive from his home to the Colorado Rockies for a hunting expedition with his buddies. Once there, this man was convinced that he was divinely inspired to kill and proceeded to gun down several of his hunting companions. His plea was also temporary insanity due to the chemicals in the lozenges.

Court-appointed psychologists for the accused in a series of gruesome murders in Oceanside, California, determined that, due to malnutrition during his early years, this man's brain could not associate his acts with society's expectations. He was deemed permanently and irremediably unfit for society due to a poor diet during his childhood.

An elderly gentleman with no history of psychiatric ailments

shot his wife and grandson. His prescribed medication had seriously altered his calcium levels in the blood, which changed a
pleasant grandfather with no history of emotional problems into a
deadly psychopath.[1]

Dr. Joyce Brothers, a popular TV and radio psychologist, has
found that much marital and family discord is due to poor diet and
hence is untreatable by psychological therapy. If nutrition is the
cause, then nutrition is the cure.

An inmate of the Central Prison in Portugal believed that his
new dietary routine had made a significant improvement in his
mental outlook on life. He was able to convince the prison officials
to provide him with food and cooking facilities for an experiment.
Twenty-two of his fellow inmates followed the program, and each
speaks of the change that proper diet has made in his behavior.[2] By
following a diet similar to the Core Diet, these people noticed
fewer flare-ups and more predictable mental and emotional performance.

What we eat can have a significant impact on our behavior, both
now and in later life.

THE PROBLEM

Mental health is deteriorating in America. This increasing trend
toward mental ailments has been called the "Great Craziness." The
President's Commission on Mental Health estimates that one out
of four people passing you on the street is suffering from some type
of emotional disorder.[3] More recent estimates put that number as
high as one-third of Americans, meaning that up to 77 million
people in this country have some form of mental illness.

Our children are affected. Hyperactivity, a condition that was
almost unknown until the last two decades, affects 10–20 percent
of today's schoolchildren.[4] Since 1950, the teenage suicide rate has
increased by 500 percent.

Mental illness often leads to substance abuse. Alcoholism costs
this country at least $8 billion each year. There are over 17 million
substance abusers in America. Another 50 million adults are ad-
dicted to tobacco products, one of the most dangerous and carcinogenic substances known.

The "Great Craziness" has increased the crime rate in this
country. More than 12 million children are arrested each year for

nontraffic crimes.[5] On any given day, over 1 million adults are on probation or parole from prison, while another 600,000 convicted felons are locked up in our antiquated prison system. For what it costs to keep someone in jail for a year, the taxpayer could send that person to Harvard University, all expenses paid, with a convertible car thrown in. Our penal system costs over $50 billion annually, with many new prisons under construction. And our prison system is not working. It neither reforms criminals nor deters crime.

Not everyone with mental illness commits a crime or abuses drugs. Nineteen million Americans suffer from severe anxiety, 14 million are plagued by severe depression, and 7 million are either schizophrenics or have the borderline version of this debilitating mental illness (called *schizoids*). These people often just suffer silently and let their human potential go to waste.

It has been said that "statistics are people with the tears washed off." Overall, the "Great Craziness" in America costs us over $250 billion annually in direct expenses.[6] And what about the indirect expenses—the fits of violence that shouldn't happen, the vague sense of uneasiness and fear that inhibits people for much of their lives, the wasted talent, the wife, child, and parent abuse that is reaching epidemic proportions in America?

No one can estimate the number of "normal" people who spend most of their years in lethargy, fatigue, and depression, which are the most common complaints heard by today's physicians. The patient says, "I don't feel well. I'm always tired, sometimes grouchy, and occasionally depressed. Can't you do something, doctor?" And the physician tries. Unfortunately, Valium, one of the most widely prescribed drugs in America, is often the doctor's "solution." But no adult ever suffered depression due to a deficiency of Valium, nor has any hyperactive child ever had a deficiency of Ritalin. And again, such drugs only temporarily mask the symptoms, rather than solve the problem.

Something very widespread is wrong with the minds of many Americans. The stress of modern life cannot explain all of this dilemma. Unquestionably, nutrition relates to the drastic increases in mental illness. The mind is no more immune to malnutrition than the body. In fact, the mind is even more sensitive to malnutrition than other organs of the body (see Chapter 9 for details on this).

In many cases, nutrition can prevent, treat, or at least improve unpredictable swings in emotions, insomnia, depression, nerve and muscle disorders, Alzheimer's disease and other types of senility, pain, headache, confused behavior, lethargy, and a host of other common mental problems.

THE SOLUTION

Earliest attempts at treating mental problems involved ostracizing the victims, killing them, drilling holes in their skulls "to let out the evil spirits," punishing them, ridiculing them, and other inhumane approaches. The horrors of Bedlam, a 13th-century insane asylum in England, are not far from the modern misdirected efforts described by Ken Kesey in *One Flew Over the Cuckoo's Nest*. Electroshock therapy, which one psychiatrist compared to kicking the TV when it doesn't work right, is still used on violent and depressed individuals. Other disturbed people simply end up in prison.

Current approaches to mental illness center around drug therapy and long-term psychotherapy. Drugs have numerous side effects and do nothing for the real problem. Psychotherapy can occasionally treat the problem, but it is a long-term, expensive process.

When you evaluate the risks and dubious benefits of the more prominent forms of treating mental illness today, you can see that nutrition is at least worth trying. The cost is low, the potential benefits are high, the risks are near zero, and the problem itself is dealt with.

This is not to say that nutrition is the cause and cure for all mental problems in America. Until recently, psychologists and psychiatrists claimed that human behavior was a result of:

- *Psychology:* "She's always been shy since her mother embarrassed her in front of her friends." Psychology is a valid explanation of behavior.
- *Sociology:* "Raised in a ghetto, what else could he become?" Our environment can strongly influence our emotional health. Another valid explanation of behavior.
- *Genetics:* "His pa was such a hellion; what did you expect that boy to turn out like?" Another valid explanation. Many men-

tal disorders and even personality traits come from the parent-to-child genetic link.

AN INTERDISCIPLINARY APPROACH

These three factors are useful and sometimes accurate indicators of why we do what we do. Yet they do not totally explain the majestic complexity of human behavior. Today, many experts in the fields of psychology and psychiatry understand the need for a much more comprehensive explanation of human behavior, an "interdisciplinary approach" to mental and emotional health that takes into account the following other factors:

Exercise

We evolved as active creatures. We function more efficiently, both physically and mentally, when we are active. Exercise can treat hyperactivity,[7] depression, anxiety, and a host of other mild to moderate mental problems.[8]

Brain Hemispheric Balance

The left hemisphere of the human brain is devoted primarily to the logical functions of science, math, language, etc. The right hemisphere is in charge of laughter, play, music, art, social appropriateness, three-dimensional recognition, and other factors that are difficult to put down as numbers or words. American society, especially our educational system, emphasizes almost exclusive left-brain development. This leads to poorly balanced brain use. By spending more time in right-brain activities, people become happier, healthier, and better adjusted.

Pollution

This is truly a critical issue. Every year, 90 billion pounds of toxic waste are dumped into our 55,000 toxic waste sites across the country. The rise in both physical and mental illness in this country closely parallels the rise in environmental pollution. In 1979, the Environmental Protection Agency estimated that pollutants and environment hazards are responsible for up to 20 percent of all deaths in this country. Matters have gotten much worse since then. Based upon that estimate, it would be quite valid to project that up to 20 percent of all mental illness is due to pollutants. Our food, water, and air are dangerously contaminated. Chemicals that can kill tenacious insects and weeds can certainly influence brain chemistry (for more on this issue, see Chapter 16).

Physical Environment

Light that does not contain the full spectrum of colors found in sunlight (malillumination), weather changes (biometeorology), noise, electromagnetic radiation (from computers, color televisions, FM transmitting towers, high-voltage lines, etc.), biorhythms, and perhaps even surrounding color can all influence the brain of some sensitive individuals.[9] Noise definitely affects behavior. These factors are promising areas that are worthy of further research.

Nutrition

The mind is an organ. Just like the kidneys, heart, and muscles, the brain has certain nutrient needs, while other substances can interfere with its normal workings. To be more specific, nutrients that affect the human brain fall into eight categories.

HOW NUTRITION RELATES TO BEHAVIOR: BIOLOGICAL NEEDS OF THE MIND

1. Energy. The brain requires a steady supply of blood glucose to function smoothly. Most other parts of the body are less selective about their fuel source, allowing carbohydrates, fats, protein, and perhaps even alcohol to be used for energy needs. The brain has established itself as one of the most finicky organs in the body when it comes to fuel usage. It will accept only blood glucose for energy.

2. Nutrients to Metabolize that Fuel. Thiamine, niacin, riboflavin, biotin, pantothenic acid, magnesium and chromium are needed to carry out the complete "burning" of that fuel. These nutrients are something like the spark that ignites the fuel.

3. Oxygen. The brain needs oxygen, delivered by red blood cells, which are built directly from the nutrients folacin, vitamin B_{12}, vitamin B_6, protein, iron, zinc, and copper. Other nutrients indirectly relate to red blood cell levels. Antioxidants, like vitamin E, protect the membranes of the red blood cells from being prematurely destroyed. Vitamin C helps the body to absorb iron.

4. The "Electrolyte Soup." The brain has been compared to a "soggy computer." Electrical conduction of nerve impulses relies on the electrolytes sodium, potassium, chloride, calcium, and magnesium, all being dissolved in a bath of water. This mixture creates low-level electricity that makes each cell in the body somewhat of a battery, like the battery in your car or portable stereo. All cells in the body depend on this critical "electrolyte soup," yet the brain is even more reliant on the proper recipe for this important solution since nerve cell functioning involves rapid changes in the "electrolyte soup."

5. *Chemical Transmission.* Nerve cells do not touch each other. Hence, the 10–13 billion nerve cells that make up the human brain must communicate by sending chemical "messages" across minute gaps. These "neurochemical transmitters" are made completely from the raw materials (precursors) found in the diet.

6. *Interfering Factors.* The brain is one of the most vulnerable organs in the human body. Drugs, pollutants, food allergies, and food sensitivities can "jam" the normal workings of the brain and should be avoided.

7. *Maintenance.* Once the brain has been built, it must be repaired regularly and maintained, like any other part of the body. Antioxidants (like vitamins A, C, and E and the mineral selenium) help to slow down the fat "rusting," or lipid peroxidation, that can occur in the fatty tissue of the brain. Folacin, B_{12}, thiamine, and zinc help to rebuild worn-out tissue and maintain the brain.

8. *Proper Development.* All creatures develop their greatest survival tool quickly in life. For humans, that tool is thinking. By age five, the human brain has grown to 90 percent of its adult weight. By age 7, the human brain is built, for better or for worse. A malnourished mind cannot be repaired once the DNA timing pattern has run its course. Brain growth is totally dependent on the nutrients that are found in the diet. A low nutrient supply while in the uterus and during the first seven years of life can irremediably retard brain development. Emotional and intellectual health suffer accordingly.

THE FUEL: BLOOD GLUCOSE

In the Andes Mountains of South America lives a tribe of Indians known as the Qolla. They are the meanest people on earth. No brag, just fact. A scientist wondered if blood glucose levels had anything to do with the Qollas' truculence. With modern laboratory equipment and a staff of nurses to assist, Dr. Robert Bolton had glucose tolerance tests performed on 66 adult male Qolla Indians. Blood glucose and relative levels of ferocity were recorded throughout the study. There was a direct relationship between blood sugar levels and degree of hostility.[10] The more rapid the decline in blood glucose levels, the more ornery that person became.

These Qollas often say that "fighting makes one feel better." Interestingly enough, when catecholamines (the stress hormones) flow through the body, glycogen stores are released to increase blood glucose levels, making a glucose-starved mind feel better again. Fighting, indeed, may provide temporary relief for the fuel-starved brain of the hypoglycemic. However, there are better ways of keeping blood glucose in the healthy range.

Why is blood glucose so important to the brain? The brain, lenses of the eyes, kidneys, and lungs operate almost entirely off blood glucose for fuel.[11] More than coincidentally, diabetics who experience abnormal blood sugar levels have a much higher incidence of blindness (eyes), psychosis (brain), and kidney failure than the healthy population at large.

Biologists know that the more primitive the life form, the more independent and adaptable that creature is. The most simplistic one-celled microorganisms can get along with a grocery list of about 5 essential nutrients. Plants need about 15. Most animals require 30 and up. Humans, at the pinnacle of complexity, need about 50. The more complex the organism, the more specific and demanding are its nutrient needs. This is not unlike society. Hermits who attempt to be self-sufficient have little time for poetry, computers, or brain surgery. Their needs are the same as their output: simple. Yet the more specialized a society, the greater the chance that each member can concentrate on his or her own expertise and enhance overall productivity. The brain is very much like a highly structured society: both have complex needs and impressive output.

Hypoglycemia is low blood sugar. It usually influences the nerve and muscle systems with such symptoms as headache, fatigue, lethargy, depression, nausea, blurred vision, and trembling muscles. Paperback books on the subject have made it sound as if anyone who wasn't happy had hypoglycemia. Not so. For almost two decades the controversy has raged about hypoglycemia. One side calls hypoglycemics hypochondriacs. The other side says that a large percentage of Americans suffer from this condition. The truth is probably somewhere in between.

Scientists at the University of California at Berkeley examined the blood glucose curves of 67 "normal" subjects. Twenty-nine of these people (43 percent) had blood glucose curves that fell below 60 mg %, which technically throws them into the category of "hypoglycemia" (mg % means the amount of glucose, expressed in milligrams, that is found in a given volume—100 milliliters, usually abbreviated as "%".) A standardized test for mental agility (SST) was given to each subject at half-hour intervals. Those subjects whose blood sugar levels stayed in the healthy range had average SST scores of 22, while the low-blood-sugar group had mean scores of 5. There was definite mental confusion in the participants who had low blood sugar levels.[12] These findings indicate that hypoglycemia could be much more common than once thought.

In this study, low points in blood sugar levels occurred two to four hours after the start. That is also significant, since blood glucose tests in the past were usually only three hours in length, which means that the patient would often experience the abnormal blood glucose levels *after* the test was over. The Mayo Clinic says that blood glucose tests should be five hours in length and should be performed when the patient is experiencing symptoms, not at some random time that is convenient only to the clinic.[13]

One common symptom of hypoglycemia is meanness. This may relate hypoglycemia to some criminal behavior. A probation officer, Barbara Reed of Ohio, testified before the Senate hearings on nutrition and mental health in 1977. From her own personal experience, she found that a certain dietary regimen controlled her hypoglycemia and her radical mood swings. She began applying this idea to the criminals left in her charge. Of the 318 people that she had dealt with in a 2½ year period, 252 tested positive for hypoglycemia according to her subjective questionnaire. Of the 252 criminals who were put on her special dietary regimen to regulate blood glucose, *none* who adhered to the program had returned to the court system.[14] A few of the questions from her subjective test follow. If you answer "yes" to five or more of these, then perhaps you need to regulate your blood sugar for more predictable levels of mental energy.

SUBJECTIVE TEST FOR HYPOGLYCEMIA

1. Does your mind go blank at times?
2. Are you forgetful?
3. Do you occasionally have difficulty with concentration?
4. Do you lose your temper easily?
5. Do you have difficulty in controlling your emotions?
6. Are you very impatient?
7. Do certain things irritate you very much?
8. Are you depressed, blue?
9. Are you nervous?
10. Are you very tense?

If you answered "yes" to five or more of these questions, it does not mean that you necessarily have hypoglycemia. You might need counseling, you might have unusual stresses in your life at this time, or other factors as explained in the "interdisciplinary approach" might be affecting you. However, answering "yes" to five or more of these questions means that an Oral Glucose Tolerance Test would be a worthwhile investment for you.

ORAL GLUCOSE TOLERANCE TESTS

How can abnormal blood glucose be diagnosed scientifically? The accepted method is the Oral Glucose Tolerance Test (OGTT), which measures the ability of your body to absorb, process, and use carbohydrates.

Case History 1. Sally M. was fed up. She went to her doctor for help. For years her quick breakfast of coffee and sweet roll had provided adequate energy to get her through work until lunchtime. Yet for the past few months, her mental and physical energies were spent by 10:00 A.M. Weakness, trembles, headache, nausea, dizziness, depression, and other problems assaulted her a few hours after a meal. She was told that she would be given an OGTT. She could eat dinner, but no snacks at night and no breakfast the next morning. The clinic would run the test in the morning. At that time, she was given a glass of sweet water (glucose solution) to drink. Blood samples were drawn from Sally at regular intervals throughout the coming three hours (time frame used by many clinics, although using five hours is more accurate). Toward the end of the test, Sally experienced all the symptoms that she felt at the office. Both her symptoms and the OGTT confirmed what her doctor had suspected: hypoglycemia. She was placed on a special dietary program to help regulate her erratic blood glucose levels.

Case Study 2. Roger B. had been finding it increasingly difficult to do his job. Fatigue was constant and almost overwhelming. He had a tremendous thirst and had to urinate often. His wounds were slow to heal. He went to the doctor for help. The OGTT was performed as described above. He tested positive for diabetes and was placed on a very specific clinical regimen designed to help regulate his blood glucose levels.

In many cases, the patient has the symptoms of hypoglycemia while the OGTT is being performed, yet by lab standards the OGTT is diagnosed as "normal." There are limitless varieties of blood glucose curves between the classical extremes just described of diabetes (hyperglycemia) and hypoglycemia. "Normal" values in the OGTT are a statistical average of the people who have taken the test in the past. These people are often overweight, underexercised, poorly nourished, overstressed, smoking, drinking, and feeling sicker than normal at the time of the test. Why else would you have an OGTT done unless you didn't feel good? So being classified as "normal" in comparison to such a curve is not a categorical clearance for a health problem.

Hypoglycemia can stem from many problems: early diabetes; intestinal, pancreatic, or liver problems; tumors in key organs; pituitary or adrenal insufficiencies; too much exercise; too little food; and on.[15]

Certain common agents can cause blood sugar levels to go into a downward tailspin. Caffeine, alcohol, tobacco, large amounts of sugar, and other agents can instigate temporary hypoglycemia in a person who would otherwise have healthy blood sugar levels. Caffeine is found in large amounts in coffee, tea, many medications, cola drinks, and chocolate. Caffeine stimulates insulin output, which then lowers blood sugar.

Eight hundred grade school children had their caffeine intake measured by scientists. Thirty of them were consuming over 300 mg of caffeine daily,[16] which is equivalent to five or six stiff cups of coffee. Nine of the 30 children who were consuming the most caffeine were diagnosed as hyperactive. This means that 30 percent of these high-caffeine children were hyperative, which is significantly above the 10–20 percent incidence that is found in the population at large. To find out if caffeine intake is a result of or a cause of hyperactivity, the same scientist performed a double-blind crossover study and found that a similar percentage of nonhyperactive children became hyperactive when given the same high doses of caffeine. In some sensitive individuals, excess caffeine can change behavior.

Alcohol also lowers blood sugar levels. Low blood sugar could be responsible for the "Jekyll and Hyde" behavioral changes that are seen in many people who drink. Hypoglycemia is also a factor in the torturous effects of a hangover. Alcoholics Anonymous (AA) meetings are often full of people who are smoking and drinking strong coffee with much sugar and plenty of sweet rolls. All of these substances (caffeine, tobacco, sugar) can cause major swings in blood sugar and thus emotions. Alcoholics may be people who have problems regulating their blood sugar levels. By stabilizing blood sugar, many people are able to reduce their affinity for alcohol.

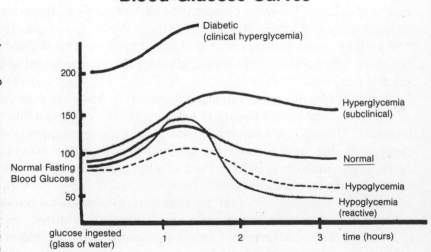

Blood Glucose Curves

A blood glucose tolerance curve is a valuable indicator of how well your body can handle carbohydrates and how sustained your mental and physical energies are.

Diets high in simple sugars can cause wild roller coaster effects in OGTT. Since sugar is quickly and totally absorbed in the intestines, it causes a precipitous rise in blood sugar, which, in some people, is followed by a precipitous fall. The net effect is a feeling of extreme fatigue or perhaps changes in behavior.

Sugar may also influence the mind in other ways. Schoolchildren aged 5–16 had their one-day diet history taken along with hair samples for hair analysis. A definite relationship emerged: the more sugar the children ate, the more cadmium their hair retained and the lower their cognitive scores.[17] Put simply, sugar makes people stupid. Another group of scientists found that the higher the intake of sugar, the lower the absorption efficiency for copper.[18] Copper is important in a variety of brain functions, including energy metabolism and creation of red blood cells for oxygen transport.

There are many different types of carbohydrate foods, and they have different influences on blood sugar curves. The most basic categories of dietary carbohydrates are (1) simple (as in easily digested and absorbed sugars) and (2) complex (as in starches that require more time and enzymes for digestion and absorption into the bloodstream). The more complex the carbohydrate is, the more digestive work will be required by the intestinal tract to absorb this food and the slower will be the rise in blood glucose. This is good. The more gradual the rise in blood glucose, the more gradual the fall will be.

Blood sugar curves are somewhat similar to business growth curves. The slope of the upside is often equal to the slope of the downside. Usually the companies that grow quickly die quickly. Companies that have a long and gradual growth phase are less likely to succumb in a short period of time. *Gradual* is the key word in trying to stabilize blood glucose levels.

The body also has different mechanisms to absorb carbohydrates. Glucose is found in table sugar (sucrose), maltose, and many other foods. Glucose is actively pumped into the blood, while fructose (as from fruits and honey) is passively absorbed into the bloodstream. This slower means of absorption through passive diffusion helps to prevent "peaks and valleys" in blood glucose levels.

Fiber is indigestible carbohydrate. Among the many benefits of fiber, it interferes with the digestion and absorption of the other foods in the gut. This is good. This interference slows the absorption of carbohydrates into the blood and provides more gradual and predictable energy levels.

Myoinositol (a.k.a *muscle sugar*) is another substance that is involved in the normal functioning of nerve cells. Most healthy people make some myoinositol in their system. In people with abnormal blood glucose levels (like diabetics), myoinositol could become an essential nutrient. When supplements of 1,000 mg of myoinositol daily were given to volunteers, the action potential of certain nerve cells improved.[19] The nerve function in diabetic patients improved significantly when even larger supplements (up to 1,648 mg daily) were given.[20] Myoinositol is probably useful for diabetics and may also be important for people with hypoglycemia (see Chapter 14 for more on myoinositol).

L-carnitine is a substance found in varying levels in a carnivorous diet and produced to a certain extent in the body. Carnitine is crucial to the proper burning of fat. Muscles, heart, and other organs will burn fat if adequate carnitine is available. The same tissues will rely more heavily on carbohydrate fuel if the carnitine supply is low. In that case, the brain may end up competing for the limited glucose supplies. Carnitine is an essential nutrient for certain stress states, including drug therapy, preterm infants, hemodialysis patients, and others with unusual metabolic needs.[21] Adequate carnitine allows people to burn fat more efficiently, thus saving blood glucose for the selective appetite of the brain.

PROGRAM TO STABILIZE BLOOD GLUCOSE

1. Eat small, frequent meals. Just when the blood glucose is starting to drop, each new meal provides a new source of carbohydrates to sustain predictable levels of blood glucose.

2. Minimize or avoid alcohol, caffeine, tobacco.

3. Minimize intake of simple carbohydrates. The average American consumes about 130 pounds of sugar per year. Cut this at least in half. From best to worst, select sweet foods from the following list: fresh fruits, dried fruits, lactose (milk sugar), molasses, honey, fructose, refined sugars (brown, white, confectioners'). Limit the intake of artificial sweeteners (saccharin, NutraSweet) to two servings daily. Pregnant women would be wise to avoid them. Artificial sweeteners have a long and tainted history.

4. Maximize intake of food high in complex carbohydrates and fiber, including whole grains, legumes, fresh vegetables, and nuts. This program works for *most* people. The few remaining people with very volatile blood sugar regulation may have to eat only high-protein foods (meat, chicken, fish, eggs, dairy, cheese) and vegetables. This program definitely stabilizes the most sensitive of systems but is required in only a small percentage of cases.

5. Exercise at least three times weekly for at least 45 minutes per session. Exercise improves blood sugar regulation and the receptivity of the cells to insulin.[22]

NUTRIENTS TO BURN THE CARBOHYDRATE FUEL

Nature has provided us with a complicated series of steps that allow us to slowly, methodically, and safely squeeze much of the available energy from foodstuffs. On paper, this complex biochemical pathway looks like a staircase, with each step bringing the foodstuff to a lower energy level and harnessing the released energy for purposes of supporting the body's processes. Energy metabolism involves the vitamins thiamine, niacin, riboflavin, biotin, and pantothenic acid. The mineral chromium is also essential to allow the glucose to get into the cell for burning. Iron and copper are involved in the final stage of electron transport. Magnesium is critical for the final formation of ATP, the "gold currency" of energy metabolism. Hence, these nutrients are the "spark" that ignites the flame in the cell furnace. Without them, the brain is one of the first organs of the body to suffer the effects of a nutrient deficiency.

"Normally," glucose tolerance progressively deteriorates with age.[23] This could provoke fatigue and changes in behavior in older adults. Yet, this "norm" does not mean that poor glucose tolerance is inescapable in the elderly. Many older Americans are riding out the tail end of an unhealthy lifestyle. Most Americans are deficient in chromium, and this situation gradually deteriorates as people age. Two hundred micrograms of chromium supplements daily improved glucose tolerance in all of the 76 normal subjects who were tested.[24] Chromium supplements also effectively treated patients with reactive hypoglycemia.[25]

Many older people live precariously on the edge of marginal thiamine status. In a study of 64 elderly patients in an English hospital, the investigators found a definite relationship between confused behavior and low blood thiamine levels.[26] Low thiamine levels can be detected in the spinal fluid, indicating a dependence of nervous tissue on circulating thiamine levels.[27] Thiamine injections given to lab animals improved their low serotonin levels (important chemical transmitters in the brain) and ended their spasms and convulsions.[28] Thiamine therapy has been tried with some success on infants who had nonfatal attacks of sudden infant death syndrome (SIDS).

Pantothenic acid is an energy nutrient that is commonly found in low supply in the American diet. Older adults receive only about one-third of the RDA for pantothenic acid,[29] while the typical adolescent is consuming less than half of the RDA.[30] Pantothenic acid is removed in wheat milling.

Thirty-three percent of elderly males and 18 percent of elderly females are consuming less than two-thirds of the RDA for riboflavin.[31] Many people might just feel sluggish when their riboflavin levels are marginally low. But a low riboflavin status can also instigate iron deficiency anemia,[32] which can become a serious problem for the brain.

The brain must have these vital "metabolite" nutrients to burn blood glucose properly. Seriously low levels of these nutrients can produce severe mental confusion. More likely in America, though, our marginal intake of these nutrients could produce subclinical symptoms of lowered mental abilities.[33]

OXYGEN

The brain is an incredibly thirsty oxygen sponge. Although comprising only about 5 percent of an adult's body weight, the brain uses up nearly 25 percent of the body's oxygen supply. Most people can live weeks without food and days without water. Yet, after only a few minutes without oxygen, the brain quickly begins to deteriorate. Red blood cells deliver this vital oxygen supply to the brain. If the blood supply is low (anemia), then you can suffer changes in emotions or intellect. Menstruating women and growing children are at great risk for anemia and the mental changes that accompany this common nutritional problem. Also, pulmonary units in hospitals are notoriously difficult to work in, since the patients' lung problems mean their brains are getting less oxygen, which makes them lethargic or hostile.

The brain demands a continuous flow of oxygen. Oxygen is delivered via red blood cells, which are built directly from the nutrients iron, copper, zinc, B_6, protein, folacin, and B_{12}. Although many people are given iron supplements for anemia, iron alone will not build red blood cells. The average American consumes half the RDA for copper. Many Americans are low in folacin and B_6. Many elderly people and those with gastrointestinal problems lose the ability to absorb B_{12}. So building red blood cells requires a more broad-minded approach to nutrition beyond just iron.

Iron deficiency can seriously influence both behavior and intellect.[34] Infants who are iron-anemic are often irritable, lack interest in their surroundings, and have abnormal physical, mental and emotional reactions. All of these symptoms improve with iron supplementation.[35]

How many Americans are anemic? Twenty-five percent of the infants with *normal* hemoglobin levels showed increases in hemoglobin with iron supplements.[36] They were soaking up these iron supplements like a dry sponge. This indicates that "normal" hemoglobin levels may be better classified as a subclinical iron deficiency. A nationwide survey conducted by the U.S. Department of Agriculture found that as many as 35 percent of American infants are iron-deficient.[37] Of over 4,000 Louisiana children studied, the average iron intake for the girls (ages 5–17) was 58 percent of their RDA.[38]

And iron deficiency is not restricted to infants, children, and poor people. Somewhere between 25 and 50 percent of menstruating women and growing children in America could be considered low in their body's iron supply. For adult men and postmenopausal women, the incidence of iron deficiency is less than half of that. Eighteen percent of the female students at Yale University were found to be anemic.[39] The three-day food record of 574 adolescents was analyzed along with various blood fractions. Although the red blood cell levels were normal in most subjects, serum ferritin (a storage form of iron reserves in the blood) was low in 39 percent of these young people.[40] One out of four of these subjects was eating adequate iron, yet had low serum ferritin.

Forty-four percent of female adolescent runners were found to be iron-deficient.[41] At least half of all runners are borderline to full-blown anemic,[42] though not enough iron is lost in sweat to justify this deficiency.[43]

However, the abundant oxygen that is brought into the body during exercise quickly destroys the wrapping (membranes) of the red blood cells. Supplements of vitamin E (450 IU daily), an antioxidant whose main job is to retard the corrosive effects of oxygen in the body, were able to increase the survival time of human red blood cells significantly.[44]

An oxygen-starved brain simply does not work well. Iron supplements have been shown to improve school achievement scores in iron-anemic children.[45] Yet it takes about three months for the body to build up hemoglobin levels from dietary iron. So it was somewhat surprising when iron supplements improved behavior, attention span, and problem-solving abilities in iron-deficient preschoolers *after only 7–10 days* of supplementation.[46] The reason for these results is that iron not only works in hemoglobin to bring oxygen to the brain but also is involved in the conversion of tyrosine to dopamine, which is a key chemical in the brain. Therefore, iron has both immediate and long-term influences on mental abilities.

Building enough red blood cells to supply the brain with oxygen goes way beyond mere iron. Vitamin E supplements have been effective in providing relief for various inherited blood disorders.[47] Fifteen renal dialysis patients were given 900 IU of vitamin E supplements daily in a blind study. Although all 15 were anemic, none showed low levels of plasma vitamin E, yet the vitamin E supplements improved the red blood cell count in 80 percent of the subjects tested.[48] Low levels of vitamin A can also lead to anemia.[49] In anemic patients for whom iron therapy was ineffective, vitamin A supplements helped to bolster red blood cell counts.[50]

Vitamin C helps to change iron into a more absorbable state in the intestines. Vitamin C deficiencies are quite common. Fifty-four anemic preschool children were given either 100 mg of ascorbic acid daily or a placebo, but no iron. The children receiving the ascorbic acid showed major improvements in their hemoglobin levels 60 days later.[51] Vitamin C and bioflavonoids together have reduced mid-cycle bleeding (ovulatory menorrhagia) in women, to help improve hemoglobin status.[52]

Are iron supplements safe? Yes. Even prolonged used of iron supplements rarely produce any iron overload,[53] though iron excess is possible in adult males, who do not have the escape valve of monthly blood loss that menstruating women have. Supplements of 10–30 mg of iron daily would be quite safe and probably helpful for nearly all people, with the lower amounts appropriate for sedentary adult males who are eating considerable amounts of iron-rich red meat. Pregnant, lactating, very active, menstruating, and growing people may need even higher supplement levels. Worldwide, iron supplements could provide cheap and significant health improvements to billions of people. Iron deficiency is so common and so pernicious in its effects on the mind and body that a number of experts have recommended that iron be added to table salt in developing countries.[54]

Vitamin B_{12} is intimately tied to the production of new cell growth, such as the making of red blood cells. Usually red blood cells have a life span of about three to four months. After major blood loss or carbon monoxide poisoning, it often takes weeks to months to build up a noticeable improvement in red blood cell levels. Yet only 24 hours after injections of vitamin B_{12}, patients with pernicious anemia (B_{12} deficiency) showed noticeable improvements in their hemoglobin levels.[55] Folacin works closely with B_{12} in new cell growth. Folacin deficiencies are common and are often reflected in anemia.[56]

Carnitine is a substance produced in the body that allows fats to be burned. In order to make carnitine, the body must have the raw materials of lysine, methionine, iron, vitamin C, niacin, and vitamin B_6. Of these nutrients, iron, vitamin C, and vitamin B_6 are in short supply in the American diet and could lead to a carnitine deficiency. When an iron deficiency was created in a group of young lab animals, it caused major changes in carnitine, fat, and carbohydrate metabolism.[57] This could influence brain functions. Carnitine deficiencies could be quite common, especially in people drinking any more than small amounts of alcohol.[58] The brain may be shortchanged in numerous ways with an iron deficiency, through low production of carnitine, dopamine, and red blood cells.

Zinc is involved in all new cell growth in the body, including making red blood cells. Zinc deficiencies are quite common in America and could be responsible for more than a small amount of anemia and poor mental function. Twenty-two young patients with sickle-cell anemia (an inherited blood disorder) were found to have low to very low levels of zinc.[59]

ELECTROLYTE SOUP

The brain is immersed in an ocean of electrolytes, not unlike the ocean in which life evolved. A nerve impulse reaches its destination by using both electrical and chemical means to travel throughout the body.

Sodium, potassium, chloride, magnesium, calcium, and water are electrolytes that create low-voltage electricity. For a nerve impulse to get from one end of a nerve cell to the other, a certain amount of electricity (action potential) is needed, which changes once the cell has been stimulated. If the "recipe" for this electrolyte soup is not followed closely, then changes in mental functions can occur.

Health care professionals who work in emergency units know that electrolytes are among the critical components that are checked when someone is admitted to emergency care. If the "electrolyte soup" is slightly off, problems can result. If it is markedly off, the patient will die quickly.

Water is a major factor in the "electrolyte soup." It has long been known that one of the first symptoms of dehydration is confusion. If the concentration of either the electrolytes or the water is changed, then the brain will not work well. Alcohol is a diuretic, invoking great fluid loss in an evening of heavy drinking. It is this dehydrated brain that cries out for mercy in the morning, with pain, confusion, and depression as likely symptoms of serious brain dehydration.

Long-term intensive exercise also causes major fluid and electrolyte loss, which can influence brain function. Two runners in the 1983 Chicago ultramarathon had to be hospitalized for water intoxication. In this 50-mile race, much sweat can be lost. Sweat is composed of considerable quantities of water and small amounts of the electrolytes sodium, potassium, chloride, and others. These runners were drinking only water (20–24 liters) and thus diluting their "electrolyte soup" by not replenishing the lost electrolytes. They each experienced stuporous and disoriented behavior, and one had a grand mal seizure from this water intoxication/electrolyte deficiency.[60] Although these two ended up in the hospital emergency room, being young and fit, neither died.

You don't have to be an athlete to get water intoxication. A 21-year-old college student was told to drink plenty of water before her hospital tests began. She did. Thirty glasses of tap water later, she began developing nausea, headache, and restlessness.[61] She was later brought to the emergency room with bizarre and confused behavior—another example of overdiluting the "electrolyte soup" of the brain.

Sailors of the great age of exploration used to speak of the insanity that would affect anyone who drank sea water in desperation when the fresh water stores were gone. Ocean water actually dehydrates people, due to its high salt content. These are all somewhat extreme examples of changing the electrolyte concentration in the body and brain. If serious problems occur when the "electrolyte soup" is seriously off, then it seems logical that moderate changes in the brain would occur if there were moderate changes in the "electrolyte soup."

And that logic is well supported. When 90 adults with hypertension were put on a low-sodium diet, no one was surprised when their blood pressure went down. However, as a bonus many reported feeling happier and less depressed and used fewer painkillers.[62] By optimizing their "electrolyte soup" with a low-sodium diet, these people found a new, more comfortable brain performance level. New data in hypertension show that deficient intake of calcium, magnesium, and potassium are probably more responsible for high blood pressure than excess sodium intake. Imbalances in the "electrolyte soup" deteriorate both physical health (as in hypertension) and mental health.

And what adds to the complexity of this issue is how all ingredients in the "electrolyte soup" are interrelated. Low levels of magnesium will instigate lower body levels of potassium and calcium.[63] Of the 50 million people with hypertension in this country, at least half are on diuretic therapy, which depletes potassium.

Low serum levels of magnesium can cause migraine headaches in some people. Magnesium supplements can help a good percentage of migraine sufferers.[64] Another possible cure for migraine headaches is feverfew, a medicinal herb that can be taken in capsule form.[65]

Caffeine causes a high urinary loss of calcium, magnesium, sodium, and chloride.[66] Many people complain of "fuzzy thinking" upon awakening, which could be due to an unbalanced electrolyte soup in the brain. Few Americans get enough clean fluids, calcium, magnesium, and potassium. Many people get too much

.sodium and chloride through salt. The net result could be an erosion of both physical and mental health.

CHEMICAL TRANSMISSION

There are roughly 13 billion separate nerve cells in an average adult brain. As stated earlier, these nerve cells come very close to one another but do not touch. Any given nerve cell may be adjacent to a thousand other nerve cells. There are perhaps a dozen different chemical communicators between nerve cells. If you take 13 billion to 1,000 permutations and take this number again to 12 permutations, then you have the possible number of storage areas for memory and behavior in the human brain. "Almost limitless" would be your answer to that math puzzle. We have virtually limitless "bytes" of memory in our brain, to borrow from computer jargon.

The gap (synapse) between nerve cells is bridged by chemical means. These "neurochemical transmitters" are made from raw materials found in the diet:

- tryptophan converted into serotonin, with the help of B_6
- tyrosine converted into either dopamine or norepinephrine, with the help of B_6, C, and iron
- Choline converted into acetylcholine
- L-glutamate converted into GABA (gamma amino butyric acid) with the help of magnesium

There are others. Neurophysiologists realize how much is yet to be learned regarding chemical communication between brain cells. Each of these neurochemical transmitters plays an important role in thought, behavior, and stress tolerance. Depression, confusion, compulsive behavior, eating disorders, substance abuse, gambling, hyperactivity, pain tolerance, Parkinson's disease, schizophrenia, and other mental problems have all been linked to abnormal levels of these vital chemical transmitters in the brain. In some cases, nutrition can improve the chemistry of the brain. In other cases, the problem is more organic and is resistant to nutrition therapy. Most drugs that work on the central nervous system attempt to block (antagonists), mimic (agonists), or enhance the production of these neurochemical transmitters.

Tyrosine supplements were able to improve stress tolerance in lab animals,[67] which makes perfect sense. When tyrosine is being diverted into norepinephrine production for stress response, there is less left for dopamine production, which is vital to normal behavior. Tyrosine supplements (6 g daily) also helped depressed patients who lacked normal levels of norepinephrine.[68] Manganese is a trace mineral that also helps the brain manufacture dopamine from tyrosine.[69] There are anecdotal reports that large doses of manganese can help treat schizophrenia[70] and tardive dyskinesia (a muscle tremor problem that is found in people who have been on long-term sedative medication).[71]

Dopamine (from tyrosine) is crucial to normal healthy emotions, thought, and muscle control. Preliminary work done at the UCLA medical school shows that hyperactive children have abnormally low levels of dopamine in their brains. Parkinson's victims also have low levels of dopamine in their brain. Dopamine itself cannot pass through the blood brain barrier, but a precursor (the drug L-dopa) can. L-dopa provides the brain with some extra dopamine precursors and a certain amount of relief for victims of Parkinson's disease. Anecdotally, tyrosine supplements have improved the condition in some patients with Parkinson's disease.

Phenylalanine is an amino acid that can be converted into tyrosine in the body. In humans, the L (*levo*, Latin for "left-handed") form of all amino acids is useful, while the D (*dextro*, Latin for "right-handed") form is normally useless. Yet D-phenylalanine apparently inhibits the breakdown of endorphins (the body's own morphinelike compound), thus becoming a potent painkilling agent.[72] Supplements of L-phenylalanine amplified the painkilling effect of electroacupuncture.[73]

Tryptophan is another amino acid that has been successful in treating pain, insomnia, and depression. In a few cases, tryptophan supplements have cured insomnia when the strongest prescription medication wouldn't.[74] Infants given tryptophan entered active and quiet sleep sooner.[75] Mother's milk is high in tryptophan. Tryptophan supplements at bedtime (1–4 g) provided relief from insomnia for 30 percent of the patients tested with no side effects in 90 percent of them.[76] In another study, 1 g of tryptophan taken at bedtime with a carbohydrate snack (bread, crackers, etc.) has been shown to be a useful sleep aid.[77] Tryptophan is likely to relieve insomnia in people who have low serotonin levels in their brain.

Tryptophan also improves pain tolerance. Thirty dental students were given either a placebo or 2 g of tryptophan daily for one week. They were then subjected to electrical voltage on their teeth to record pain threshold. Although the tryptophan did not reduce pain perception, it did significantly raise the pain threshold.[78]

In a double-blind study, 20 men were given either a placebo or tryptophan supplements. The tryptophan provided significant sedative effects without interfering with normal alert performance.[79] This should be good news for the people who find that most sedatives are nearly incapacitating when driving or at work. Tryptophan supplements also provided relief from depression in a double-blind study using 115 patients. More importantly, tryptophan induced no side effects, unlike the heavy sedative hypnotic drugs that were also tested against depression.[80]

Tryptophan can also be converted into niacin, a crucial energy vitamin, on a very inefficient 60-to-1 ratio. Given the choice between thinking (tryptophan to serotonin) and living (niacin for energy metabolism), the body chooses living, and the mind can suffer extraordinary discomfort in a niacin deficiency. At least 10 percent of all patients in mental institutions in America at the turn of the century were there due to a niacin deficiency, which produces mental illness symptoms in the condition called *pellagra*. Due to this interaction between niacin and tryptophan, scientists have found that supplements of nicotinamide (a version of niacin) given with tryptophan enhance the effectiveness of the tryptophan by slowing the rate at which the liver breaks down tryptophan.[81] Niacin supplements by themselves act as a mild tranquilizer for some people,[82] probably by sparing the tryptophan in the brain for more serotonin production.

Serotonin levels may even be linked to compulsive gambling. Some very current research by Dr. Robert Custer at the National Institute of Mental Health estimates that many of the 2.5 million compulsive gamblers in this country have abnormally low levels of serotonin in their brains. The nutritional relevance of this is yet to be discovered.

Tryptophan and tyrosine are converted into their active brain chemicals through the assistance of vitamin B_6. B_6 is another crucial nutrient for thought. The Nationwide Food Consumption Survey examined over 40,000 Americans and found that nearly 40 percent of us eat less than two-thirds of the RDA for B_6. A study of

583 adolescent females found that the average person was consuming only 60 percent of the RDA for B_6.[83] Supplements of B_6 have been able to reverse problems in tryptophan metabolism.[84] Tardive dyskinesia can be prevented and sometimes even treated with high-dose B_6 supplements.[85]

Carpel tunnel syndrome (CTS) is a common problem of numbness and a tingling sensation in the hand and wrist region. Surgery is the favorite approach to CTS in American health care. Yet, B_6 supplements (100–300 mg daily) have effectively treated CTS.[86] In a more recent double-blind study, 100 mg of vitamin B_6 daily cured CTS in 27 out of 28 patients.[87] Perhaps because of the role that B_6 plays in producing neurochemical transmitters, supplements of B_6 were able to almost totally eliminate the nerve and muscle problems that accompany excess MSG intake.[88]

In Chapter 2, we talked about a mother who discovered that B_6 helped her autistic son. In four different double-blind experiments on 60 autistic children, scientists found that large doses of B_6 (up to 1,000 mg daily) coupled with magnesium (up to 500 mg daily) provided relief from many of the symptoms of autism.[89] When B_6 and magnesium were used individually, they were marginally effective. Yet coupled together, B_6 and magnesium had an amazing synergistic action against autism. High doses (25 mg and up) of B_6 will degrade the drug L-dopa quickly and thus would not be advised for people taking L-dopa.

Choline is converted in the brain into acetylcholine, which is an important chemical bridge between nerve cells. Choline is also produced in the body to some extent, so it is not considered an essential nutrient. Yet various stress stages of life can probably move choline from the "nonessential" into the "essential" category. This explains why choline and lecithin (the best source of choline) have been successful in treating various nerve and muscle disorders. Preliminary evidence shows that choline supplements may be able to improve memory.[90] Choline supplements helped the short-term memory in some Alzheimer's patients[91] and improved the overall condition of Alzheimer's patients in another study.[92]

Since lecithin is the richest source of choline, it should not be surprising that lecithin supplements have been as successful as choline in some studies. Lecithin helps tardive dyskinesia, a muscle tremor condition.[93] Lecithin has achieved some success in treating other conditions involving nerve and muscle degeneration, like

Tourette's syndrome, Friedreich's ataxia, Huntington's disease, and myasthenic syndrome.[94] Unfortunately, the lecithin sold on supermarket and health food shelves may not be as pure and useful as the quality lecithin that was used in these laboratory experiments, says Dr. Wurtman at MIT.[95] You can find 55 percent pure lecithin from some vitamin purveyors. This grade of lecithin should be good enough to elicit results as mentioned above.

Glutamic acid is an amino acid (found in high-quality protein foods) that may form GABA in the brain. GABA is one of the more ubiquitous of all the neurochemical transmitters. Glutamine readily crosses the blood brain barrier to make more GABA available for mental functions. Wine has been shown to help promote better sleeping habits in retirement homes. A deficiency of GABA can cause mild insomnia.[96] Potatoes and wine are among the foods that contain preformed GABA. Some research indicates that glutamine problems may be the beginning of such brain ailments as Huntington's disease.[97] Supplements of glutamine have been used against schizophrenia[98] and to reduce the cravings for alcohol in laboratory animals.[99]

Vitamin C is involved in the production of serotonin. A group of older dementia patients were found to have very low levels of vitamin C in their blood plasma and white cells. When investigators gave only 50 mg of vitamin C daily to a group of these senile dementia patients, their blood levels of ascorbic acid rose 500 percent.[100] (For more details on mental vigor in the older adult, see Chapter 9.)

Enkephalins are internally produced substances that provide us with pain relief and pleasure.[101] Endorphins (*endo* for "inside," *orphin* for "morphine") are one of the better researched enkephalins. Scientists discovered this substance when trying to unlock some of the mysteries of intensive heroine addiction. Heroine, morphine, and cocaine activate these sites of pleasure in the brain. Too much activation from drug abuse can deaden these areas. Some drug abusers lose (at least temporarily) the ability to experience pleasure. Meditation, exercise, and certain pleasurable experiences are able to trigger the release of endorphins for a euphoric experience. Even the placenta contains some endorphins, indicating nature's readiness to provide some pain relief during childbirth. Some drugs, alcohol, perhaps tobacco, and even eating experiences may be able to evoke an endorphin experience.

Endorphins provide some clues about people who are substance abusers or who have eating disorders. Copper is involved in the production of enkephalins. Copper intake in America is roughly half of the RDA. Researchers fed 24 male subjects low-copper diets and found a closely tied drop in the levels of enkephalins that were produced in the brain.[102] Binge eaters (bulimics) have been found to have lower levels of endorphins.[103] Cocaine abusers are much more likely to have an eating disorder.[104] There may be a link between compulsive behavior (eating disorders or substance abuse) and abnormally low levels of brain chemicals. Perhaps poor nutrition leads to low endorphins, which spurs that person toward drugs or binge eating. Perhaps nutritional supplementation can change the unfavorable chemical environment in the brains of overeaters and substance abusers. Perhaps. This field is very new.

Taurine is an unusual amino acid. Taurine prefers to participate in reactions, like nerve excitability, rather than tissue construction projects like most other amino acids. (Taurine is examined more in depth in Chapter 11.) Taurine seems to be an essential nutrient for rapidly growing brains and is found in mother's milk, but not cow's milk or most infant formulas.[105] When genetically susceptible animals are raised on taurine-deficient diets, they develop epilepsy.[106] Oral supplements of taurine showed a definite but mild ability to reduce convulsions in human epileptics.[107] It would be interesting to find out how many victims of epilepsy were not breastfed.

There are some topical agents that can help relieve pain in certain conditions. DMSO (dimethyl sulfoxide) is a liniment that was first used on sore muscles in people and animals. DMSO has shown some ability to reduce pain, when it involves muscles and joints.[108] Topical use of aloe vera can provide some pain relief from skin burns.[109] Topical application of bioflavonoids was able to reduce the pain of bites, stings, and oral surgery with a potency comparable to topical cocaine.[110] Oral supplements of bioflavonoids were able to reduce headache pain without the usual stomach irritation that is found with aspirin.[111]

AVOID INTERFERING FACTORS

Computers are sensitive and potentially productive machines. Dust, humidity, changes in voltage, and temperature can all seriously influence computer functions. The brain is more sophisticated and less sensitive than a computer. But there are some similarities. Psychoactive drugs, food sensitivities, food allergies, and pollutants can cause a normal, healthy brain to go awry.

Drugs are a significant interfering factor. Of 191,400 state prison inmates questioned, 43 percent said they had been drinking at the time of their criminal act.[112] A poll taken by the U.S. Bureau of the Census in 1974 found that 26 percent of all state prison inmates were under the influence of drugs other than alcohol at the time of their crime. This means that up to three out of four crimes are committed while the delicate machinery of the brain is under siege from some type of drug.

Alcohol is an unusual agent since it is both a potent drug and a nutrient by virtue of its 7 kilocalories per gram. Forty-six percent of all homicide victims brought to the coroner's office in Los Angeles county had detectable levels of alcohol, while 30 percent were legally drunk.[113] Half of all fatal auto accidents are caused by alcohol or drugs. Alcohol can make a person the killer or the victim. Much of child and wife abuse occurs under the influence of drugs or alcohol. Psychoactive drugs include amphetamines ("uppers"), barbituates ("downers"), hallucinogens (LSD, PCP), alcohol, and opioids (cocaine, morphine, heroin). The mind does not work well when bludgeoned with interfering factors like drugs.

Food sensitivities were first suspected as a cause of mental disorders in the late 1960s. In addition to the thousands of intentional and unintentional additives, there are thousands of other naturally occurring components in foods that are only beginning to be isolated and understood. Any one of these substances could cause brain changes in certain sensitive individuals. (Food sensitivities and food allergies are covered thoroughly in Chapter 8.)

As much as 25 percent of the population suffers from migraine headaches. Alcohol (especially red wines), chocolate, and certain processed cheeses contain tyramines, which can provoke these excruciating headaches.[114]

Since the brain is composed primarily of fatty tissue, special fatty acids could play a role in mental health. Seventy-seven percent of migraine headache sufferers were found to have unusually high rates of platelet aggregation (sticky blood cells that clot easily).[115] Fish oil contains EPA and DHA, which are special fats that can thin the blood and prevent this clumping from occurring.

These clumping blood cells could somehow create the agony of the migraine headache.

Or there may be some other means by which these fatty acids work in mental health. Cod liver oil supplements (2–6 tablespoons daily) provided noticeable improvement in the emotional disorders of eight psychiatric patients within six to eight weeks.[116] Modern diets contain less than one-fifth of the EPA that more natural and primitive diets used to contain. It would be interesting to find out how many migraine sufferers also have a family history of circulatory problems since these "sticky" blood cells are also prone to plug up the circulatory system. Since cod liver oil contains high levels of vitamins A and D, one teaspoon daily is the maximum dosage that should be taken for long periods of time without requiring some type of medical supervision.

Allergies also can cause headaches or major behavioral changes.[117] Proteins from food can be absorbed intact into the bloodstream, only to be attacked by a hypersensitive immune system, which turns on its own body in an autoimmune response. If the brain is attacked by the immune cells, swelling can occur, with radical shifts in emotions and intellect. More evidence is mounting that many childhood ailments, including bedwetting, asthma, skin and sinus problems, migraines, and hyperactivity can be caused by food allergies[118] (see Chapter 8 for more information).

An alarming array of pollutants also could influence mental health. Certain common metals, like lead, aluminum, cadmium, and mercury, can jam the normal workings of the brain. Lead is a heavy metal that may have contributed to the downfall of the Roman Empire, since the Romans used lead for drinking containers and water conduits. When lead gets into the brain, it sits on the receptor sites in the nerve cells, thus blocking neurochemical transmitters from doing their job. Lead toxicity is especially tragic in growing children, since their higher metabolic rate takes the lead into the body more quickly and deposits the lead in the vulnerable and rapidly growing brain. Up to one-third of all inner-city children have lead levels that may interfere with normal thought and emotions. A study in Boston of over 11,000 infants compared the amounts of lead found in the umbilical cord at birth with the amount of leaded gasoline sold in the area. The *relationship* between the two amounts remained constant. As the sale of leaded gasoline went up and down, so too did the levels of lead in the umbilical blood.[119] Chicago has banned the sale of leaded gasoline within the city limits. A new study from Harvard University found that levels of lead that were once considered harmless actually seriously reduce mental and physical abilities in humans.[120] Selenium competes with lead for absorption sites, so diets that are high in selenium absorb less lead.

The highest lead sources are polluted air (leaded exhaust from leaded gasoline) and industrial pollutants in the water and food supply. Smaller amounts of lead are found along the seam in canned food, in the plug in canned milk, and in dolomite tablets of calcium and magnesium.[121]

Cadmium is found in industrial pollution, canned foods, tobacco products, and other places. Mercury is an industrial pollutant in addition to being the solvent of choice to make tooth fillings (amalgams). Some dentists question the safety of using a poisonous metal in the mouth. Cadmium, mercury, and other toxic minerals could influence mental performance.

Aluminum is found in very high concentrations in the brains of Alzheimer's victims.[122] Alzheimer's disease is the most prevalent type of senility in Western society. (Aluminum and Alzheimer's disease are discussed in the section on mental vigor in Chapter 9.)

Aspartame is a relatively new artificial sweetener that contains the amino acid phenylalanine and is sold as NutraSweet or Equal by Searle Labs. Exorbitant amounts of NutraSweet have provoked epileptic-like seizures in people who were consuming two gallons of NutraSweet-flavored beverages daily.[123] In spite of 517 consumer complaints against aspartame, the Food and Drug Administration still considers aspartame to be safe.[124] *Something* in aspartame when consumed in ridiculous amounts can irritate the brain chemistry in some sensitive individuals.

There are probably many other substances that could cause havoc in the brains of certain people. That should not be too surprising. With many thousands of artificial agents added to our food supply; many thousands of questionable pollutants found in our water, air, and food; and thousands of other chemicals naturally found in food, there is a distinct possibility that one of these agents could antagonize certain sensitive individuals. Very few of these substances have been in the evolutionary scheme of mankind for more than a few decades. That is the proverbial wink in the eye of time. Pollutants, drugs, alcohol, caffeine, toxic metals, additives, and other substances can distort the normal chemical workings of a healthy brain.

MAINTENANCE

The brain, like all other parts of the body, must be repaired continuously. Vitamin B_{12}, folacin, zinc, and thiamine are important repair nutrients for the brain. Free radicals are produced in the normal course of life functions and can quickly destroy living tissue. Antioxidants, like vitamins A, E, and C and the mineral selenium, can all slow down oxidation in the brain. Since poor maintenance of the brain usually surfaces in later years, this topic is discussed thoroughly in the section on mental vigor in Chapter 9.

Vitamin B_{12} and folacin deficiencies could occur in older people, those with poor gastrointestinal health, those abusing alcohol,[125] those using long-term drugs,[126] vegetarians, and people under considerable stress. Also, dietary surveys find that about 40 percent of Americans do not even get two-thirds of their RDA for folacin, disregarding the complexities of absorbing it. For centuries, the dreaded pernicious anemia (B_{12} deficiency) was noted for slowly killing many older people. As humans age, the ability of the intestines to perform the juggling act of absorbing B_{12} often diminishes. The ability of the body to absorb folacin also diminishes as humans age.[127] The results of poor folacin and B_{12} status can be a slow mental deterioration. Some people may need injections to bypass the hindered absorption routes. Folacin has been successful in treating a variety of polyneuropathies (nerve disorders).[128] Folacin is also crucial to the reproduction of healthy DNA chromosomes. Injections of folic acid (50 mg daily, 125 times the RDA) reduced the incidence of damaged chromosomes in Down's syndrome children from 33 percent to 1 percent. Improvements in the behavior and appearance of Down's syndrome children were also noted in this study.[129] The same results have been seen in a recent follow-up study.[130] High-dose, broad-spectrum vitamin supplements have been able to improve the IQ of Down's syndrome children by an average of 10 points.[131]

There are other substances that influence brain maintenance. Scientists are only beginning to understand the role of trace minerals in brain growth and repair.[132] Orotate is a product that eventually becomes one of the nucleic acids. Supplements of orotate have been used to treat pernicious anemia (B_{12} deficiency.)[133]

Orthomolecular Psychiatry

It has been proven that some people are born with higher-than-normal needs for certain nutrients. Without the high-dose nutrients that these people need, various physical and mental problems set in. The benefits of high-dose supplements on Down's syndrome and autistic children are just two examples of genetic errors that probably increase the need for certain nutrients.

Professor Linus Pauling was one of the founders of the orthomolecular ("the right amounts of nutrients supplied to the cells") theory.[134] Orthomolecular psychiatry is an exact science that should only be practiced by qualified health care professionals. Orthomolecular psychiatry does not work in even a majority of mental patients. But if only 10 percent could be saved from the agony of mental illness and the stupor of drugs, then the effort would be worthwhile. Although this field is relatively new and very controversial, the risks are near zero, the benefits are many, and the costs are negligible when compared to long-term psychotherapy.

BRAIN DEVELOPMENT

All creatures develop their survival skills as early as possible in life. An African wildebeest can run with its mother only three hours after its birth. Speed is that creature's edge on survival. Humans rely on intellect for survival. The brain grows fastest early in life to allow each of us to be independent as soon as possible. By age five, the human brain has grown to 90 percent of its adult weight. By age seven, the brain is built, for better or for worse.[135] Perhaps you have noticed the disproportionately large heads on children. If the brain is not fed properly while in the uterus and during the first seven years of life, then the underdeveloped brain will be permanently and irremedially stunted.

This great waste of human talent occurs in millions of people around the world each year. Low food supply to children produces an ignorant adult, who has little to offer in job skills and gives no thought to family planning, has more children than can be fed, and whose children get the same low subsistence living, which perpetuates the vicious cycle, ad infinitum.

Spiritual possession rituals occur almost exclusively in regions of severe food poverty.[136] An adult brain that is underfed now and

was poorly nourished during development years is more susceptible to mental trances that are interpreted as spiritual possession.

Since most of you readers are probably older than seven years of
age, there is little that you can do about this part of your own brain
function. But there is much that a pregnant woman and her husband can do to nourish their child's brain to its fullest potential
(Chapter 11 contains the details on how to build an optimal brain
through optimal nutrition). There is a very definite timing mechanism built into the DNA machinery for brain growth. If the ideal
supply of nutrients is not present at the right time, then the brain
will not live up to that person's genetic potential.

NUTRITIONAL SUPPLEMENTS
DIETARY GUIDELINES

To maximize intellectual and emotional health, follow the Core
Diet, with the following special emphasis:

1. Minimize exposure to food additives, tyramine foods (e.g.,
sharp cheddar cheese and red wines), high-sugar foods, and caffeine.

2. See the chapter on food sensitivities and allergies for more
details on salicylates and other food factors that can influence
behavior.

3. Drink 5–10 cups of clean fluids daily.

4. Eat plenty of plant food for the potassium.

DAILY SUPPLEMENTS TO ADD TO YOUR
CORE PROGRAM

Vitamins
  Vitamin A   +10,000 IU
    (beta-carotene)
  Vitamin E   +200 IU
  Thiamine   +20 mg
  Riboflavin   +20 mg
  Niacin   +100 mg
  Vitamin B_6 +50 mg
  Vitamin B_{12} +100 mcg
  Folacin   +400 mcg
  Vitamin C   +2,000 mg
  Pantothenic acid   +50 mg

Minerals
  Calcium   +400 mg
  Magnesium   +200 mg
  Zinc   +15 mg
  Iron   +10 mg
    (women and children only)
  Copper   +2 mg
  Manganese   +7 mg
  Chromium (yeast)   +200 mcg
  Selenium (yeast)   +200 mcg

Quasi vitamins
  Choline   +2,000 mg (for memory, Alzheimer's, or muscle trem-
        ors)
   or as lecithin   +6 tablespoons daily
  L-carnitine   +500 mg
  EPA   +1,000 mg
  Myoinositol   +1,000 mg
  L-tryptophan   +2,000–6,000 mg (for insomnia, depression, or
          pain tolerance)
  L-tyrosine   +2,000–6,000 mg (for depression or stress)

11
THE REPRODUCTIVE SYSTEM
Making Healthy Babies

Pregnancy is one of the most common events in life, yet it is still one of the most miraculous. By the union of egg and sperm, a unique human being has been started. All the information needed to build and maintain this new human is encoded on the DNA molecule, which is invisible to all but the best microscopes. This fertilized egg will then begin the rapid cell division that eventually results in an adult of about 60 trillion cells. Nutrition relates intimately to this process of creating a baby. All of the raw materials needed by both mother and fetus come from the mother's diet. Breastfed infants continue their dependence on mother's diet as their sole source of nutrient intake.

Not long ago, the accepted thought was that babies were either healthy or not healthy. No shades of gray between these extremes were considered. If the infant bore no obvious signs of defects, then he or she was considered healthy, and all was well. That doesn't make good logical sense. Health is not like a light switch: either on or off. Health is a continuum, with limitless shades of disease, ill health, and decent health in between the extremes of death and optimal health. A mother may have smoked, drunk "socially," eaten poorly, and not exercised and said that her children were all

240

perfectly "normal." So obviously, this nutrition thing must not be important. Or is it?

Many nonnutrition factors contribute to the health of a baby: smoking, drugs, alcohol, age, infectious diseases (like German measles and herpes), genetic background, health care, hygiene, stress levels, past performance in childbearing, and so on. Yet nutrition is one of the most important factors that determines the outcome of pregnancy.

HOW NUTRITION AFFECTS THE BABY'S HEALTH

During World War II, both Holland and Leningrad were starved by the Nazi troops. The Dutch women had some increases in problems of delivery and smaller infants, and there were significantly fewer births, since many abnormal fetuses spontaneously abort. Yet the Russian women who were pregnant during this starvation era showed a major deterioration in the quality and quantity of babies produced. The stillbirth rate was twice normal. Prematurity increased by 41 percent. Many of the children who lived had low vitality, poor suckling ability, and reduced disease resistance.[1] The Dutch women fared better due to their better diets before the siege, indicating that nutrient reserves are important. The Russian women lived on the brink of starvation even before Hitler's troops came, so these women had no nutrient reserves to draw from in order to make healthy babies. Their starvation diet disastrously affected the outcome of their pregnancy. Hence, nutrition relates in two ways to pregnancy: (1) nutrient reserves, or what was eaten yesterday, and (2) current nutrient intake, or what is eaten today.

It's obvious that starvation influences the outcome of pregnancy, but what about those "shades of gray"? A classical study published in the *Journal of Nutrition* in 1949 compared the quality of the mother's diet and the outcome of her pregnancy. The study found a direct relationship between quality of diet and quality of infant. The better mother's diet, the greater her chance of having a healthy infant.

There are definitely shades of gray in the continuum of infant health. The Darwinian theory of survival does not recognize the states of "ideal" health or fulfillment of genetic potential. Those that survive to reproduce will pass on their characteristics. Many people will survive pregnancy, but few are given the best nutrient environment in which to thrive.

A study in rural Guatemala followed the course of 138 children from the prenatal stage through eight years of age. Those children who were provided with supplemental nutrition before and after birth showed more interest in their environment, were more explorative, and more involved in competitive games, and had greater persistence in doing frustrating tasks, better motor impluse control, and greater initiative than their unsupplemented but "normal" peers.[2]

The *Handbook of Nutrition*, written by the American Medical Association in 1951, states, "Life histories of patients and studies of their personalities have shown that the earliest effects of nutritive deficiency are not found first in severe physical ailments, but rather in the mental depression, nervous instability and other forms of personality changes."[3] In many people, low intellectual achievements and unstable behavior could be caused by marginal nutrition during developmental years.

Trace elements also play an important but poorly understood role in the building of the human brain.[4] An area of New Guinea has marginal levels of iodine in the soil and therefore also in the diet. Investigators gave one group of pregnant women injections of iodized oil and a control group injections of saline (saltwater) solution. Although the children born to the unsupplemented women were "normal" and without defects, the children of the iodine-supplemented mothers later scored much higher on all tests of manual dexterity and motor coordination.[5] Normal nutrition produces "normal" children. Better nutriton produces "better" children, in both mental and physical parameters. This study shows us again that there are limitless levels of nourishment and that each stage may bring incremental improvements in the physical and mental well-being of that child.

What does iodine deficiency have to do with a wealthy nation like America? In spite of seemingly adequate iodine intake, 23–36 percent of the 9- to 15-year old children in rural Kentucky were found to have goiter (clinical iodine deficiency).[6] No one could explain why, since iodized salt allegedly wiped out goiter in America. Nor can anyone predict how many children have marginal health due to a less detectable level of iodine deficiency.

In a Canadian study, 325 infants were followed from birth through age three. Infants who received regular nutritional supplementation had fewer illnesses and gastrointestinal upsets than the unsupplemented group.[7] A professor at Northwestern Medical School in Chicago found 16 infants who had been diagnosed with the elusive "failure to thrive" syndrome, which is a common label for sick infants in the U.S. Fifteen of these children had marasmus (severe calorie deficiency), while the 16th child had both marasmus and kwashiorkor (severe protein deficiency).[8] Although all of the children had been admitted to a modern, big-city hospital, none had been given a nutritional analysis. One physician finds that many children who are not growing adequately are also not eating well.[9] He suggests that, before anxious parents jump into growth hormones for their small children, they should try nutrition counseling. Ironically, nutrition is rarely considered, although it seems like such a blatantly obvious and simple solution to many health woes in America.

Scientists at UCLA found that supplements given during pregnancy lowered the risk for premature delivery, spontaneous abortion, and low-birth-weight infants.[10] In the same study, the women who were given zinc in their supplements had markedly fewer hypertensive problems of edema, high blood pressure, eclampsia, and toxemia.

Most of us have "normal" physical and mental health. But how much better could our minds and bodies perform if given more than just survival nourishment during early growth years? Returning to that mother who boasted that she didn't follow all of these nutrition rules during pregnancy and her kids turned out all right, is "all right" good enough for your kids? Could they have been more vigorous, more resistant to disease, more intelligent, more rational, and just generally "better" if ideally nourished? The answer is "probably yes."

If all of this is so, then the best-fed kids should also grow the tallest. So shouldn't the biggest children also be the brightest? In a nation of such mixed ancestry as America, that is not necessarily true. But in a country where the people are more homogeneous in their genetic background, such as India, that theory should apply. In a study of 250 children, ages four and five, from rural and urban homes in India, the tallest children scored the highest in IQ tests.[11]

Height and weight as well as head, arm, and chest circumference were accurate predictors of intellectual abilities.

Researchers provided groups of pregnant lab animals with varying levels of folic acid and/or vitamin C. The group that was receiving the Recommended Daily Intake (RDI) for both folic acid and vitamin C had an average size and number of pups per litter with a small percentage of defective pups lost. Supplements of four to five times the RDI for vitamin C and folic acid increased the size of pups, number in each litter, and reduced the number of defective pups lost. Nutrient intake levels that had no effect whatsoever on the mother had devastating effects on the viability of the newborn pups. Supplements of folic acid reduced embryonic deaths, while supplements of vitamin C increased the size and weight of the pups.[12] When you consider that roughly half of all conceived human fetuses will spontaneously abort before coming to term, this study begins to mean something to human pregnancy. Of live human births, approximately 1 out of 100 infants will require some type of special care for a handicap, illness, or defect.[13] Some of this high infant mortality and birth defect rate may stem from "normal" nutrition.

Sixty-five percent of all infant deaths occur in neonates who weigh less than 5.5 pounds (2.5 kg) at birth.[14] Small babies are not as well prepared to survive on their own. Nutrition is *the* most crucial factor in getting that fetus to adequate weight. Weight is a prime indicator of fuller organ development and viability. Yet nutrition is still considered a secondary topic in many clinics and hospitals.

Optimal nutrition could probably *eliminate* some infant health problems and signficantly *reduce* the incidence of others. A little time and money spent on nutrition during these critical foundational years could save money, pain, tears, and lost potential later on. A mother's diet while pregnant may dictate whether her child will later develop diabetes.[15] After age seven, the brain is built.[16] Good or bad, the quality of the brain and its ability to live up to its genetic potential are based to a large extent on the quality of the diet for those first few years of life. We must feed these young people well. Malnutrition in developmental years can permanently and irremedially erode IQ and behavior.

HOW COMMON IS MALNUTRITION IN PREGNANT WOMEN?

Of 76 healthy pregnant women examined in one study, 78 percent had at least one glaring vitamin deficiency, if not more.[17] Over half of the women in this study took supplements containing folic acid and iron, with few taking any supplemental zinc. Since both iron and folic acid compete with zinc for absorption, supplements of iron and folic acid can make a marginal zinc deficiency even worse. In spite of taking nutritional supplements, there were common deficiencies of folic acid; vitamins C, A, B_6, and B_{12}, and niacin among the 174 pregnant American women who were examined in another study.[18]

Vegetarians can be healthy, nourished people. Yet they must be very nutrition-wise, especially during pregnancy and lactation, lest their marginal deficiencies register as full-blown problems in their young. Zinc, protein, B_{12}, iron, B_6, copper, and other nutrients must be conscientiously searched out in the vegetarian diet. Some pregnant American women cannot afford good nutrition. For others, apathy or ignorance may limit their nutritional support of pregnancy.

Pica is the compulsive eating of non-foods, like clay, paint chips, etc. Pica causes malnutrition, since these people fill up on non-foods. Pica also may be the result of malnutrition, since scientists think that pica is related to the pregnant woman's higher needs for iron, zinc, and other nutrients.[19]

Physicians found that various vitamins existed in different ratios between mother and fetal blood supply, indicating that some vitamins and minerals can literally be pumped into the placenta, while others can only passively diffuse. For some nutrients, the mother's blood supply offers the fetus only what can be spared. Hence, mother may be reasonably healthy, yet have precious little nutrients left over for the developing baby. This could lead to problems at delivery and later on for this growing human.

WHAT OPTIMAL NUTRITION CAN DO FOR INFANT AND MATERNAL HEALTH

1. Nearly eliminate certain major birth defects, like spinal bifida and fetal alcohol syndrome.

2. Extend gestation by at least one week while also encouraging fetal growth. This longer gestation improves organ development, which increases the viability of the newborn infant.

3. Reduce the frequency of spontaneous abortions and other problems of delivery.

4. Markedly lower incidence and severity of maternal health problems that risk the birthing procedure, like hypertension, edema, preeclampsia, and toxemia.

5. Eliminate certain health risks to mother, such as osteoporosis, infections, colds, hemorrhoids, gallstones, and premature tooth loss. These problems could occur in the mother after the infant scavenges on mother's marginal nutrient supply.

6. Raise the physical, intellectual, and emotional health of most infants several steps beyond "normal."

It requires about $200 to provide good nutrition supplements to a woman throughout her pregnancy and lactation. It costs about $100,000 to keep a premature infant in intensive care for a month. It costs several million dollars for the government to provide lifetime institutional care for defective infants. Healing nutrients are both humane and cost-effective. What are we waiting for?

How various nutrients can contribute to infant and maternal health is detailed on the following pages.

PROTEIN AND CALORIES

The most important risk factor in neonatal health is size. As mentioned, 65 percent of all newborn deaths occur in neonates under 5.5 pounds (2.5 kg) at birth. A small infant is more likely to occur in women who smoke, drink excessively, gain too little weight, or have twins.[20] A small baby is usually somewhat underdeveloped. The lungs, kidney, liver, immune system, and other vital functions are not ready to make that infant independent of its mother's womb. Of all the raw materials needed to build a healthy baby in the uterus, the bulk items of protein and calories are the most critical.

Fetal development is the primary period in a human being's life when new brain cells are being developed. A low-protein diet during this phase stunts the number of brain cells and produces a smaller brain.[21] This smaller brain has a different behavioral response and is less tolerant of its environmental changes.[22] A smaller brain also has a lower learning capacity and may have certain emotional quirks that do not surface until later in life. A low-protein diet during pregnancy will even induce poor cold adaptation in the infant.[23]

How many extra kilocalories and how much extra protein should a pregnant woman consume? How much weight should she gain? For many years, health care professionals recommended that women gain minimal weight during pregnancy, because this would produce a small baby; which would be easier to deliver. The objective of this plan was to provide less pain and risk for the mother and less effort for the physician. Yet the same baby that was

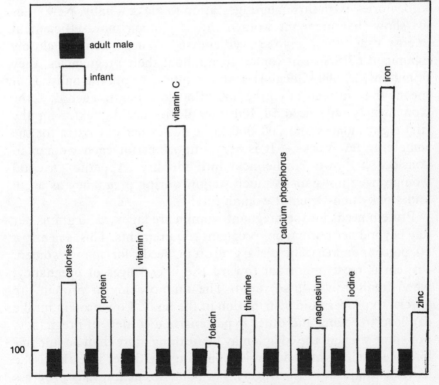

Relative to their body weight, an infant has impressive nutrient needs. Per unit of body weight the nutrient needs of a 3-month-old infant are far greater than the average adult male.

SOURCE: Hamilton, E., et al., NUTRITION: CONCEPTS AND CONTROVERSIES, p. 413, West Publishing, St. Paul, MN, 1985

easy to deliver often was difficult to keep alive, due to underdeveloped organs. Depending on the mother's size and the father's size (which are both influential in predicting the infant's size), the mother should gain between 20 and 30 pounds by the delivery date. Even women who are overweight are still encouraged to gain at least 15.4 pounds (7 kg).[24] Mothers should go on a weight reduction program *after* the baby has been nursed, not while it is totally reliant on mother's diet for crucial raw materials.

The RDA for energy for the pregnant woman is an extra 300 kilocalories per day beyond her normal intake. Yet that estimate is based on the premise that pregnant women need roughly 80,000 kilocalories extra throughout gestation to make a baby. New studies show that pregnant women may be much more efficient at energy usage than anyone ever guessed. When scientists closely examined 67 Scottish women throughout their pregnancies, they found only 20,000 kilocalories were required to build a baby. That means that, instead of eating 300 kilocalories extra each day, the woman may only need 50–100 kilocalories per day extra for the first eight months and 200–300 kilocalories per day extra for the remaining few weeks.[25] It is very important for each woman to consider her own biochemical individuality. A petite Oriental woman need not gain as much weight during pregnancy as a tall and stocky non-Oriental woman might.

Protein needs for the pregnant woman are an extra 30 grams per day beyond her normal nonpregnant requirements. This is nearly a 50 percent increase in dietary protein needs for many women. Protein is most important toward the later stages of pregnancy, when fetal growth is so rapid. The amino acids in protein are crucial to proper fluid distribution in the body. Low-protein intake can lead to edema and other hypertensive disorders of pregnancy. For some women, the edema may be nothing more than an uncomfortable swelling in their ankles (pushing the finger into the tissue leaves an imprint of the finger). For some women, it may progress into dangerously high blood pressure or a high loss of protein in the urine. These women are at great risk of having difficult deliveries. Preeclampsia and eclampsia are conditions that often follow the hypertensive problems of pregnancy. Eclampsia can involve convulsions, coma, and even death during delivery. A high-quality, high-quantity protein diet is one way to guard against these problems.

By eating optimal amounts of protein and kilocalories during pregnancy, assuming that food is reasonably dense in other nutrients, the mother has taken a major step toward ensuring the health of the baby and herself.

ZINC

Zinc is probably the most versatile of all the minerals in the human body. Zinc is a component of at least 80 different enzyme systems, involving DNA replication, protein growth, and many other functions.[26] The body has many ways to store various nutrients, including calories, protein, iron, calcium, and others. Yet there is no way to "stockpile" zinc for periods of great demand, like pregnancy. Zinc is important for both maternal and fetal health, but it is in low supply in the American diet.

Pregnant women with marginal zinc stores are more likely to have:

- a Caesarian birth or smaller infant.[27]
- an infant with lower weight, less muscle mass, higher serum glucose, larger liver, elevated liver glycogen and liver fats.[28]
- a smaller, less healthy baby with various complications at delivery.[29]
- an infant with a smaller-than-genetic-potential brain.[30]
- toxemia and/or an infant with birth defects.[31]
- any of the hypertensive disorders of pregnancy (edema, proteinuria, toxemia, eclampsia).[32]
- a growth-retarded infant who is also more likely to die in infancy.[33]

Low levels of zinc slow down the ability of the body to utilize protein for growth.[34] Zinc deficiencies are common in children with retarded growth.[35] These zinc deficiencies are not isolated to war-torn starvation areas of the world. Growth retarded children in Denver[36] and Baltimore were found to have a very high incidence of zinc deficiencies.[37]

Not only is zinc intake important, but the balance between zinc and other nutrients is also crucial. As mentioned earlier, both iron and folacin seem to compete with zinc for intestinal absorption sites. The greater the folacin[38] or iron[39] intake, the less zinc will be absorbed. Most prenatal nutrition supplements used throughout the last two decades have contained large amounts of iron and folacin, with little or no zinc. Hence, some of these supplements, due to their poor design, may make a bad situation even worse. When investigators looked at 450 women in Ohio receiving normal medical care and routine vitamin and mineral supplements (high in folacin with little or no zinc), they found high folacin levels in the body to be a *risk* factor in a poor outcome of pregnancy.[40] Of 53 nursing women studied, 98 percent of those not taking a zinc supplement were getting less than two thirds of their RDA for zinc.[41] Twenty-nine percent of these unsupplemented women were getting less than one third of the RDA for zinc.

Fetal Alcohol Syndrome (FAS) is a collection of abnormal physical and mental traits that are common in infants born to alcoholic mothers. Ten of the 31 heavy drinkers (32 percent) who were followed in one study gave birth to infants with blatant FAS.[42] More subtle infant defects also are caused by alcohol.

Since alcohol uses up body zinc stores, it is possible that heavy drinking merely worsens a marginal zinc deficiency. There are striking similarities between the offspring born to alcoholic mothers and those born to zinc-deficient mothers. Zinc supplements during pregnancy may be able to mollify some of the effects of moderate drinking on the developing fetus.[43]

Both zinc and iron are commonly low during fetal and infancy stages of life.[44] Of the 24 pregnant women in one study, only those taking supplements of zinc and copper had adequate serum levels of these two trace minerals.[45] Preterm infants, especially those fed exclusively on breast milk, need zinc supplements in order to maintain adequate serum zinc levels.[46] It is important that copper, iron, folacin, and zinc arrive in a reasonably balanced formula in the diet of a pregnant woman. Excess of one can create a deficiency of another.

Supplements of 28 milligrams daily of zinc showed no adverse effects in human studies.[47] Zinc levels are very influential on cell divisions, such as occur in pregnancy.[48] When zinc concentrations are optimal, cell division occurs normally. When zinc supplies are low or excessive, cell division slows down or becomes more error prone. Zinc supplements also were able to reduce the rate of spontaneous abortion and birth defects in one study.[49] And in a variety of ways, zinc influences brain development.[50] So, depending on the quality of the woman's diet, she should take zinc supplements of 10–30 mg daily while pregnant and lactating. This is a perfectly safe range.

The average American is at least marginally if not significantly deficient in zinc.[51] Since the RDA for zinc for a pregnant woman is 20 mg daily, and the average woman consumes only 10 mg, a supplement containing at least 10 mg of zinc would be highly recommended during pregnancy. Zinc supplements are probably needed for the lactating woman, too. In 23 breastfeeding women studied, the mean zinc intake was less than half of the RDA.[52] In order for a lactating woman to get the RDA of zinc in her diet, she would have to consume 4,500 kilocalories of normal American food per day. That is just not practical or recommended. Nature shows us the importance of zinc with human milk containing special proteins that enhance zinc bioavailability to the nursing infant.[53]

Once weaned at six months to one year of age, the infant can be given nutritional supplements in liquid drop form containing 5 mg of zinc daily. Ten milligrams of zinc supplements during childhood and 15 mg during adolescence would continue this nutrition protection program.

FOLACIN

Although the RDA for all nutrients increases when a woman becomes pregnant, only the need for folacin *doubles*. Folacin is a key nutrient in new cell growth, such as occurs in fetal development and infancy.

Folacin deficiencies are quite common in pregnancy.[54] Folacin supplements can often alleviate the anemia problems that pregnant women encounter, even when extra iron intake does no good. Folacin is important in making new red blood cells.

Neural tube defects (NTD) are one of the most common birth defects known.[55] Two out of every 1,000 live births have NTD (a.k.a. spinal bifida) in which the brain or spinal cord is not well developed or is even outside of the body. Many of these infants die. It was once thought that neural tube defects were an inherited disorder that could not be treated or prevented, short of genetic counseling. Yet some keen minds noticed that poor people had a much greater incidence of NTD, and diet and hygiene became suspected causes of NTD. By reviewing records, investigators found a strong relationship betweeen poor diet and higher rate of NTD.[56] Irish people living in Boston had a much lower NTD rate than Irish people living in Ireland.[57] Hence, the theory that NTD was totally inherited was ruled out.

A study of Welsh women found that NTD occurred almost exclusively in women who ate almost no green vegetables, salad, or fresh fruits. Women who had NTD infants often lived off of convenience foods, white bread, sugar, and fried foods.[58] At the same time, three French studies covering 310 pregnant women found a definite link between the levels of folacin in the pregnant woman's blood and the outcome of the pregnancy. Low folacin often led to preterm or low-birth-weight infants.[59] Researchers gave a multivitamin supplement to over 1,000 women who were at high risk to have an NTD baby. The supplements dropped their risk seven-fold when compared to unsupplemented women.[60]

Several hundred other women who had NTD infants were gathered into another study. Of the women who received nutrition supplements, 185 became pregnant. Two-hundred-sixty-four of the women who did not receive supplements later became pregnant. The recurrence of NTD infants in the unsupplemented control group was 11.5 percent, while the supplemented group had only 0.6 percent recurrence of NTD.[61] This means that unsupplemented women had a 1,900 percent greater chance of having an NTD baby than the supplemented mothers.

In a 5-year double-blind study involving 905 Welsh women, those who had previously given birth to an NTD infant and who took their nutritional supplements had zero recurrence of NTD. Of those high risk women who were given a placebo, 6 gave birth to another NTD baby.[62] In other words, folacin supplements nearly *eliminated* NTD among high risk mothers.

Yet, ever the skeptics, scientists immediately planned other studies to corroborate these findings. Many other health care professionals and scientists questioned the ethics of trying to get more results when so much was already known. If more studies were mounted, then many NTD infants would be born that could have been avoided.[63] How much evidence is needed? That's exactly what the women in the new studies were asking themselves. As of June 1984, doctors at 27 different medical centers had agreed to participate in further tests involving folacin and NTD. Yet 25 percent of the women who were recruited into the study declined to continue. Two thirds of these women dropped out because they felt that the evidence warranted taking supplements rather than diddling with another study.[64]

Overall quality of diet, especially folacin, riboflavin, and ascorbic acid, has also been related to NTD.[65] Folacin requires some minor "digestion" in the intestines, as well as activation in the body in order for the active version of folacin to be available for new cell growth. Some people do not activate folacin well.[66]

Folacin is probably related to other defects of fetal growth. Eighty women who had already given birth to cleft palate and harelip infants were given multivitamin supplements. Two-hundred-twelve other women who also had conceived cleft palate and harelip infants would not accept the supplements and therefore served as controls. Only one percent of the supplemented group had recurrent harelip infants, while 7.4 percent of the unsupplemented group (15) had harelip infants.[67] Not taking supplements increased the risk by over 700 percent.

In one study, folacin supplements taken during pregnancy increased the average length of gestation by one week, with major improvements also noted in the height and weight of the newborn.[68]

Most prenatal supplements provide at least the RDA of folacin for pregnant women (800 mcg), if not more. Folacin supplements are essential during pregnancy and lactation to minimize risks and provide optimal health to mother and child.[69] Folacin is so critical to the outcome of pregnancy, and is so easy and cheap to add to food, that many areas of the world have considered fortifying some common food product with folacin, just as Americans add iodine to salt.[70] Such supplements would probably become a very cost-effective prophylactic against serious and expensive birth defects.

VITAMIN B_6

Since vitamin B_6 is essential for protein metabolism, and since protein need goes up dramatically during fetal development, B_6 is a critical nutrient during pregnancy.[71]

Many American women are low in their intake of B_6. A study of pregnant women conducted by the U.S. Department of Agriculture found that the mean intake of B_6 in pregnant women was roughly half of the RDA. Lactating women were consuming less than two thirds of the RDA for B_6.[72] And the RDA may be hazardously low for pregnant and lactating women. For instance, in one study there was not enough B_6 present in the infants' milk until the mothers were taking supplements containing 20 milligrams of B_6 (eight times the RDA).[73] Follow-up studies found the same results: that the RDA for B_6 in lactating women does not provide enough B_6 in breast milk.[74] Although none of the infants at the lower intake levels showed any overt clinical symptoms of B_6 deficiency, can we be sure these low levels of B_6 in breast milk are adequate to provide for optimal growth in the infant? Many drugs, including oral contraceptives, increase the body's need for B_6. Pregnant women who were also taking a drug to treat tuberculosis (isoniazid), had their B_6 requirements skyrocket to 50 mg, which is 20 times the RDA.[75]

Some of the typical problems of pregnancy may be due to marginal intake of B_6. Due to the demands of pregnancy, many women develop prediabetic symptoms (i.e., fatigue, thirst, frequent urination, and poor wound healing), which then go away shortly after childbirth. Supplements of B_6 have been used to improve carbohydrate tolerance in pregnant women and eliminate these prediabetic symptoms.[76] Some infants have an inborn error of metabolism that raises their needs for B_6. Without large doses of B_6, these infants go into convulsive seizures and die.[77]

Injections of B_6 (100 mg) in newborn infants were shown to enhance the oxygen transportation ability of the newborn's blood significantly.[78] Supplementation of vitamin B_6 during pregnancy and lactation is important for the optimal health of both mother and infant.[79]

OTHER B VITAMINS

Biotin is a B vitamin involved in energy metabolism and other functions. The blood levels of biotin drop off noticeably in pregnant women and continue to dwindle throughout gestation.[80] This may mean a need for more biotin in the diet during pregnancy. Few vitamin companies put biotin in their products, since it costs about $7,000 per kilogram or $3,180 per pound. Yet supplements containing 300 mcg daily of biotin (the USRDA) could be a wise investment for the expecting mother.

A B_{12} deficiency can lead to brain damage in the vulnerable developing infant.[81] Since vitamin B_{12} is found primarily in animal foods, vegetarians are at risk for low levels of B_{12}. However, a few plant products like spirulina (ocean plankton), tempeh and miso (fermented soy products), and lactobacillus bacteria (found in live cultured yogurt), and brewer's yeast are decent sources of B_{12}.

ALCOHOL AND CAFFEINE

Alcohol is not nutritious. But, by virtue of its seven kilocalories per gram, it *is* a nutrient. The most harmful effects of short-term alcohol excess (i.e., the hangover) can eventually be reversed in the adult. Not so in the pregnant woman. Alcohol is a fetal toxin. It poisons the cell differentiation process that is turning a fertilized egg into a complete, miniature human being. In the last decade, Fetal Alcohol Syndrome (FAS), has become a widespread, recognizable cause of abnormality in infants. Thirty to 70 percent of all children born to heavy-drinking mothers (five–six drinks/day) will have blatant FAS.[82] FAS is the third leading cause of birth defects in America. FAS infants often have a flat, blank-looking face. The upper lip is thin, and the body is hairier than in other infants. They cry more often. The list of physical and mental defects that can accompany FAS is extensive.

Alcohol has long been known to affect pregnancy. Roman and Greek mythology referred to it. In Carthage, newlywed couples were forbidden from drinking wine on their wedding night in order to avoid bearing a defective child. The Bible (Judges 13:7) states: "Behold, thou shalt conceive and bear a son, and now drink no wine or strong drink." In 1834, a report to the British House of Commons noted that infants born to alcoholic mothers had "a starved, shrivelled, and imperfect look."[83] At the turn of the century in America, a higher rate of abortion was noted among alcoholic mothers. Are there shades of gray in between blatant FAS and perfect health? How much alcohol is too much? Can small amounts also do harm?

In one study, 144 social-drinking pregnant English women (ages 19–35) were followed from two months of gestation to term. All were in good health. None were alcoholics or smokers. By consuming only one drink per day, these social drinkers decreased the average birth weight of males by 225 grams, or about 1 pound.[84]

The female infants were apparently unaffected by this moderate alcohol intake. Other health care professionals suggest that one drink per day might be safe.[85] Abstinence would be the safest route. Short of that, one drink daily sipped slowly with a meal would minimize the risk to most well-nourished (especially in zinc levels) pregnant women.

Similar effects have been seen with caffeine. When pregnant lab animals were fed caffeine that would equal 12–24 cups of coffee daily for humans, 20 percent of the pups were born with partial absence of toes.[86] At caffeine intake that would equal two cups of coffee daily, the rat pups had retarded bone development. A Belgian study found that 23 percent of the human mothers who gave birth to abnormal babies had consumed eight or more cups of coffee daily.[87] Compared to the population at large, this means that heavy coffee drinking or the coffee drinker's lifestyle (tobacco, sugar, etc.) increases risks for a defective baby 20- to 200-fold. Human studies find that moderate (two or fewer cups daily) coffee intake does not increase the risk for blatantly abnormal human infants.[88]

Yet scientists asked the same question about coffee that they had about alcohol: "Are there finer shades of infant impairment from moderate coffee drinking?" Pregnant rats were given injections of caffeine that would resemble moderate coffee drinking in humans. Although there were no apparent differences in the caffeine pups, all pups were studied for the next seven months. The pups of the "coffee drinking" mothers avoided the center of the testing apparatus and spent more time in the corners and more time grooming.[89] These caffeine pups were more timid and less adventuresome. Somehow the coffee had subtly influenced voluntary motor activity and behavior, although no obvious defects were present. The moral of the story with respect to coffee and alcohol is: "Less is better, and none is best."

CALCIUM AND MAGNESIUM

Probably the greatest risk *to mother* during pregnancy is the various forms of hypertensive disorders that strike: high blood pressure, edema, toxemia, protein in the urine, preeclampsia, and eclampsia. Five to 10 percent of all American pregnancies are affected by one of these disorders, which account for 50,000 maternal and fetal deaths annually. When any of these hypertensive problems are present during pregnancy, the risk of a difficult and dangerous delivery increases.

Researchers at Johns Hopkins University find that a higher calcium intake lowers the risk for eclampsia during pregnancy,[90] which makes perfect sense. Recall the role of calcium in lowering blood pressure in nonpregnant adults (see Chapter 5). A pregnant woman is adding about 30 percent extra blood and nearly 50 percent extra fluid to her body, which creates quite a strain on her kidneys' filtration abilities. Extra calcium during pregnancy can reduce the risk of toxemia.[91] Extra calcium in the diet also can inhibit the abnormal rise of blood pressure that often occurs during pregnancy.[92]

Low calcium intake during pregnancy also results in the growing fetus robbing the mother's blood supply of calcium, which depletes maternal bone stores and may lead to osteoporosis later in life. So, not only is the developing infant's health dependent on mother's diet, but *mother's* health is also dependent on her diet.

Magnesium must be in balance with calcium in a one-to-two ratio. Magnesium supplements have also been quite effective in treating preeclampsia in pregnant women.[93] Magnesium deficiency causes spasms in the placenta and umbilical cord, which explains why intravenous magnesium has been very effective in preventing premature labor.[94] Magnesium also is important to proper muscle relaxation.

Forty percent of Americans consume less than two-thirds of the RDA for magnesium. For pregnant women, the need for magnesium goes up nearly 50 percent, meaning that nearly all pregnant women get too little magnesium.

IRON

Iron anemia is another common problem of pregnancy and infancy. The woman's blood volume increases by 33 percent, some for herself, some for the placenta, and some for the circulatory system of the developing infant. In low socioeconomic groups, about 30 percent of the infants are anemic, with another 25 percent being iron-deficient.[95] One out of four infants with normal hemoglobin levels show an increase in hemoglobin when given iron supplements. This finding indicates that perhaps "normal" hemoglobin for infants is slightly anemic. Behavioral and intellectual changes occur in the iron-deficient infant. Nine- to 12-month-old infants without iron anemia, but with iron deficiency, were given intramuscular injections of iron and retested seven days later for mental development. These infants showed major improvements in their test scores after iron supplementation.[96]

Iron-deficient infants also are often irritable and lack interest in their surroundings. Anemic infants are tense, less active, more fearful, and less responsive to their environment. Often, only two to four weeks of iron therapy can drastically improve the behavioral problems of iron-deficient infants.[97] Iron is involved not only in bringing oxygen to the brain but also in the construction of important brain chemicals, like serotonin, dopamine, and noradrenaline. Iron supplements (15–60 mg daily) are recommended for all pregnant and lactating women.[98] Since the iron found in breast milk is much more available than that in infant formula, breastfed infants of well-nourished mothers may not need iron supplements until six months of age.[99]

IODINE

Iodine is a trace mineral involved in thyroid function. Thyroid output regulates basal metabolism, which increases by about 25 percent toward the end of pregnancy. When a pregnant woman or an infant suffers from iodine deficiency, the results can be permanent and irremedial cretinism: an intellectual idiot. Marginal deficiencies of iodine may create children with lower motor coordination and manual dexterity.[100] In regions of China where iodine deficiencies are common, the children *without* iodine deficiency often have poor hearing, which could be a result of marginal iodine intake.[101]

As mentioned earlier in the chapter, a large percentage of "normal" schoolchildren in the U.S. have been found to have clinical goiter.[102] But why anyone but the most destitute of Americans would have a blatant iodine deficiency is something of a mystery. Not only is salt iodized in America, but iodine-based detergents used in the dairy industry have bolstered milk products to become very rich sources of iodine.[103]

SELENIUM

Selenium is a very important trace mineral involved in slowing oxidation throughout the body and also stimulating the immune system. Selenium is a potent protector against harm from pollutants. Pollutants are likely responsible for a sizeable percentage of slight to severe birth defects in America. Selenium is in marginal supply in the American diet. Selenium from specially cultured brewer's yeast is a particularly potent form of selenium, passing into the breast milk more readily than inorganic versions of selenium.[104]

VITAMIN D

Vitamin D is responsible for directing calcium metabolism, which goes on at a very rapid pace throughout fetal development. The infants of women who did not use vitamin D supplements had low calcium levels in their blood, and many had defects in their tooth enamel.[105] In a double-blind study using 18 American infants, those given vitamin D supplements had much higher bone mineral content at 12 weeks of life than those who were given a placebo.[106] Either regular sunshine exposure or vitamin D supplements are probably mandatory for both pregnant and lactating women.

Vegetarian mothers and their infants who live in sun-poor areas are at great risk for developing rickets.[107] Even in the sun-drenched regions of the Middle East, well-intentioned mothers are hiding their babies from the sun and creating epidemic proportions of rickets in their infants.[108] Rickets is also very common among Canadian Indians.[109]

A teaspoon of cod liver oil daily for the pregnant and lactating woman can provide 1,120 IU of vitamin D, 11,500 IU of vitamin A, and appreciable amounts of the special fatty acids EPA and DHA. Do not take excessive amounts of these fat-soluble vitamins A and D, however, especially when pregnant.

VITAMIN A

Vitamin A is intimately involved in cell differentiation, skin integrity, disease resistance, and other functions. Deficiencies of vitamin A are common in the U.S.,[110] and low vitamin A levels may be related to the lung problems that premature infants have. Sixty-two percent of the 91 preterm infants examined had blatant vitamin A deficiencies.[111] RDA-level supplements of vitamin A were not able to improve the condition of these distressed infants.

Preformed vitamin A from animal foods can be toxic to the pregnant woman and may even cause birth defects.[112] One woman was taking 150,000 IU of vitamin A daily for several months for her acne. Through ultrasound examination, her fetus was determined to be deformed and was terminated.[113] Toxicity from the plant version of vitamin A, beta-carotene, is unlikely. And even normal commercial baby foods can provide impressive amounts of beta-carotene. One 10-month-old infant was brought to the hospital with orange discoloration of her skin. She was experiencing beta-carotene overdose from her food supply. She had been fed two jars of baby food daily, primarily pureed carrots, and thus was getting 8–10 times her RDA for vitamin A.[114] Though beta-carotene does not present nearly as many risks as vitamin A does, pregnancy is no time to experiment with megadoses. Keep vitamin A intake under 20,000 IU daily and beta-carotene under 50,000 IU while pregnant.

VITAMIN K

Vitamin K is involved in blood clotting and possibly other functions. Most people get plenty of vitamin K, compliments of their intestinal bacteria, which produce it. Since infants are born with sterile guts, they have no intestinal bacteria or vitamin K, and hemorrhaging can be a real hazard in neonates. Intravenous vitamin K given to the infant shortly after birth protects them from such a risk. Oral doses of vitamin K for lactating mothers will provide much needed vitamin K in the breast milk.[115] Giving oral doses of vitamin K (0.5 mg) at birth is now common practice in most U.S. hospitals.[116] Vitamin K supplements were also able to relieve the nausea of pregnancy in some women.[117]

VITAMIN C

Vitamin C is one of the nutrients that is actively pumped from the mother's bloodstream into the placenta for fetal use. When researchers examined 200 nursing mothers, they found a six-fold variation in the levels of vitamin C in their blood and a two-fold difference in the levels of C in their milk.[118] Some people are more efficient than others at using their vitamin C supplies. These scientists remarked, ". . .marginal intake [of vitamin C] in lactating mothers is more common than assumed for a well-nourished population."

Pregnant women often develop hemorrhoids, which are an indication of fragile blood vessels. When 200 mg daily of rutin (a bioflavonoid) and 500 mg of vitamin C are provided to these women, the hemorrhoids usually clear up quickly.

Levels of vitamin C decrease in the woman's blood as pregnancy progresses, which indicates that more C is needed in the final stages of rapid growth. Oral contraceptives also increase the need for vitamin C. Many women go straight from the high vitamin C needs of birth control pills into the higher vitamin C needs of pregnancy. And many get a cold, which often hangs on throughout pregnancy, indicating that a nutrient need is not being satisfied. One thousand milligrams daily of vitamin C during pregnancy and lactation will nutritionally protect both mother and infant, while posing no risks to either.

Once again, don't experiment with excessive doses during pregnancy. In one study, pregnant women taking large doses (usually at least 5,000 mg daily) of vitamin C gave birth to healthy babies, who soon thereafter developed symptoms of scurvy.[119] These infants had been raised in a fetal environment of large doses of vitamin C and had been forced to suddenly accept much smaller portions of vitamin C. As a result, deficiency symptoms set in. Supplements of vitamin C in progressively smaller doses completely remedied the problem for these infants.

Do things gradually, both in life and in nutrition. You need to warm up and cool down before and after your exercise. You also need to gradually change dietary habits to allow the body to accommodate these transitions.

SPECIAL FATTY ACIDS

Americans definitely eat too much fat. Yet we also eat the wrong kinds of fats. Certain fatty acids are mandatory for human health, and there is a direct relationship between the types of fats found in mother's diet and the types of fats that the fetus will receive.[120] One type of fat, linoleic acid, is found in plant oils like corn, soy, and safflower oil and is a known essential nutrient. The linoleic acid of sunflower oil was used effectively to treat the hypertension of pregnancy.[121]

The fatty acids eicosapentaenoic acid (EPA) and docosahexaenoic acid (DHA), which are primarily found in fish oils, are now thought to be essential nutrients in human nutrition. These special fats provide the raw materials to build prostaglandins and cell membranes, all of which are very important to the developing infant.

But some people may not be able to make enough of these special fats from the essential fatty acid of linoleic acid. And with 60 percent of the fats in America being hydrogenated and thus losing their special fatty acid capabilities, some pregnant women and their developing infants could be suffering from deficiencies of various types of special fatty acids.

Seventy percent of the human brain is fatty tissue. Certain fats, like DHA, play integral parts in the early development of the brain. DHA is found primarily in brain tissue, mother's milk, and fish oil. The retina of the eye and sperm also contain some DHA. When nursing mothers were given supplements of fish oil, the levels of DHA in their milk rose quickly and dramatically.[122] When the body takes on a substance so readily, it often indicates that subsaturation levels were there to begin with. Animals raised on diets deficient in DHA develop impaired vision or retarded mental functions. While breast milk has varying small amounts of DHA, infant formulas have none. Since DHA is found in very low levels in the American diet, and DHA serves a vital role in brain development, fish oil supplements could be important during fetal growth and infancy. A teaspoon of cod liver oil and a teaspoon of linseed oil daily in the pregnant woman's diet would probably provide some very important fatty acids for the developing fetus.

Gamma linolenic acid (GLA), often called evening primrose oil, is another unique fat that may be important in fetal development. GLA has been used to treat the hypertension of pregnancy,[123] as well as preeclampsia.[124]

CARNITINE

Carnitine is a substance that is crucial to the fat-burning process. We eat some carnitine through animal foods, or we make some carnitine within us, but few people probably make saturation levels of carnitine.

Reye's syndrome is an inflammation of the brain that is most common in children who are recovering from a viral infection, such as chicken pox. Carnitine has the ability to trap some of the toxic compounds that are produced in Reye's syndrome that can lead to fatty infiltration of the liver.[125] Carnitine is poorly produced by newborn infants and is found in near zero levels in formulas.[126] Many scientists feel that carnitine may be an essential nutrient for newborns and definitely is an essential nutrient for preterm infants.[127] Without adequate carnitine, the body develops problems in burning fats, which carries over into abnormal protein and carbohydrate metabolism.

VITAMIN E

Infants are born with precariously low levels of vitamin E. Premature infants have even smaller vitamin E stores. Premature infants often have difficulty breathing on their own and are placed in oxygen tents. Vitamin E is an antioxidant nutrient. With low levels of the antioxidant vitamin E and exposed to concentrated oxygen intake, and above-normal amounts of the oxidizing oxygen in their blood, premature infants are at serious risk of going blind as the oxygen attacks their retina (retrolental fibroplasia, or RF). Each year, 1,300 infants lose some of their vision, and another 250 infants lose most of their vision due to this condition. In a controlled study with premature human infants, oral vitamin E (100 mg/kg of body weight) significantly reduced the severity of RF in all treated infants.[128] These physicians were so impressed by the effectiveness of vitamin E that they recommended vitamin E therapy for all premature infants exposed to oxygen-rich environments. When injections of vitamin E were used in premature infants, a lower rate of brain hemorrhaging (intraventricular hemorrhage) was also found by researchers as an added bonus.[129]

However, there is some question about the safety of the synthetic derivative injections of vitamin E that were developed to treat some premature infants. Oral therapy of natural vitamin E, in contrast, has been found to be quite safe and effective in raising plasma tocopherol (vitamin E) levels.[130] More than coincidentally, early breast milk has high levels of vitamin E, which slowly subside as time goes on.[131]

SMOKING

Smoking is a major risk for the developing fetus. In over 30,000 California women studied, premature infants were 20 percent more likely to occur in pregnant women who smoked a pack of cigarettes daily than in those who did not smoke. Smoking mothers were 60 percent more likely to have a premature infant (born after less than 33 weeks of gestation).[132] Smoking women are 100 percent more likely to have a small (less than 5.5 pounds) infant, which is a major risk factor in infant sickness and death.[133] Nicotine from cigarettes lowers the production of prostacyclin, a potent hormonelike substance that is essential to health, in the human uterus during pregnancy.[134] Cigarettes also seriously reduce the levels of vitamin C and other nutrients in the body of the pregnant woman. Smoking women are much more likely to give birth to an infant with cleft lip and palate.[135] The damage from tobacco products could be in the toxins that they bring or in the prostacyclin and nutrients that they destroy.

In a study of over 12,000 pregnant Boston women, investigators found that heavy coffee users smoked three times as much as women who did not use coffee or tea, and these coffee drinkers also weighed more.[136] So it may be the overall disastrous lifestyle of some people that creates the problems in pregnancy: smoking, coffee, overweight, no exercise, etc.

AFLATOXIN

Aflatoxin is a deadly substance that is produced by certain microorganisms that are living on improperly stored legumes and grains. Peanuts and beans that are stored in damp climates are very likely sources of aflatoxins. In adults, aflatoxins can cause liver damage. In pregnant women, aflatoxins may cause mental retardation in the newborn.[137] A region of rural Georgia has nearly twice the rate for mental retardation as the nation at large. The diet of women in that area may contain high amounts of aflatoxin, which could account for the high rate of mental retardation.

SALT AND SUGAR

A woman's taste buds do change during pregnancy. Pregnant women have a stronger yearning for salt, probably due to the increased sodium needs during fetal development.[138] Therefore, pregnant women must be careful that these taste bud changes do not chaffeur them into eating high-salt junk foods rather than nutritious foods.

Large amounts of refined sugar are probably not good for the pregnant woman or her unborn child. Pregnant lab animals were fed diets high in either cornstarch, refined sugar, or unrefined sugar. Eighty-five percent to 100 percent of the pups from the unrefined-sugar group survived, compared to only 30–75 percent survival rate in the refined sugar and cornstarch groups.[139]

BREASTMILK

For millions of years, nature has been perfecting and refining an infant formula that is specifically tailored to the needs of human infants. That formula is mother's milk. Nobody does it better, though many have certainly tried. Breastfeeding is a major health advantage to both mother and infant. Nutrition experts at Cornell University in New York have predicted that infant mortality in underdeveloped nations would be doubled if infants were not breastfed.[140]

And yet, probably not long after Eve's first child, women were wondering if alternatives to nursing were available. The Louvre in Paris has a relief painting depicting a woman holding a nursing bottle with one hand and a stick to stir the formula in the other hand. This picture was found in a palace in the Tigris and Euphrates river basin and is considered to have been painted around 888 B.C., making infant formulas nearly 3,000 years old.[141] Alternatives to breastfeeding were most consistently presented to royalty and aristocrats because they allowed these mothers more freedom in their "royal" schedules. The earliest attempts to feed human infants some type of animal milk resulted in a 95 percent mortality rate.[142] The poor hygiene of milking a dirty and dung-clad goat or cow made animal milk nearly lethal to human infants. But since people are attracted to the practices of the wealthy, the trend away from human milk continued, in spite of these early disastrous attempts.

The incidence of Americans nursing their young hit a nadir in the 1950s and 1960s, with only 11 percent of mothers nursing for at least six months. With renewed awareness of the advantages of breastfeeding, this trend has since reversed itself. By 1969, 19 percent of white women and 9 percent of black women were nursing. By 1980, those numbers had risen to 51 percent of whites and 25 percent of blacks.[143] Women who are better educated, wealthier, and living in the western U.S. are more likely to nurse than others.

Advantages to the Infant

The case in favor of human milk for human babies would fill a textbook the size of the New York phone directory. For the first 10 days after birth, a thin milk called *colostrum* is produced. Though lower in nutrient density, this early milk is incredibly rich in immune bodies.[144] The newborn infant has been living in the semisterile environment of the mother's womb for roughly nine months. Now it is time to face the nonillions of pathogenic organisms that inhabit our planet. Through lactation, women are able to bestow their accumulated adult disease resistance upon their newborn infants. A major threat to live births is infection. With the vast arsenal of immune factors contained within mother's milk, the baby has a very good chance of avoiding many infections.[145]

Breastfeeding also helps to lower the likelihood of the infant's developing allergies now or later on in life.[146] Nursing reduces the chance of overfatness in the infant, since the baby suckles until satiated and then quits. With bottle feeding, mothers have a tendency to encourage the infant to finish the bottle, which may add fat cells that can make weight control a lifetime battle.

Breastfeeding also costs less. The La Leche League, a group of women who encourage other mothers to nurse, has estimated that one year of nursing saves about $500 over infant formulas. Nursing is convenient and very sanitary, while the same cannot always be said for infant formulas.

Mother's milk is always the right temperature and concentration, with no chances of errors in mixing. Infants have died from consuming too concentrated a mixture of formula.[147] Many infants in Third World countries have died from starvation due to overly diluted formulas.

The nutritional advantages of mother's milk are almost overwhelming. The quantity and quality of human milk are suited to human needs, rather than cow's milk for calves' needs. There are substances in human milk that help the infant's immature digestive tract to break down protein.[148] Human milk contains more lactose, less sodium, more cholesterol, more essential fatty acids, high absorption efficiency of the vitamins and minerals, ideal zinc to copper ratio, less phosphorus, twice the efficiency of calcium absorption, less strontium, less trace element impurities, and more selenium than cow's milk or formula. With the shape of the human nipple and the mouth exercises that are required to nurse, the breastfed infant is more likely to have proper mouth and tooth formation. Each of these points is a nutritional advantage of breastmilk.

Higher cholesterol levels than formula or cow's milk may not seem like an advantage of breastmilk—formula manufacturers didn't think so either, and they omitted the cholesterol with the boast that their product was superior. Not so. Breastfed infants have lower rates of heart disease. Cholesterol is the precursor to form the fatty wrapping (myelin sheath) around all nerve cells and to make vitamin D for calcium metabolism, bile salts (for fat digestion), and part of all cell membranes. Cholesterol is essential to all humans and particularly critical to growing infants.

Infants with bilirubinemia, a jaundice condition that can jeopardize the vulnerable growing brain, were given 300 mg of orotate daily. Orotate is a substance not required in the diet, but made in the body. There was a 700 percent reduction in the number of orotate-treated infants who had to have blood transfusions.[149]

With each new discovery about human milk, this wondrous compound becomes more impressive:

- Formulas contain more aluminum, which could become toxic to an infant with poor kidney filtration abilities, than human milk.[150]

- Choline is important to brain development and function. A unique array of choline precursors are found in human milk, providing the infant as much choline as is found in an adult's diet.[151]
- Taurine is a maverick amino acid that is found in high levels in early human milk and is thought to participate in the growth of the brain and sense organs.[152] In animal studies, taurine-deficient diets have been linked to vision and growth problems. In genetically susceptible lab animals, taurine-deficient diets produced epilepsy. Taurine is now considered by some noted scientists to be essential for infants.[153]

Advantages to the Mother

Nursing creates a substance in mother's body (oxytocin) that causes her abdomen to contract, which quickly shrinks her understandably distended figure back into normal shape. Breastfeeding also requires about 700–800 kilocalories daily, which is equal to running about 9–10 miles per day. Although nursing mothers are encouraged to consume an additional 500 kcal per day to provide energy and raw materials for their milk, these women will still be able to lose weight. Nursing also is a marginally effective means of birth control, since *most* women do not ovulate while lactating. Also, mothers who nurse have a lower incidence of breast cancer.

Limitations of Breastfeeding

Are there any limitations or special notes of caution with breastfeeding? Yes. Breastmilk is produced in the mammary glands of the breast. The raw materials to produce milk come from the mother's diet. Thus, the quality of mother's diet will be reflected directly in the quality of the milk that she is producing. A well-nourished mother can properly nourish her infant with nothing but breast milk for up to 12 months.[154] However, most studies find that the average Amerian diet needs supplements in order for the infant to receive high-quality breast milk.[155] As previously mentioned, B_6 supplements of 5–10 times the RDA are required in order for the nursing mother to provide enough B_6 in her milk.[156] *Premature* infants do not get enough riboflavin from normal mother's milk.[157] In famine-stricken regions of the world, breast milk can be low in quality and quantity, thus not only starving the infant, but also draining emergency nutrient supplies from the malnourished mother.

Also, with respect to at least some nutrients, the quality of milk declines as mother continues to nurse. Forty mothers who nursed beyond seven months had their milk evaluated on a monthly basis. Concentrations of zinc, calcium, vitamin B_6, and vitamin C decreased over the months.[158] Levels of folacin remained unchanged up to 25 months into breastfeeding. Magnesium began decreasing only after 18 months. This fading quality of milk may be due to a dwindling supply of mother's nutrient reserves, or to changes that take place in mammary glands, or to nature's assumption that other foods besides milk will be introduced after six months. When mother's diet is marginal, the quality of her milk is marginal.[159]

Rest and emotional support are very important for the nursing mother. Stress can dry up breast milk production as fast as malnutrition. The active ingredient in certain foods (like onion, garlic, coffee, and others) can pass into the breast milk and change the flavor of the milk and may cause irritation in the infant. A mother also may express a food allergy through her breast milk. When a group of lactating women with colicky babies stopped drinking cow's milk, one-third of their colicky babies got better.[160] In some cases, mother's diet can affect the infant's behavior through unknown factors that are passed in breast milk.

Most physicians and nurses agree that a mother who wants to breastfeed can do so. Very few women actually have physical limitations. Sore breasts can be treated with a topical application of vitamin E (one gelatin capsule of 400 international units) after each feeding.[161] When mother is working out of the home, she can pump her breasts and give this milk to the babysitter and thus still provide her infant with some of the advantages of breastfeeding.

NUTRITIONAL RECOMMENDATIONS
DIET FOR PREGNANT WOMEN

Follow the Core Diet with the following special modifications:

Dietary Guidelines
1. Consume often: whole grains, fresh fruits and vegetables, low-fat dairy, meat, fish, and poultry. Beyond mother's normal needs, an extra 10 g daily of protein is required during the first trimester of pregnancy; in the last two trimesters, add 30 g per day. During early pregnancy, an extra 50–100 kilocalories daily are

needed; in the later stages of pregnancy, energy needs increase by an extra 200–300 kilocalories daily. Plan on gaining 20–30 pounds by term (36–40 weeks after conception).

2. Avoid: tobacco, alcohol, caffeine, all but the most essential prescription drugs, any illicit drugs, food dyes, MSG, poorly stored beans and nuts, bizarre eating behavior (pica), weight reduction attempts.

3. Minimize: consumption of sugar, artificial sweeteners.

DAILY SUPPLEMENTS TO ADD TO YOUR CORE PROGRAM

Vitamins
Vitamin A   +10,000 IU (2,000 RE)
(beta-carotene)
Vitamin D   +400 IU
Vitamin E   +200 IU
Vitamin K   +100 mcg
Vitamin B_6 +20 mg
Vitamin B_{12} 100 mcg
Folic Acid   +400 mcg
Biotin   +300 mcg
Vitamin C   +1,000 mg

Minerals
Calcium   +600 mg
Magnesium   +300 mg
Zinc   +15 mg
Iron   +30 mg
Copper   +2 mg
Iodine   +150 mcg

Quasi vitamins
Carnitine   +500 mg
EPA   +1,000 mg
(also contains some DHA)

FOOD INTRODUCTION PROGRAM FOR THE FIRST YEAR OF LIFE

1. Breast milk exclusively until at least 6 months and longer if mother and infant so desire. Gradually wean to cup by age 12 months.

2. At 6 months, one feeding per day of iron-enriched rice cereal, or mashed potato pudding with milk and fruit juice. Live cultured yogurt can be served.

3. At 7 months, pureed green and orange vegetables, such as squash, peas, and carrots. Introduce only one new food per week to note for allergic reactions.

4. At 8 months, pureed fresh fruits.

5. At 9 months, pureed meats or other foods high in protein and iron for vegetarian families. Egg yolk can be cooked into the cereal or mashed potato pudding.

6. At 10 months, chopped finger foods. Avoid raisins and other similar foods that can be aspirated.

7. At 12 months, wean to cup. Many foods may be chopped and served from the dinner table, which hopefully is loaded with nourishing foods. Children learn more by example than instruction.

12
THE REPRODUCTIVE SYSTEM
Libido, Potency, Fertility, Premenstrual Syndrome

"A man comes to me, suffering from cancer, TB, or many other dangerous diseases, and, in addition, he is impotent. He says, 'Doctor, fix up the impotency and let the cancer go hang.'"
"Doctor" John Romulus Brinkley

Food, water, air, sleep, and sex are our basic physical needs—not necessarily in that order of importance. Sex is many things to many people. It can be adult play time, intense emotional bonding, reproduction of the species, physical release, and more. But many things can go wrong in sex:

- *Impotence* in the male can be due to psychological problems, hormonal imbalances, nutritional deficiencies, or even obstructed blood vessels.
- *Infertility* in the male can be caused by low sperm count, clumping of sperm, or reduced sperm vitality. In the female, infertility can be due to no egg or an unviable egg, blocked ovarian tubes, or a high-acid uterine environment that kills the sperm.
- *Premenstrual syndrome* is linked to the woman's regular ovulatory cycle. PMS has both physical and emotional symptoms that disrupt the woman's life and the lives of those around her.

Healing nutrients can help some of these sexual problems.

272

IMPOTENCE

If prostitution is the world's oldest profession, then impotence is probably one of the world's oldest diseases. Impotence clinics have moved from practicing questionable techniques in dingy back rooms to today's scientific approaches that are used in the most respected clinics.

Is modern man more sexually vulnerable, or are people just beginning to accept a problem that was once hushed? Whatever the case, it is unfortunate that the nutritional solutions found in this chapter are rarely offered at even the most sophisticated impotence clinics.

There are many possible explanations for male impotence. Disease (like venereal diseases), drugs, tobacco, alcohol, and psychology are nonnutritional explanations for impotence. Also, it has been said that "sexual performance depends more on what's between your ears than on what's between your legs." Very true.

Few American men seem to be intimidated by the prospect of heart disease, in spite of roughly one million American deaths each year from circulatory disorders. But many of the same men are terrified by the idea of impotence, or the inability to produce an erection. Yet, the same plugged-up vessels that cause a heart attack can also cause a flaccid penis. Researchers examined 440 men, age 40 years old and older, all with impotency. Ninety-two percent of these patients were found to have at least two major risk factors toward heart disease. Eighty percent were found to have definite occlusions in various blood vessels in the body.[1] Vascular obstructions could cause their impotence. The penis is an intricate maze of tiny blood vessels with valves to trap the blood when an erection is to be produced. Clogged vessels could hamper both heart contractions and penis erections.

Another sexual dysfunction that relates to the blood vessels is hypertension. At least half of the 50 million hypertensive people in this country are on some type of medication to lower their blood pressure. In many males, this medication seems to have the side effect of impotence (see Chapter 5 for more on how to maintain healthy blood pressure without drugs).

The average American eats one half to two thirds of the recommended intake for zinc, which is involved in making sperm, the matrix fluid that the semen is carried in, and the male hormones for sexual desire. Artificial kidney machines are inefficient at recycling zinc as they attempt to filter the blood of the dialysis patient. From 48 to 80 percent of male renal dialysis patients experience impotency.[2]

Twenty healthy hemodialysis patients were given either 50 mg of zinc acetate daily or a placebo. The 10 treated patients experienced significant increases in their testosterone (male hormone) levels and sperm count.[3] These patients also reported an improvement in potency, libido, and frequency of intercourse.

Mild zinc deficiency can lead to a low sperm count.[4] Zinc supplements can increase the sperm count and testosterone levels in "normal" healthy people who have only a mild zinc deficiency.[5]

As children enter the chrysallis of adolescence, their "normal" serum zinc levels increase, in both males and females,[6] indicating that sexual maturation requires impressive amounts of zinc. Zinc supplements may relieve impotence in some men. Taking 50 mg of zinc gluconate daily for two months will either improve sexual abilities or prove that something else was the problem.

MALE FERTILITY

Arginine is an amino acid that is involved in the making of sperm. Thirty-nine percent of 178 men with low sperm levels experienced major improvements in their sperm count when given arginine supplements, and 13 pregnancies resulted.[7] These impressive results were produced by 10–20 grams of L-arginine daily for three months.

Often, male infertility is due to sperm clumping. When more than 20 percent of the sperm clumps, that person is labeled "infertile." In a study of 35 men with at least 33 percent sperm clumping, 1,000 mg of ascorbic acid daily for three weeks gave these men a 14-fold increase in their serum ascorbic acid levels and a 67-percent drop in sperm clumping. Now, only 11 percent of their sperm clumped.[8]

Carnitine is found in high levels in sperm. Carnitine supplements were able to improve the motility and fertility of the sperm in some patients.[9]

FEMALE FERTILITY

Serious malnutriton is known to erode sex drive and the ability to reproduce. When women fall below about 10 percent body fat, they cease menstruation. The body seems to be saying, "If there isn't enough food available to sustain a pregnancy, why even start one?" Certain animals will reabsorb an abnormal fetus, rather than just rejecting it and wasting the nutrients in the material. Humans do not have this option. So, pregnancy during sessions of unpredictable food intake can be hazardous to both mother and child. In underdeveloped nations, thinner women also begin menopause earlier.[10] Fertility in women can be a direct result of their nutritional status.

Too much or too little vitamin A can seriously affect a woman's menstrual pattern. An extreme excess of beta-carotene (vitamin A) can cause disturbances in menstrual rhythms.[11] Yet vitamin A supplements can reduce the flow and discomfort of heavy menstrual periods.[12]

In women with unexplained infertility, vitamin B_6 supplements provided a high conception rate.[13] B_6 is also valuable for relieving the symptoms of PMS, as will be explained later. B_6 can apparently help to stabilize the erratic flow of both progesterone and estrogen, which are two key female hormones. In other words, B_6 can help the woman who wants to get pregnant to do so and help the woman who doesn't want to get pregnant to experience a more comfortable estrus cycle.

GENERAL SEXUAL NEEDS

Sexual problems can stem from a poor attitude, which can be a result of malnutrition (see Chapter 10 for more on how to deal with that issue). Sex problems can also be caused by low energy levels, which can be caused by poor nutrient status (see Chapters 4 and 18 for more on that). Obese individuals often experience lost libido, lower potency, or just plain no willing partners (see Chapter 13 to treat that problem). Diabetes, hypertension, and vascular disease can infringe upon normal sexual abilities (see Chapters 5 and 14 for more information). Much of sexual problems can be psychological. With an interested and interesting partner, the mind is more likely to be an eager participant in regular sex. Venereal diseases can lead to sexual dysfunctions. See your physician for more on this issue.

PREMENSTRUAL SYNDROME

In the late 19th century, Lydia Pinkham offered her 30-proof concoction of alcohol and herbs as a solution to "female complaints."[14] She made a fortune. Her product is still manufactured outside of the United States for her devoted customers. For the vast majority of mankind's history, women who have "female complaints" have been ignored, misunderstood, heavily sedated, or labeled hypochondriacs by a predominantly male medical group. No longer. In 1984, a woman in Great Britain pleaded temporary insanity for murdering her husband due to her premenstrual syndrome (PMS). She was acquitted. The hormonal changes taking place in the PMS woman can indeed provoke radical mood swings and aggression.[15]

PMS is both serious and widespread. The hormonal deficiency of progesterone that often accompanies PMS has been shown to increase the risk of breast cancer by over 540 percent.[16] In many people, proper nutrition can seriously reduce the symptoms of PMS. In some people, nutrition can literally be the cure.

Symptoms of PMS usually begin about 10–14 days before the onset of menstruation, although timing varies considerably among women. Symptoms can include radical mood swings, tender breasts, acne, fluid retention, weight gain, binge eating (especially on sweets, salt, and chocolate), insomnia, depression, awkwardness, and fatigue.[17] Many women go to their doctors because they feel they are "going crazy," only to find out that PMS is their problem. For many women, just knowing that others share the same experience provides some encouragement. Somewhere between 30 and 60 percent of healthy menstruating women have some degree of PMS. Not only is PMS common, but it often appears to be an indicator of other health problems. Over half of the PMS patients studied were found to have some other female abnormality, including endometriosis (a condition of uterine cells growing elsewhere in the woman's pelvic area) and fibroids.[18] No one knows exactly what causes PMS. Current best guesses are a hormonal imbalance, a nutritional problem, or a psychosomatic condition. PMS is definitely linked to the woman's hormonal tides that instigate ovulation.

Physicians and scientists began to wonder why the well-nourished healthy woman was much less likely to suffer from PMS. Since that initial curiosity, many nutritional links to PMS have been found. The intake of caffeine directly influences the prevalence and severity of PMS.[19] Caffeine intake (coffee, tea, cola, chocolate) is also a risk factor in fibrocystic breast disease.[20] Supplements of vitamin E can help this breast condition. Seventy-five women with fibrocystic breast disease and PMS were given vitamin E (alpha tocopherol) in double-blind fashion. After two months of therapy, in varying levels of intake, 300 international units of vitamin E daily proved to substantially relieve breast tenderness and other symptoms of PMS.[21] A follow-up study found the same results.[22]

Vitamin B_6 also shows great promise as an effective treatment for PMS. Twenty-one of 25 PMS patients given 500 mg of B_6 daily in sustained-release form had signficant relief of their symptoms.[23] B_6 was also effective in preventing PMS fluid retention, weight gain, and acne.[24] (See Chapter 19 for more on acne.) Avoid excessive B_6 intake, since large doses of B_6 (as low as 200 mg daily) for long periods of time (months) may cause reversible nerve damage in some people.[25] Doses of 50–150 mg of B_6 daily will help most women without presenting any risk.

Oral glucose tolerance curves change during the PMS phase in many women.[26] Yet hypoglycemia does not cause PMS, nor does PMS cause hypoglycemia. Hormonal rhythms probably cause the change in glucose tolerance. Sugar does play a role in this condition, though. Many women report an irresistable urge to binge on high-sugar and high-salt foods during their PMS phase. The ensuing weight gain could be from the extra calories consumed or the fluid retention via the high salt intake. Sugar also causes a loss of magnesium from the body, which is definitely related to PMS. Sugar also stimulates the production of greater amounts of insulin, which promotes fluid retention. Complex carbohydrates slow the passage of glucose into the blood and lower the insulin response.

Dietary fats can influence PMS. Animal fats encourage the production of arachidonic acid and then the prostaglandin PGF, which in turn will discourage the production of progesterone (the female hormone).[27] This may worsen PMS. A diet high in polyunsaturated plant oils contributes much linoleic acid, which is converted in the body to gamma-linolenic acid (GLA) for the production of prostaglandin PGE. This seems to help PMS. A high-meat diet has also been found to alter normal hormonal and menstrual cycles in women.[28] GLA, a.k.a *evening primrose oil*, has been tested as a treatment for PMS, and initial results were good.[29] Yet follow-up studies did not have the same sterling results. The jury is still out regarding any benefits that GLA may confer on PMS patients.

Magnesium has several roles in treating PMS. Magnesium is one of the nutrients involved in converting dietary linoleic acid to linolenic acid, which can alleviate PMS symptoms.[30] Zinc, vitamin C, and niacin are also involved in this essential fatty acid conversion process. Magnesium helps to regulate levels of brain dopamine, a vital chemical for balanced thought and emotions. By consuming excess calcium, magnesium intake could be reduced, since these two minerals compete for absorption sites. In one interesting study, a group of chronic female criminals consumed an average of twice the milk of noncriminal females.[31] Milk has much calcium and negligible magnesium. Subclinical magnesium deficiencies are common among Americans, with women consuming an average of 250 mg, compared to the USRDA of 400 mg.[32] PMS often mimics a magnesium deficiency, causing various problems in the nervous and muscular systems.

Tyrosine is an important amino acid that provides the raw materials for dopamine and noradrenaline (two vital chemicals for thought and emotions) in the brain. Low levels of tyrosine have been found in depressed patients.[33] Up to 6 g daily of L-tyrosine have been effective in clinical trials in treating certain types of PMS depression.

There are many nutrients that relate to the onset and severity of PMS. There is no one nutrient that is the "magic bullet" against PMS since different women have differing nutrient deficiencies. In a double-blind study, a broad-spectrum vitamin and mineral supplement was quite effective in treating many PMS patients.[34]

Two-thirds of the alcoholic women studied could relate their drinking bouts to their menstrual cycle.[35] Not only can alcohol create or worsen nutritional deficiencies, but it is also a depressant and lowers blood sugar.

Lead prevents estrogen (the important female hormone) from binding to its receptor sites in the body. Lead toxicity is becoming a growing concern in the U.S., from leaded gasoline emissions, lead-seamed food cans, lead in the water supply, lead paints, and industrial pollutants. Lead toxicity is more likely to occur in urban areas and could definitely be a factor in some cases of PMS.

The favorite nonnutritional treatment for PMS is progesterone, followed by estrogen, lithium carbonate (for psychotic symptoms), aspirin for aches, diuretics for fluid retention (probably overused), and bromocriptine danazol for breast swelling. Exercise is unquestionably the cheapest, most effective, and least risky method of treating PMS. It reduces stress, helps you lose weight, regulates appetite, and provides major relief for other symptoms.

Placebo treatment improves as much as 53 percent of PMS patients,[36] so it is important to provide psychological support for the PMS sufferer in addition to optimal nutrition.

NUTRITIONAL RECOMMENDATIONS FOR PMS

DIETARY GUIDELINES

1. Emphasize regular exercise.

2. Minimize consumption of alcohol, tobacco, caffeine, sugar, and salt.

3. Lower your intake of meat products.

DAILY SUPPLEMENTS TO ADD TO YOUR CORE PROGRAM

Vitamin B_6 +50 mg
Vitamin E   +100 IU
Magnesium   +500 mg
Chromium   +200 mcg
 (from yeast)
GLA   +300 mg
EPA totaling   +5,000
L-tyrosine   +3,000 mg

13
EATING DISORDERS
Obesity, Anorexia, Bulimia, Pica

"Then I tried the Chinese restaurant diet . . . all you can eat with one chopstick."

Robert Orben

When most people picture someone suffering from malnutrition, they see a starving child with protruding ribs and the look of death in his or her eyes. But malnutrition actually can be caused by an excess, a deficiency, or an imbalance of nutrients. Right now, the most prevalent form of malnutrition in America is overfatness; too many calories. Most creatures spend most of their lives in constant pursuit of food. Yet today most Americans have transcended this hand-to-mouth subsistence. We have access to more food than ever before in history. This newly acquired privilege may take some getting used to. Food has become more than just biochemical nourishment for many Americans. It has become a reward, an emotional retreat, the glue to bind a social gathering, oral gratification, the epicenter of family occasions, isolated stabs at pleasure in an otherwise unpleasant life, and an emotional outlet for an entire attic full of psychological problems.

OVERFATNESS

According to the height-weight tables developed by the life insurance companies, about 40 percent of Americans are over-

280

weight. According to new "percent body fat" standards, that percentage would about double. After all, the *quantity* of body weight is not nearly as critical as the *quality* of body weight. Some people may look decent in clothes and be relatively normal in comparison to the height-weight tables, yet they are overfat from lack of exercise. Hence, *overweight* is being replaced with *overfat* as a more accurate description of people whose percentage of body fat is too high.

Overfatness is a major health risk. Make no mistake about it. Obese individuals are at a much higher risk of developing hypertension, stroke, kidney failure, cirrhosis of the liver, appendicitis, hernia, gallstones, back problems, and auto accidents. (Obese individuals often have poor spatial orientation and coordination. This increases their chances of getting in a car wreck.)[1] Overfatness increases the risk of colon, breast, prostate, and endometrium cancers.[2] Heart disease risk is doubled, and the risk for diabetes is quadrupled for overfat people. Obese people are usually sick more often, live less vigorously, and die sooner. The image of the jolly corpulent person living a continuous belly laugh is a myth. Overfat people are more prone to depression.[3] Altogether, obese people have enormous health problems to face. Obesity is a deep rut to escape from, yet the potential benefits make the effort most worthwhile.

Overfatness is considered to be the easiest condition to diagnose and the most difficult condition to treat. That is only partly true, because it's not always obvious that someone has a weight problem.

The most common means of detecting overweight has been the bathroom scale. For many decades, people have awakened to the morning ritual of weighing themselves. This is usually a very bad way to start the day. For most people, the scales provide continuous reinforcement of their worst fears. And the scales are not really an accurate indicator of the quality of body weight. Some people can actually gain weight on a successful diet. By exercising and eating properly, they may lose weight to a point where the heavier muscle mass begins replacing the lighter fatty tissue. Although the news on the scale is depressing, that person looks better, feels better, is healthier, and has accomplished his or her goal of improving the quality of body composition. Thus, percent body fat is a better method of determining who has a weight problem.

There are numerous means of determining percent body fat. Since fat floats and lean mass doesn't, underwater weighing is the standard of accuracy. Since lean mass conducts electricity and fat doesn't, measuring electrical resistance is also accurate. Since approximately half of all body fat is in the skin region and is there to insulate the body thermally, skinfold thickness can also be an accurate assessment of percent body fat.

The most practical home method is the skinfold measurement. Note, however, that men and women deposit their body fat in different regions. Measure the thickness of a pinch of skin just above the hip bone for men or women, or on the back of the arm (women) or mid-thigh (women). If this skinfold is less than an inch in thickness, you have done well in your fitness program, or perhaps you are successfully starving yourself in anorexia. If the skinfold thickness is one to two inches, it is time to reactivate your interest in proper eating and exercise. If the skinfold thickness is greater than two inches, then "red lights" are flashing on your dashboard. Heed the warning signs before it becomes too late. Overfatness can be a deep pit to climb out of.

CAUSES OF OVERFATNESS

Genetics plays a role. Children of two obese parents have an 80 percent chance of becoming obese themselves. Overfatness may be an inherited vulnerability.[4] Obese children chew their food less and eat faster.[5] Some people are very calorie-efficient and hence more likely to store their food calories as body fat.[6] A study of over 6,000 adults found that obese individuals did *not* eat more than their normal weight peers, even when exercise levels were taken into consideration.[7] Because of the variability in fuel efficiency, the dogmatic expression "3,500 kilocalories equals a pound of body fat" should be used more as a guide than as an inflexible law.

The sodium potassium pump is a mechanism in all body cells that regulates the concentration of electrolytes inside and outside of the cells. The difference in electrical potential between inside and outside the cell is what creates low-level electricity, or the "battery" of each living cell. How efficiently this pump works can influence how likely someone is to store excess food calories as body fat.

Vanadium is a trace element that may direct the sodium potassium pump. Human foods contain even lower vanadium concentrations than the amount that resulted in a vanadium deficiency in lab animals.[8] Thus, a marginal vanadium deficiency may retard the efficiency of the sodium potassium pump and essentially lower the fuel burning rate for that person. The net effect might be unexplainable weight gain, which resulted from eating too much junk food. Vanadium is found primarily in plant foods and unrefined foods.

Yet, in most instances, the greater the amount of additional fatty tissue on that person, the *higher* his or her basal metabolism.[9] Thus, for most people, rotundity is not caused by an economical metabolism.

Obese individuals have 18–25 less trytophan circulating in their brain, which could create depression or even changes in eating habits through low serotonin levels.[10] Obese people have a lower tyrosine-to-norepinephrine conversion rate in the brain, which could also lead to altered behavior.[11] Cocaine abusers have a higher-than-normal incidence of eating disorders.[12] The question then arises, "Do the changes in brain chemicals cause the overeating, or does the overeating cause the changes in brain chemicals?" Could it be that certain brains are more prone toward addictive behavior? If not food, then would drugs, alcohol, or gambling be their outlet? No one knows yet. But many people with eating disorders do have a different chemical environment in their brain that could be responsible for changes in thought and appetite. (See Chapter 10 for more information on how nutrition can influence the brain chemicals that encourage healthy thought processes.)

There is a constant discussion among scientists about which has a greater influence: nature (genetics) or nurture (lifestyle, such as diet and exercise). Lifestyle definitely influences weight problems.[13] Social and psychological factors play important roles in one's girth. Children are greatly influenced by their parents. In families where regular activity and proper eating habits were encouraged, pre-school children had better nutrition habits and were slimmer and more active.[14] In studies involving over 100,000 people, low-income people (especially women) were much more likely to have a weight problem than wealthy individuals.[15] There is also a strong relationship between hours of TV watched and incidence of obesity.[16] TV viewing burns almost no calories and encourages continuous trips to the refrigerator.

Do not be discouraged if you have developed bad eating and lifestyle habits. Your parents probably thought that they were doing their best. Take charge of your habits today and change them for the better. Others have done it. Why not you?

Many people are overfat because they have no idea of portion control. On diet histories, men underestimated their calorie intake by an average of 500 kilocalories daily, while the women missed the mark by an average of 900 kilocalories daily.[17] When you consider that the average American adult only needs about 1,500 to 2,500 kilocalories per day to maintain their weight, these portion control oversights become significant. People who overeat may have a quicker stomach emptying time, thus making them hungrier sooner.[18] In some cases, overfat people do not eat more than others, but they do drink more alcohol than others. Alcohol is high in calories.

The "set point" theory says that there is a weight at which your body would like to be. Have you ever noticed that weight can be lost easily and quickly up to a certain point? Then the weight clings to your body like a long-lost child. That weight (or plateau) may be your body's set point, which is based on your genetic build, the number of fat cells built throughout your childhood, and your current diet-exercise program.

The *only* safe way (drugs and surgery are the risky alternatives) to lower your body's set point is through exercise. Then your body finds a new, lower set point that is equally easy to maintain. Without exercise in a weight reduction program, people are fighting their body's set point, and the body retaliates by inflicting great fatigue and a ravenous appetite on the well-intentioned dieter. Losing weight below your body's set point is both difficult and borderline futile. Only exercise can lower your set point.

Nutrition obviously has a great deal to do with weight problems. Although fat in the diet does not have to be stored as fat in the body, there is great metabolic ease in this simple conversion process. It takes energy to change excess dietary protein and carbohydrate into stored fat, while the switch from dietary fat to stored body fat is quick and energy-efficient. The average American eats 50 percent more fat than is recommended. Studies with both animals[19] and humans confirm that high-fat diets promote overfatness in the body.[20] High-fat diets in animals also produce a much lower metabolism and higher fuel efficiency.[21] For many reasons, vegetarians have only one-third the risk of overfatness when compared to meat eaters.[22]

Vitamin A deficiency (not uncommon in America) causes low thyroid output, which slows the metabolic rate to a crawl and encourages the storage of fat.[23] Vitamin A supplements were able to return thyroid output to normal flow in some patients.

SOLUTIONS TO THE PROBLEM

Exercise. Less than 5 percent of all people in an unstructured weight loss program will be able to keep their weight off. Exercise is absolutely mandatory for quick and permanent weight loss.[24] Some people think that they can take a pill or a shot or sit on an electrical device to lose weight without any effort. They are only deceiving themselves.

Exercise elevates basal metabolism to burn stored fat more quickly and allow you to eat more without gaining weight. Contrary to what the average person might think, the exercise should not be done at maximum exertion. When the body is getting enough air, it uses mostly fat for fuel. This is exactly what the corpulent person wants. Yet during times of insufficient air intake (when you are gasping for breath), much more carbohydrate is burned. If you can carry on a running (no pun intended) conversation, then you are not moving briskly enough. But if you are too winded to talk at all, then you are burning more carbohydrates than stored body fat. Your exercise should be vigorous enough that you can just barely talk during it.

Behavior Modification. Many people have accumulated an endless list of bad habits that encourage overfatness: eating in front of the TV, eating while depressed or bored, eating all the table scraps to avoid wasting them. Behavior modification programs teach people a lifestyle that changes these fat-conducive habits.[25]

Physical Environment. Another interesting phenomenom of weight gain is ambient temperature. Humans exposed to cold air lose weight faster.[26] The body must use some calories to "stoke the furnace" and keep the body temperature close to normal. You don't need to shiver your way through the winter in order to take advantage of this easy weight loss principle. Just turn the thermostat down a few degrees. The equatorial climate of some homes encourages a steady accumulation of fat.[27]

Nutrition. Nutritional solutions to overfatness are many. The most obvious one is to eat less food overall. Calories do count. An excess of fat, carbohydrate, protein, or alcohol will result in an accumulation of body fat. Yet there is a limited capacity to store excess carbohydrates as body fat.[28] The most crucial of these macronutrients is dietary fat. A low-fat diet will produce quicker and more long-lasting weight loss. Yet small amounts of fat in each meal help to prevent quick stomach emptying and also help to release a substance (cholecystokinin) that signals appetite satiety to the brain.[29] Each meal should contain a small amount of fat, with about 20–30 percent of total calories in the diet coming from fat.

There is a certain thermic effect (raising of body heat and burning of excess calories) that occurs after each meal. Researchers found that this thermic effect is higher after eating a carbohydrate-rich meal than after a fat-laden meal.[30] Other studies find that only obese subjects show a reduced thermic response to high-fat meals.[31] This means that some people should be particularly cautious about keeping their fat intake low.

Thyroid output regulates the rate at which your body burns its fuel. The thyroid could be compared to the set screw on an automobile carburetor. Thyroid output is reduced when food intake is reduced, and thyroid output increases during feeding, especially with high-carbohydrate meals.[32] People who eat very little red meat (vegetarians, lacto-ovo-vegetarians, fish and poultry eaters) have a lower average percent body fat, and their diets better comply with the Senate Dietary Goals of eating.[33]

"Nibbling" versus "gorging" is another key issue in weight maintenance. Eating five or six smaller meals each day, rather than the conventional one or three large ones seems to slow down the fat storage mechanism. Laboratory animals that are fed less food for a week, then fed normally again, will gain fatty tissue much faster than would be expected.[34] Once the food supply becomes undependable, as happens in occasional fasting, the body becomes more inclined to store more body fat for a portable pantry to draw from. The typical American eats no breakfast, a small lunch, and a huge dinner. Many dieters ride the roller coaster of starvation followed by binging. This meal pattern is perfectly conducive to fat storage and poor health. Nibblers are less likely to have weight problems than gorgers.[35]

Also, the more food that is consumed at a meal, the more the gastrointestinal tract adapts to encourage body fat storage.[36] When you consider the evolutionary design of humans, this principle makes sense. During periods of bountiful food, there would be no need to store fat, since that creature is eating on a regular basis. Yet, when the shadows of autumn grow taller, and the food becomes less available, and the meals get further apart, it's time to engage the fat storage mechanism to accumulate calories for the coming winter.

This weight gain effect is even more obvious in some animals. Many predatory creatures kill their prey and then gorge themselves because it may be some time before another meal is encountered. A perfect survival tool of nature would be to provide creatures with more efficient fat storage during times of gorging or undependable food supply. In a study of over 2,000 men and women, there was an inverse relationship between the number of meals eaten each day and the risk of obesity: the more meals eaten, the lower the chance for weight problems.[37] Gorging, both in logical theory and in proven laboratory experiments, adds body fat more rapidly than nibbling.

Several years ago, about 50 avid dieters died on what was appropriately entitled "The Last Chance Diet." This diet involved a collagen (jello-like) solution that was to be consumed as the exclusive food source. Collagen is nearly pure protein, but it is lacking in several essential amino acids. This diet also neglected to incorporate a balanced vitamin and mineral supplementation program. The cause of death for these dieters was electrolyte imbalance, tissue wasting of the heart, or thiamine deficiency. All of these causes indicate that it was a poorly designed formula for supporting human life. But some people really need to see quick weight loss results lest they lose their zeal for the whole idea of reducing.

There are well-designed powdered protein formulas available today that can be quite useful in stimulating quick and safe weight loss. As long as you consume at least 600 kilocalories per day with a well-designed formula, weight loss can be safe and rapid.[38] By consuming two "meals" of these diet mix drinks and then one meal of regular low-calorie food for a total of 600 kilocalories daily, you can have quick, safe, painless, and long-lasting weight loss.

It is crucial on a very low-calorie program to maintain ideal protein intake, usually around 50–70 g per day. When calorie intake does not meet the calorie needs of the body, not only does weight loss occur, but the body begins to scavenge its protein stores to manufacture its own carbohydrate source. This scavenging can lead to lean tissue wasting and even shrinkage of the heart until it can no longer pump.

There have always been "gimmick" diets available to the public. A favorite category of the "gimmick diets" is the low-carbohydrate approach (e.g., Atkins, Stillman, Air Force, Last Chance). These low-carbohydrate diets are able to "trick" the body into losing water weight quickly.[39] Low-carbohydrate diets cause initial water loss that has the dieter overjoyed—until the weight all returns in a week or so. What the dieter is trying to lose is excess stored body fat, not lean muscle tissue or water.

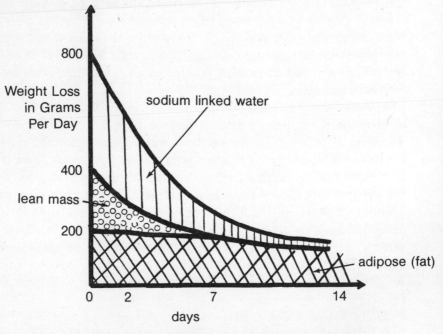

High protein "quick weight loss" programs can be very deceiving. The idea of a "diet" is to lose fat. As you can see, the high protein diet loses almost entirely water weight, which can quickly return once the body has adjusted to this abnormal nutrient intake.

SOURCE: Apfelbaum, M., Clinics in Endocrinology and Metabolism, vol. 5, no. 2, p. 417, July 1976

Fiber is a "wonder nutrient" in the weight control game. It fills you up, not out, by providing oral and intestinal satiety without calories. Twenty obese and nonobese human subjects were observed over a five-day period as they were fed meals of high- or low-fiber foods. Subjects were allowed to eat until full. On the high-fiber/low-calorie-density diet, all subjects ate about 1,570 kilocalories per day. The low-fiber/high-calorie-density diet required 3,000 kilocalories each day to provide the same full feeling in the same subjects.[40] It took an average of 33 percent more time for the subjects to eat their high-fiber meals. There was no difference in the oral satisfaction ratings for each type of diet. Both diets were rated "very good" in taste. In other words, high-fiber foods allow you to spend more time at the dinner table and to eat the same amount of food with equal satisfaction, yet with only half of the calories.

Carnitine is another "wonder nutrient" that could make weight reduction just a bit easier. Carnitine is the shuttle mechanism to get fats into the cell furnace. This step is often the bottleneck in fat burning.[41] Most people operate at subsaturation levels of carnitine; hence, carnitine supplements usually improve their ability to burn fats more efficiently.[42] Not only does carnitine help to burn fat, but it helps to maintain blood sugar levels while fasting. Japanese medical students were placed on a two-day fast. Some of the students were given injections of 200 mg of L-carnitine, while the others were given a placebo. The fasting students who were receiving the carnitine maintained ideal levels of blood glucose, while the other group had blood glucose levels that were less than two thirds of the carnitine group.[43] Thus, carnitine can keep blood glucose levels up throughout a weight reduction program, which means the dieter's physical and mental energy levels would be high throughout the normally lackluster dieting period. Carnitine keeps fats burning more efficiently while also maintaining ideal blood glucose levels.[44] Carnitine should also prevent the hunger pangs that often hamper the efforts of even the most dedicated dieter.

OTHER TYPES OF EATING DISORDERS

Modern America has added several new members to the category of eating disorders: anorexia, bulimia, and pica. Anorexia is found predominantly among upper-middle-class young white females who are subconsciously attempting to starve themselves. One-third of all anorexics die from their condition. Around 1 percent of high school and college women meet the criteria for anorexia. Bulimia is a bizarre binge-then-vomit pattern that starts off as the ultimate diet for many women of high school and college age. Bulimia is found in about 30 percent of all high school and college age women.[45] "Eat all you want without gaining weight," promise their friends. Yet the physical and psychological effects of bulimia are far-reaching. Bulimia is dangerous in itself yet often leads to anorexia, which is potentially fatal. Pica is the compulsive eating of nonfood items. It is found in nearly 25 percent of the population.[46]

These are all common and harmful conditions that can be treated in part with a nutritional approach. In the majority of instances, however, eating disorders stem from emotional problems and cannot be treated with nutrition alone.

Bulimia is more difficult for outsiders to detect than overfatness. The key symptoms of bulimia include common sessions of binge eating, often followed by self-induced vomiting; awareness that the victim's habits are not normal; fear of no control over the victim's situation; depression and self-beratement following these binge sessions.

Close friends and family may notice that the bulimic manages to maintain a trim shape in spite of a healthy performance at the dinner table. They may also notice that this thin person, usually female, excuses herself from the dinner table shortly after the meal and always goes to the bathroom. An observant person may detect the lingering stench of vomit in the bathroom after the bulimic has made her "postmeal deposit." Eventually, bulimics can develop discolored teeth from their continuous exposure to stomach acid. The bulimic is often irritable, jittery, and very orally oriented. Whether it's nail biting, smoking, drinking, or gum chewing, there always seems to be something in the bulimic's mouth.

Anorexia is characterized by an intense fear of becoming obese, which does not diminish as weight is lost. Anorexics often starve themselves through food restriction, while some overexercise until they look like skeletons. Many lose 25 percent more of their body weight. People who are overfat, bulimic, and anorexic often have a distorted self-image. They do not see themselves as other people and the mirror see them.[47]

Pica is characterized by strange eating habits. Often clay, laundry soap, buttons, and paint chips become attractive edibles to pica sufferers. Pica is most common in children, pregnant women, and other people who are likely candidates for malnutrition via their increased nutrient needs. Low levels of zinc, iron, magnesium, calcium, and other nutrients can trigger pica.

A favorite pica food of pregnant women is red clay from the southeastern United States. This clay is coincidentally loaded with iron; hence its red appearance. Pregnant women have been known to develop an irrepressible urge to eat up to a quart of clay each week during pregnancy. There have been numerous case studies of pregnant women who showed the effects of the clay intake. One woman went into labor, yet the infant did not drop into the birth canal as usual. Upon taking x-rays, the physicians found her bowels were totally impacted with clay which obstructed the movement of the baby. Once this clay was removed, the birthing process was able to proceed. Another woman had her clay pica detected by her dentist. Clay has an abrasive ability on the enamel of the teeth. Chewing clay is not unlike chewing fine sand. The dentist noticed the wear on this woman's enamel, and she readily admitted to eating a shoebox full of clay each week during each of her seven pregnancies. Pica is a serious problem, especially for the pregnant woman and growing child. Usually, high-potency, broad-spectrum nutrition supplements will relieve this intense yearning to eat nonfoods.

Zinc deficiencies can play a key role in bizarre eating behavior. One of the functions of zinc is to help maintain a healthy appetite. So it should not be too surprising that:

- Zinc supplements have been shown to be effective in improving the appetite and attitude of anorexics.[48]
- Many of the symptoms of anorexia are also the symptoms of zinc deficiency.[49]
- Zinc supplements improved the appetites of children who were "picky eaters."[50]
- Many pica victims are deficient in zinc.[51]
- Common zinc deficiencies in the elderly often produce a poor appetite and reduced taste sensitivity.[52]

Zinc deficiencies are common in this country, and they may play a role in each of the eating disorders described in this chapter.

As in cases of overfatness, social and psychological factors play roles in these eating disorders. Families of bulimics and anorexics are less involved, less supportive, more isolated, conflictual, understructured, and detached than the families of normal healthy controls.[53] And our modern media helps many young people develop unrealistic expectations for themselves. Television role models seem to eat continuously on the screen and paradoxically maintain svelte figures. This is unrealistic and confusing and can lead to eating disorders.

People with eating disorders often claim to have an obsession to eat. Are they different, or are they just lacking in common restraint? Perhaps there is a reason for their eating obsessions. Bulimics have been found to have lower levels of circulating endorphins, which are the body's internally produced morphinelike pleasure compounds.[54] Copper deficiencies are common in the U.S. and can result in low endorphin levels in the brain.[55] Perhaps food becomes the surrogate endorphins for bulimics.

NUTRITIONAL RECOMMENDATIONS FOR LIFETIME WEIGHT CONTROL

Follow the core program, minus 10 percent fat in the diet.

DIETARY GUIDELINES

1. Replace the lost fat in the diet with high-fiber foods such as whole grains, legumes, fruits, and vegetables. Allow yourself as much of these foods as you would like. It is nearly impossible to avoid losing weight on a high-fiber diet, no matter how much of these good foods you eat.

2. Eat small, frequent meals. Have a snack every two hours. Tell yourself that there is no need to binge since another meal is right around the corner. If you have the insatiable urge to "cheat," allow yourself one day a week to do so. The nutritional impact will be much less if you limit your "off" times to once a week, rather than eating high-fat and high-sugar junk foods throughout the week.

3. Have a large bowl of homemade vegetable soup before each meal. Then have your small entree. Warm fluids blunt the appetite more impressively than many prescription drugs.

4. Emphasize unprocessed plant foods as much as possible.

DAILY SUPPLEMENTS TO ADD TO YOUR CORE PROGRAM

L-carnitine   +2,000 mg
L-tyrosine   +4,000 mg
L-tryptophan   +4,000 mg

14
THE ENDOCRINE SYSTEM
Diabetes

It's called the "silent killer." Many people who are in the early stages of diabetes do not even know that they have it. Many diabetics are unimpressed with the deadly potency of their disease, and they often fail to comply with their medical program. Diabetes almost seems innocuous as a disease in America. After all, only 35,000 Americans each year have "cause of death" listed as diabetes. Yet deaths from diabetes are much like the tip of the iceberg. Experts estimate that 100,000–350,000 Americans actually die from diabetes-related causes. Diabetics are much more vulnerable to many diseases. Compared to the average person, diabetics have 25 times the incidence of blindness, 3 times the rate of heart disease, 17 times the rate of kidney failure, 5 times the gangrene incidence, and a much higher risk for impotence, skin lesions, psychosis, and other problems.

WHAT IS DIABETES?

Diabetes is an insidious disease in which glucose, the body's preferential fuel supply, is denied entrance into the body cells due to a problem with insulin supply. This simple defect gives rise to all sorts of problems. Since the body cells need fuel and are denied access to the rising tide of blood glucose that waits outside the cells, the fat stores are mobilized, and the bloodstream becomes a freeway jammed with fats. Protein is another alternative energy source that the diabetic system begins to take advantage of. Protein, from lean tissue and organs, begins to find its way into the furnaces of the body's mitochondria. This is not unlike burning your fine walnut desk in the fireplace to keep warm. As a last resort, this is acceptable to maintain life. As a long-term process, it is disastrous.

Also, diabetics do not heal well from bruises and cuts. The blood vessel walls favor glucose for fuel. Without it, they often wither and allow gangrene to set in. Although most areas of the body are somewhat flexible in what fuel they can use, the lens of the eye, nerve tissue (including the brain), lungs, kidney, and vascular walls are almost totally dependent on blood glucose for energy. Understandably, these areas of the body are particularly vulnerable to damage in the uncontrolled diabetic. Blindness, kidney failure, heart disease, and psychoses are all more prevalent in the diabetic.

Also, insulin does more than just open the cellular door for glucose to pass through. Insulin promotes protein synthesis, wound healing, disease resistance, and the production of certain brain chemicals. As a consequence, the diabetic is subject to muscle wasting, poor wound healing, more infections, and constant fatigue.

In the diabetic, there is abundant glucose in the bloodstream, yet little gets into the body cells where it is needed. The kidneys have the responsibility of filtering much of this excess glucose out of the blood. The urine becomes saturated with sugar, so the body attempts to dilute the urine with extra water. This explains why two key symptoms of diabetes are excessive thirst and excessive urination. In 1,500 B.C., the Greeks used a phrase for diabetes that means "running through a siphon."[1] The Indians called it the "honey urine" disease. In the 17th century, the English called it the "pissing sickness." *Diabetes mellitus* literally means "sweetness running through." An old term for juvenile diabetes was interpreted as "melting down of the flesh." These expressions are astoundingly observant and correct. (Incidentally, *diabetes insipidus* is a different disease, which involves losing excess amounts of bodily fluids.)

HOW MANY PEOPLE HAVE DIABETES?

The incidence of diabetes mellitus is on the upsurge in the developed nations of the world. From 1965 to 1973, there was a 50 percent increase in the number of diabetics per capita in this country. Five percent of Americans, or nearly 12 million people, are clinically diagnosed as diabetic. Millions of other people are undiagnosed or borderline diabetics. Currently, the incidence of diabetes is increasing by 6 percent per year, which means that it is doubling every 15 years. One out of five people born today will develop diabetes sometime in their lifetime. The quality and quantity of life is threatened by diabetes. Healing nutrients can prevent some cases of diabetes and reduce the damage done in other diabetics.

CAN DIABETES BE CURED?

In some cases, yes. As mentioned early in this book, in one study 10 adult male aborigines with diabetes left the city and returned to their former native lifestyle of hunting and gathering. They were all in their early 50s and overweight, but neither obese nor insulin-dependent. Once in their native environment, they made no efforts to lose weight, yet they lost an average of 18 pounds over the seven-week period. Their diet was high in animal meat, yet low in fat (only 13 percent of the total calories) since wild game animals are better exercised than fattened domestic herds. Plasma triglycerides fell to one-fourth the original level. Fasting blood glucose levels fell to half the original levels, bringing glucose levels into the normal range. (Fasting blood glucose is the amount of sugar, or glucose, found in the blood after a fast, such as in the morning before breakfast. This is an important indicator of the body's ability to maintain a healthy blood glucose level.) Glucose tolerance curves and insulin response improved significantly. In essence, after seven weeks in their native lifestyle of better diet and more exercise, these 10 diabetics were "cured."[2] In another study, well-managed, very-low-calorie diets (300 kilocalories/day with 30 g of protein) were able to rapidly lower the serum lipids and improve glucose tolerance in a group of adult (type II) diabetics.[3]

Although diabetes was once thought to be caused only by an insulin deficiency, there is another category of diabetics who make plenty of insulin, but their insulin is not as effective as it should be.

This is called insulin-resistant diabetes and most often occurs in overfat adults. These people are good candidates for significant improvement through nutrition.

Adult diabetics who are non-insulin-dependent have a good chance of improving and perhaps even curing their diabetes through the program found in this chapter. Diabetics who are insulin-dependent have little or no insulin output and are not nearly as receptive to these nutritional approaches as people who can make at least some insulin.

WHAT CAUSES DIABETES?

Diabetes can be caused by many things: overweight,[4] allergies,[5] malnutrition in early developmental years,[6] viruses, genetics,[7] vitamin or mineral deficiencies, and others. Diabetes is probably one symptom with dozens of different causes.

Obese individuals have a 400 percent greater chance of developing diabetes. Just losing weight can often "cure" diabetes in the obese adult who is not dependent on insulin. See the chapter on eating disorders for more on how to lose weight. Exercise enhances the body's receptivity to insulin, and a lack of exercise can bring on diabetic symptoms.

A diet high in sugar or refined carbohydrate foods may bring on diabetic symptoms. As foods are refined and processed, the body is able to absorb the sugars present more efficiently, which increases the glycemic index of foods. This is bad for most people and disastrous for diabetics. Refined foods, like rice bubbles, corn flakes, and instant potatoes, create higher "peaks" and lower "valleys" on blood glucose curves.

Diabetics who are more conscientious about tracking their diet and smoothing out the peaks and valleys of their blood glucose curves will experience far fewer problems with nerve and eye damage.

HOW IS DIABETES DIAGNOSED?

Diabetics have abnormally high blood glucose levels, which are best detected through a blood test called the *oral glucose tolerance test (OGTT)*. The OGTT is fully explained in Chapter 10, since the brain is so totally dependent on blood glucose for fuel.

Diabetics are taught to look for the symptoms of low blood sugar (hypoglycemia), which include sweating, headache, trembling, and hunger; and also the symptoms of high blood sugar (hyperglycemia), which include increased thirst, frequency of urination, weakness, and nausea. Yet six different studies found that diabetics react uniquely to abnormal blood sugar levels.[8] "Classical" symptoms of high or low blood sugar are not valid in many people. Diabetics should instead be taught to monitor their blood glucose levels regularly and make mental notes of their symptoms when the levels go above or below their acceptable range.

HOW CAN NUTRITION HELP?

Weight control can improve many a diabetic condition (see Chapter 13 for more on that subject). There are also specific nutrients that can improve glucose tolerance.

CHROMIUM

Chromium can be a key nutrient in the prevention and management of certain types of diabetes. Deficiencies in chromium will lower the effectiveness of insulin in both animals and humans.[9] Chromium works in the large molecule called *glucose tolerance factor*, or GTF, to assist insulin in allowing glucose into the cells. Most Americans consume between 25 and 33 mcg of chromium daily, while the minimum acceptable level of intake is 50 mcg.[10] Even one-third of all diets designed by registered dietitians fall short of this 50 mcg minimum.[11] Refined foods are often stripped of their chromium.

As we age, the cumulative effect of a marginal nutrient intake leaves many people bankrupt of their chromium stores. Coincidentally, older adults often have diminished glucose tolerance that, if compared to younger normal people, would be considered diabetic. In a variety of other studies with normal older Americans, chromium supplements almost inevitably produced improved glucose tolerance curves.[12] The chromium supplements also produced higher levels of HDLs, which are protective against heart disease.[13] See the section "Unique Nutrient Needs" in the chapter on aging for more information on chromium.

Supplements of greater than 200 mcg of chromium daily may

provide some improvement for glucose tolerance in adult diabetics.[14] Six adult diabetics were given brewer's yeast supplements, and their blood glucose and insulin levels were monitored. The chromium-rich brewer's yeast improved insulin sensitivity in all six subjects as demonstrated by lower fasting blood glucose and lower insulin requirements.[15] In another study, 43 diabetic men received either inorganic chromium, brewer's yeast with GTF, brewer's yeast without GTF, or a placebo in a double-blind format. After four months of treatment with the supplements, one of the groups (ketosis-resistant) showed improved insulin output with GTF brewer's yeast.[16] In another report, a diabetic woman had her many symptoms and side effects "cured" after being given intravenous chromium.[17]

Something in GTF or the chromium that is found in GTF, or some other mysterious factor in brewer's yeast, is able to improve glucose tolerance in many people. Researchers find that some people are not able to make enough of their own GTF from dietary chromium.[18] Hence, for some people, GTF may be an essential vitamin, with deficiency symptoms surfacing as hypoglycemia, lethargy, or adult-onset diabetes.

Most Americans could benefit from chromium supplements of 200 mcg daily. Some people may need the added benefit of high-chromium brewer's yeast. Chromium is one of the least toxic of all essential minerals. Supplements providing up to 1,000 mcg of chromium daily would pose no threat and might provide some benefit to certain high-risk people, like hypoglycemics and diabetics. Chromium deficiency does not cause most cases of diabetes. But chromium deficiency probably accelerates the course of diabetes. Chromium supplements improve almost everyone's glucose tolerance and often improve the erratic blood glucose curves of the diabetic or hypoglycemic.

COMPLEX CARBOHDYDRATES AND FIBER

For many years, diabetics were strictly prohibited from eating much carbohydrate. Instead, they were fed diets high in protein and fat, which usually accelerated their journey toward heart disease. That has changed. Good scientific data show us that a diet high in complex carbohydrates and fiber will improve the glucose tolerance of diabetics.[19] This new type of diet has been credited with lowering insulin needs in diabetics by an average of 25–50 percent.[20] This means emphasizing fresh fruits, vegetables, whole grains, and legumes (beans). Most national diabetes associations from the developed nations now support this more effective dietary control of diabetes. Yet there are still plenty of health care practictioners who have not been able to abandon the old diabetic treatment diet.

Nutritionists have long observed that vegetarians are less likely to get heart disease, diabetes, cancer of the colon, and obesity. In a 21-year study of 26,000 Seventh Day Adventists, scientists found that vegetarians had half the incidence of diabetes when compared to nonvegetarians.[21] Vegetarians usually eat much more complex carbohydrate and fiber and much less fat than nonvegetarians. The average American eats a diet of 46 percent carbohydrates, with nearly 40 percent of those carbohydrates coming from sugar. When diabetics are given diets of up to 75 percent complex carbohydrates with minimal refined sugar, many are able to wean themselves of insulin completely.[22]

Studies in India using over 18,000 diabetics have proven that diets that are high in complex carbohydrate (providing 67 percent of energy) and high in fiber (about 52 g/day) reduced fasting blood glucose by 32 percent *in only one week*.[23] A high-fiber diet lowers the diabetic's risk for blindness from retinopathy.[24]

Each food is digested and absorbed at a different rate, which yields a unique glucose tolerance curve. The more gradual the OGTT curve from a food, the better it is for people, especially diabetics. Researchers examined the glucose tolerance curves of 62 commonly eaten carbohydrate foods in human subjects. The foods were rated as follows, with best listed first: legumes (beans), dairy products, fruit, cereals and biscuits, breakfast cereals, vegetables.[25] Lentils at breakfast were able to improve glucose tolerance in human subjects *by the time the next meal arrived*.[26] Of all grain products tested, glycemic responses from best to worst were whole rye kernels, whole wheat kernels, bulgur, pumpernickel bread, whole-meal rye bread, whole-meal wheat bread, white bread.[27]

Table sugar probably worsens the symptoms of diabetes measurably.[28] As a matter of fact, when 19 adults were fed various diets, high sugar intake deteriorated blood glucose curves *even* in people eating an otherwise very nourishing diet that was low in fat and high in fiber.[29] The more refined or ground up a food is, the more available are the carbohydrate contents, and hence the more radical the blood glucose curve will be. This is just another reason to eat foods in as close to their natural state as possible.

Fiber is basically indigestible food matter and is found almost exclusively in plant foods. There are many different types of fiber, including the insoluble forms of cellulose, hemicellulose, and lignin and the soluble forms of pectin, mucilages, and gums. Although all fiber has certain health benefits, soluble fibers seem to be most beneficial for diabetics. High-fiber diets in general are impressively effective in improving blood glucose control in diabetics.[30]

Twelve grams of supplemental guar gum or pectin were able to improve glucose tolerance in *healthy* humans.[31] When both diabetic and nondiabetic subjects were fed muffins supplemented with 12 g of xanthum gum daily, improvements were noted in fasting glucose, glucose tolerance, serum lipids, and gastric emptying rate.[32] In another experiment, 9 healthy people, 20 noninsulin dependent diabetics, and 2 people with impaired glucose tolerance were given either a placebo or a granola-type bar fortified with guar gum. The guar gum helped to stabilize glucose tolerance when eaten either alone or with a meal in both healthy and diabetic subjects.[33]

Pectin is known to slow the emptying rate of the stomach,[34] which is good. This provides a more gradual infusion of carbohydrates into the blood stream and a more gradual drop in blood glucose as insulin takes over. Although wheat bran supplements were able to drop blood fats by as much as 46 percent, wheat bran was not able to improve glucose tolerance curves noticeably.[35]

Both diabetics and "normal" people can profit by eating a diet high in complex carbohydrates and fiber. Diabetics show improved glucose tolerance when their diets are particularly high in carbohydrates (60–70 percent) and supplemented with 12 g of guar gum or pectin daily.

CARNITINE

One of the main health risks to diabetics is the flood of fats that come racing through the arteries, ready to replace the impaired glucose fuel supply. Diabetics experience serious problems with excess fat in the blood (a.k.a *heart disease*) and excessive fat byproducts throughout the body (a.k.a *ketosis*). Since carnitine is so crucial to proper fat metabolism, supplements of carnitine can reduce the health risks of poor fat metabolism in the diabetic.

Supplements of L-carnitine have been successful in lowering ketosis in humans.[36] Carnitine injections in healthy students on a fast were able to keep their blood glucose levels near normal.[37] In another study, large doses of carnitine (750 mg/kg of body weight/day) for two weeks improved both the hearts and overall conditions of the diabetics.[38]

Carnitine is nontoxic. Up to 3,000 mg daily can be taken quite safely. Human subjects taking up to 26,000 mg of L-carnitine daily experienced only mild diarrhea. Supplements of at least 1,000 mg of L-carnitine daily would improve the condition of many diabetics and substantially reduce the risks for heart disease.

ANTIOXIDANTS

Vitamin E and selenium can be of great value in lowering health risks for the diabetic. Supplements of 2,000 IU of vitamin E daily were able to lower platelet aggregation (a major risk factor in heart disease) and also lower serum glucose levels in diabetics.[39] In diabetic animals, vitamin E supplements were able to enhance the production of prostacyclin, a beneficial prostaglandin that lowers heart disease risks.[40] In another study using diabetic animals, vitamin E supplementation was able to bring serum triglyceride levels back to normal while preventing the buildup of lipid peroxides (destructive fatty by-products) in both the blood and liver.[41]

In a variety of diabetic test animals, supplements of vitamin A, especially as beta-carotene, improved wound healing and increased disease resistance.[42] These researchers at Albert Einstein College of Medicine in New York felt that ". . . supplemental vitamin A . . . will be especially useful in preventing wound infection and promoting wound healing in surgical diabetic patients."

When noninsulin-dependent adult diabetics were given 500 mg of vitamin C daily for 12 months in a double-blind study, their serum lipids dropped markedly.[43] These scientists speculated that the extra vitamin C helped the body convert cholesterol into bile salts for fat digestion, which then allowed the body to rid itself of cholesterol through the feces.

VITAMIN B₆

One of the many functions of vitamin B_6 in the body is to regulate the breakdown of glycogen into blood glucose and to stabilize glucose tolerance. Roughly two out of five Americans are considered to be deficient in B_6. Deficiencies of B_6 can lead to impaired glucose tolerance, which could be misinterpreted as diabetes.[44] Supplements of B_6 are able to clear up the "diabetes" in these B_6-deficient individuals.[45] Other researchers have found that supplements of B_6 can reduce the insulin requirements in genuine diabetics.[46]

Pregnant women often develop diabetic–like symptoms, due to the insulin demands of supporting an extra life within. B_6 supplements have also been effective in improving this temporary diabetes of pregnancy (a.k.a. *gestational diabetes*).[47]

ZINC

Zinc plays a key role in various phases of insulin production. Insulin is even stored as a zinc crystal in the pancreas. When experimental animals are fed zinc-deficient diets, they develop impaired glucose tolerance.[48] About one out of four human diabetics studied had low blood levels of zinc as well as high urinary excretion of zinc.[49] Many of the side effects and complications of diabetes are strikingly similar to the effects of a zinc deficiency, including poor wound healing and increased susceptibility to infections. It is ironic that one of the more proven therapies for diabetes is a high-fiber diet, which has been shown to worsen a zinc deficiency by binding zinc in the intestines and carrying it out with the feces. Hence, diabetics who are on a high-fiber diet may be even lower than normal Americans in zinc status. The average U.S. intake of zinc is roughly one half to two thirds of the RDA.

QUASI VITAMINS

Myoinositol is a nonessential nutrient that is both found in the diet and made in the body. Myoinositol is made in the body from glucose and is very similar in structure to glucose, which should be a clue as to why diabetics can be helped with supplements of myoinositol. Diabetics are extremely vulnerable to a painful and debilitating nerve degeneration called *peripheral neuropathy.* Myoinositol has been successful in treating this condition. When blood sugar is high and myoinositol levels are low, nerve degeneration begins.[50] Other investigators found that supplements of 1,000 mg of myoinositol daily improved the nerve function in diabetics.[51] When 20 diabetics were provided with myoinositol supplements of 1,648 mg daily, all reported improved sensory nerve functions.[52] Myoinositol is a safe supplement, with no side effects reported in humans taking up to 3,000 mg daily.[53]

Researchers in Berlin fed 6.8 g of cod liver oil daily (about 1/2 tablespoon) to diabetic patients. After only two weeks of this supplementation, there were measurable drops in heart disease risk factors.[54] The active ingredient in cod liver oil that helped these people is probably EPA, which is thoroughly reviewed in Chapter 5. Although EPA is helpful to many people, it may be a conditionally essential vitamin for diabetics.

Lipoic acid is a nonessential substance found in liver and brewer's yeast and also produced in the body. Lipoic acid has a critical role in burning carbohydrates, another hint why this substance may be particularly useful to diabetics. Using 100–200 mg of lipoic acid supplements daily, scientists in Germany were able to reduce the pain and improve the condition of diabetics with nerve damage (peripheral neuropathy).[55] Since nerve cells are almost totally dependent on carbohydrate metabolism for their fuel supply, this relationship makes sense.

Bioflavonoids are plant compounds that help out in photosynthesis. Bioflavonoid supplements were able to prevent the painful and sometimes blinding buildup of fluids in the eyes of diabetics.[56]

Coenzyme Q works in a crucial intersection of energy metabolism. Vitamin E protects CoQ from destruction and hence has a role in energy metabolism. Supplements of CoQ were able to lower blood glucose and ketone levels in human diabetics.[57]

Arginine is an amino acid that is not currently considered to be essential in the diet. That idea is being challenged briskly. Perhaps the human body cannot make enough arginine, considering all the functions that arginine performs internally. Supplements of arginine in laboratory animals have been able to improve glucose tolerance, reverse lean tissue wasting, and improve immune functions.[58] All of this could be quite important to the human diabetic.

ROOTS AND HERBS

Ginseng, an herb extract from a root plant native to the cool climates of northeast Asia, is neither useless nor dangerous when taken in reasonable levels of less than 500 mg daily. Scientists in Europe and Asia have pursued experiments with this ancient medicine. Ginseng has been shown to *raise or lower* the blood sugar levels in humans.[59] Two hundred to 500 mg daily of standardized ginseng could be valuable to those with erratic blood sugar regulation.

Fenugreek is a leguminous herb used widely throughout India, north Africa, and the Mediterranean region. Fenugreek has been scientifically shown to lower both blood glucose and insulin levels. In a controlled experiment, 25 g of fenugreek seeds (about 1 ounce), and/or 5 g of gum (fiber), and/or 150 g of fenugreek leaves were given to both normal and diabetic human subjects. The seeds and gum of fenugreek were able to lower the insulin and blood glucose levels by as much as 42 percent.[60] This makes fenugreek more effective than most prescription drugs, without the expense or risk involved in drugs. Fenugreek seeds can be sprouted and eaten regularly as a tasty portion of salads.

MEAL PATTERNS

Humans evolved as "grazers" rather than the meal eating "gorgers" that we have become. In both animal and human studies, having three to six smaller meals each day improves glucose tolerance and lowers fats in the blood.[61]

ALCOHOL

Alcohol can be a serious problem for diabetics, since alcohol lowers blood sugar levels. The British Diabetic Association has endorsed a program that restricts alcohol intake for diabetics to three drinks or less daily. High-carbohydrate drinks, like beer and sweet wines, are discouraged.[62] Alcohol also tends to raise levels of fats in the blood, which the diabetic could do without.

EXERCISE

Diabetics should exercise regularly and briskly, dedicating at least 45 minutes per session three times weekly once they are in condition. Exercise has been shown to help stabilize blood glucose, lower fats in the blood, and increase the sensitivity of the cells to the insulin available.[63]

NUTRITIONAL RECOMMENDATIONS
DIETARY GUIDELINES

Follow core diet. Lose body fat until there is roughly one inch of skinfold thickness just above the hip bone. Obesity increases blood glucose problems. Losing weight is often a miraculous "cure" for adult-onset diabetes. Exercise vigorously and regularly. Choose a fun sport.

DAILY SUPPLEMENTS TO ADD TO YOUR CORE PROGRAM

Vitamins
  Vitamin A   +15,000 IU
   (beta-carotene)
  Vitamin E   +600 IU
  Vitamin B_6 +50 mg
  Vitamin C   +1,000 mg

Minerals
  Zinc   +15 mg
  Chromium (yeast)   +600 mcg
  Selenium (yeast)   +200 mcg

Quasi vitamins
  L-carnitine   +2,500 mg
  EPA   +2,000 mg
   or cod liver oil   1 teaspoon
  Coenzyme Q   +60 mg
  Lipoic acid   +200 mg
  Bioflavonoids   +500 mg
  Myoinositol   +1,600 mg
  Ginseng   +500 mg
  L-arginine   +10 g
  Pectin or guar gum   +12 g

15
THE SKELETAL SYSTEM
Osteoporosis and Arthritis

Only the highest forms of life have bones. Bacteria, plants, jelly-fish, and other boneless creatures are severely limited in their movement and support. Bones give us an internal framework, extensive locomotion and strength, opposing indexes for manual dexterity, a storage silo of certain minerals, and an impressive "crash helmet" for our brain. Of the 206 bones found in the human body, half are located in the hands and feet.

Without bones, humans would be relegated to slithering around for survival morsels of food. With bones, we become advanced creatures. Yet bones can break, become hollowed and brittle (osteoporosis), become soft and poorly formed (rickets), create indescribable pain by pinching nerves, or have inflamed endings for painful movement (arthritis). This chapter is dedicated to maintaining your skeletal system as a positive force in your life. The two most prevalent problems with the human skeletal system are osteoporosis and arthritis.

OSTEOPOROSIS

It is being called "a 20th-century epidemic." An English physician has commented that orthopedic hospital units are so full of osteoporosis patients that they remind older physicians of the plagues from the earlier part of this century. The story is all too common: "You must come to the hospital! Mother (or Grandma) has broken her hip." Osteoporosis is basically a slow and pernicious hollowing out of the skeletal system. While normal bones can break, osteoporotic bones can shatter like a pane of glass. This leaves the surgeon with the challenging task of reassembling and bolting together many thin bone parts. Osteoporotic bones do not heal as quickly as healthy bones, either.

Osteoporosis afflicts at least 20 million Americans. It causes 1.3 million bone fractures annually in America, costing $3.8 billion. At least one out of three people age 65 and older have some form of the disease. Seventy percent of the 1 million bone fractures occurring in women 45 years and older are due to osteoporosis.[1] The incidence of hip fractures has doubled in the last 28 years.[2]

The average woman loses one-fourth of her skeletal mass from age 30 to 70. You have probably noticed that many women literally shrink in height and stature as they age. Older women lose an average of 8 inches in height, compared to 2 inches for older men.[3] Some women even develop a "humped" back, which can be an indication of even greater bone loss. Although osteoporosis is not fatal, one-third of all victims die within a year from complications arising from the original bone break.

BONE FORMATION

We come into this world with very flexible skeletal systems composed primarily of cartilage, like the divider in your nose. This flexibility allows us to develop an amorphous shape and pass through mother's narrow birth canal. A cross section of a flexible bone looks something like the honeycomb matrix of a bee hive. Shortly after birth, calcification of the bones begins. *Mineralization* is the process by which calcium and phosphorus salts begin filling in these honeycomb chambers in the bones. If a person is nourished properly, bone mineralization continues into early adulthood. Sometime in the third or fourth decade of life, the bones begin to reverse this flow of minerals. Aging is an unavoidable risk factor in osteoporosis. Although it seems difficult to stop this bone loss altogether, it can be slowed down significantly. Osteoporosis is quite preventable.

WOMEN AND OSTEOPOROSIS

Osteoporosis mostly occurs in women. Four times more women than men are afflicted. This disparity is due partially to the female hormone estrogen, which keeps calcium in the bones. Once menopause sets in, the estrogen flow begins to dry up. Mothering and breastfeeding encourage the flow of estrogen and hence fortify the woman's bones. Yet a low calcium intake during baby-making and milk production will instigate a draining of the woman's bone stores. Thus, motherhood can be a plus or a minus in osteoporosis, depending on the mother's diet. Also, women are more likely to be involved in fad diets, fasting, and other dubious dietary programs. These diets can chip away at bone stores.[4] For some women, a physician may need to prescribe estrogen. Calcium needs drop from 1,500 mg daily to 1,000 mg while on estrogen therapy. However, be aware that estrogen therapy increases a woman's need for vitamin B_6 up to 150 times the RDA to 250 mg daily.[5]

The RDA for calcium for older adults is 800 mg. There is considerable support among scientists for raising this RDA to 1,500 mg for older women.[6] In a recent study of women ages 49–66, 70 percent consumed less than 800 mg of calcium daily. Thirteen percent of the women consumed less than 400 mg. Thus, the vast majority of women are consuming one-half to one-third of their calcium requirements.

RISK FACTORS IN OSTEOPOROSIS

Another group that seems to be at high risk for osteoporosis is that of male alcoholics. Forty-seven percent of the male alcoholics studied had measurable bone loss. Even 31 percent of the *young male* alcoholics studied had osteoporosis.[7]

Other risk factors include a diet that is excessively high in fat, fiber, protein, or processed food. Dietary fat (especially saturated animal fats) mixes with calcium in the intestines to form insoluble soaps that are carried out of the system in the feces. Phytates from grain fiber can bind calcium and make it unabsorbable. Excess protein creates an unusual calcium flow out of the body through the urine.[8] One group of researchers found that all human subjects had a healthy calcium balance regardless of calcium intake (from 500–1,400 mg daily) but only if protein intake was kept low.[9] The average protein intake in America is about 100 grams daily, though most adults need only 50–80 g, depending on size and other factors.

Excess aluminum—aluminum is found in antacids, aluminum cookware, and in salt and other packaged products as an anticaking ingredient—can encourage osteoporosis.[10]

Inadequate stomach acid (achlorhydria), a common problem in older adults, also lowers efficiency in absorbing calcium.[11] In addition, in a hot dry climate, an active adult can lose a considerable amount of calcium in sweat. Worry and tension can cause both lowered calcium absorption and increased calcium loss.[12] Genetics may also play a role. A definite familial link in osteoporosis was found in 26 mother/daughter pairs.[13]

The trace minerals fluoride, manganese, and copper, all involved in the hardening of bones, are also important in preventing osteoporosis.[14] Areas with fluoridated water have a lower incidence of osteoporosis.[15] Unfortunately, the typical American diet is low in manganese and fluoride and contains only half the RDA for copper.

Excess smoking and caffeine intake can also accelerate bone loss.[16]

One of the more important nonnutrition factors in osteoporosis is exercise. During regular exercise, the skeleton fortifies itself against the stress caused by gravity. Without activity, the skeleton slims down to a minimum.[17] "Use it or lose it" is the often-repeated phrase of biologists. Sedentary lifestyle strongly encourages bone mineral loss.[18] One of the true obstacles to long-term space travel is the bone draining effects of living in a weightless environment. After only a few months in space, astronauts can lose up to 25,000 mg of bone calcium.[19] Exercise can both prevent and treat osteoporosis.

DETECTION OF OSTEOPOROSIS

One of the real dilemmas in osteoporosis is detection. X-rays cannot "see" osteoporosis until one-third of the bone mass is gone.[20] At that point, serious damage has already been done. New techniques, such as double photon densitometry and CAT scan of the spine, can detect osteoporosis earlier. Due to the high-priority calcium needs of all muscles (e.g., the heart) and nerve tissue (e.g., the brain), the body has an amazing feedback system designed to keep blood calcium levels adequate in spite of poor calcium intake.

Grand theft of the bone stores will silently proceed when calcium intake is inadequate. Thus, blood calcium tests are deceiving, since the body has artificially kept calcium blood levels high in spite of dwindling bone stores and low dietary intake. Occasional muscle spasms and minor irritability may be the only indications that a person is not getting enough calcium in the diet. One of the first bones to be robbed is the jawbone, which then erodes the anchor for tooth foundations. Hence, a symptom of advanced osteoporosis can be premature tooth loss.

THE IMPORTANCE OF BALANCED MINERAL INTAKE

The bones are fortified mainly with calcium and phosphorus. Since phosphorus is found in all foods and many food additives as phosphoric acid, calcium becomes the key limiting mineral in bone fortification. One gram (1,000 mg) of calcium daily can halt or even reverse osteoporosis in humans.[21] Yet minerals must be balanced in the diet and in the body. The ideal ratio of calcium to phosphorus to magnesium would be 1:1:0.5. When the calcium to phosphorus ratio goes above 1:1.25 or higher in phosphorus, then most other efforts to prevent osteoporosis are likely in vain.[22] The average calcium-to-phosphorus ratio in the U.S. and Canada is about 1:1.6, with 300 mg of phosphorus daily coming from food additives alone.[23] Most Americans consume far too much phosphorus from meats, colas, and processed foods and too little magnesium and calcium. Since magnesium intake in America averages about one-half to three-fourths of the recommended intake,[24] and calcium intake averages about one-half to two-thirds of recommended levels, you can see why osteoporosis is so common in America.

Even calcium intake in early developmental years is important. Apparently a well-fortified skeleton can better resist the onslaught of demineralization as a result of aging. One study found that older women who used to (but no longer do) drink milk had a higher average bone density than women who never were serious milk drinkers.[25] Forty-five percent of total adult skeletal mass is formed during the growth spurts of adolescence.[26] Since only one out of seven teenage girls consumes 100 percent or more of the RDA for calcium, more effort should be made to tell young people about the need to fortify the bones, lest they seriously regret it in the coming decades.

Although dolomite is a cheap calcium supplement with an ideal two-to-one calcium-to-magnesium ratio, it also contains alarming amounts of toxic heavy metals, like lead, arsenic, mercury, and aluminum.[27] Calcium lactate is a well-absorbed form of calcium yet it also can cause intestinal upset in people who cannot digest milk sugar.

Hard water contains significant amounts of calcium and magnesium, which form white crystals on your teakettle and prevent the efficient laundering of clothes. Many people buy a water softener to exchange sodium ions for these calcium and magnesium ions. That's OK for the teakettle and clothes, but not for your health. The added sodium in soft water can elevate blood pressure and heart disease risk, while the hard water can provide up to 375 mg of calcium per liter of drinking water.[28] By connecting your water softener only to the hot water system in your house, you can have the best of both worlds: soft water for clean clothes and dishes, and hard drinking water for better health. For comparison's sake, milk provides about 288 mg of calcium per cup. Most people would need about a quart of milk per day or its equivalent from other calcium sources in order to satisfy their calcium needs.

Although dairy products are a good source of calcium, they are not a panacea against osteoporosis. Cow's milk has a calcium-to-phosphorus ratio of one to five.[29] Some experts have advised against using milk as a primary calcium source to prevent osteoporosis. However, other studies show that low-fat milk is an excellent and well-absorbed calcium source for all who can tolerate milk.[30] The dairy industry has a tendency to oversimplify the role of milk in osteoporosis, making it sound like its product will prevent or cure the condition. It won't. A minimum of 30 million Americans are lactose-intolerant and therefore unable to digest milk sugar.[31] Yogurt can be a well-tolerated, calcium-rich alternative for these people.[32] Up to 10 million other Americans have a milk allergy. Thus milk is good for many people, bad for some, and no "magic bullet" against osteoporosis for anyone.

Recently, calcium antacids have been recommended as a source of calcium for women. This is ludicrous. Antacids change the pH (acid/base balance) of the stomach and intestines, making them more alkaline, which markedly alters the digestion efficiency of most enzymes and reduces the amount of calcium in particular that will be absorbed. Overdosing on these antacid calcium tablets can cause milk-alkali syndrome (a change in stomach pH combined with calcium overload).[33] Also, if people mistakenly take *aluminum-based* antacids, not only would they absorb less calcium (since aluminum and calcium compete),[34] but they would reduce digestive efficiency from diluted acid levels, *and* they might also run a higher risk for Alzheimer's disease via aluminum toxicity. However, pregnant women have higher calcium needs and often experience an acid burning stomach. For pregnant women, calcium-based antacids are an ideal solution to two problems.

Since many minerals compete in the intestines for sites of absorption, calcium excess may cause a deficiency of other minerals. High-dose calcium supplements have been found to lower iron absorption.[35] Calcium also interferes with zinc absorption, which is another mineral in short supply in the American diet.[36] Calcium excess may be excreted via the kidneys as calcium-based kidney stones, say some experts.[37] Calcium absorption efficiency is increased with vitamin C, lactose (milk sugar), and acid foods. There is a wide discrepancy in the ability of humans to absorb calcium. In one study of healthy postmenopausal women, the percentage of calcium absorbed from food ranged from 7 to 68 percent.[38]

Vitamin D is mandatory for the absorption and use of calcium, but older adults are often low in vitamin D intake.[39] And even if their intake of vitamin D is adequate, the vitamin must still be activated by both liver and kidney, but liver and kidney function in many people deteriorates as they age. In a double-blind study of elderly English women, vitamin D supplements of 2,000 IU daily (five times the RDA) significantly raised circulating levels of vitamin D and also improved calcium absorption.[40] No harmful side effects were noted in this two-year study. Other researchers have found that 1,500–2,000 mg daily of calcium combined with 14,000 IU of vitamin D daily (35 times the RDA) provided effective treatment in reversing osteoporosis.[41] Although vitamin D was once thought to be found only in a few animal foods, there are now some recognized plant sources (dark green leafy vegetables) of this precious vitamin.[42] One teaspoon of fish oil daily for its vitamin D and special fatty acid content also may be very effective at preventing the bone erosion of osteoporosis.

At the very least, osteoporosis can immobilize people for a few months. At its worst, osteoporosis can begin an avalanche of health problems that lead to death. Osteoporosis is quite preventable and possibly treatable through healing nutrients.

ARTHRITIS

If the entire populations of New York, Chicago, and Los Angeles were suddenly stricken with a debilitating disease, there would be an outcry from the public and action from both scientists and politicians. Twenty million Americans—the combined population of those cities—are so afflicted with arthritis that they need medical care, yet only about $20 million annually is spent on research for this disease.[43] Ten percent of the world's population and 25 percent of Americans have some degree of arthritis. About 4 million Americans are disabled by the disease. Twice as many women as men are affected. The Arthritis Foundation puts the cost of arthritis in America at $25,000 per minute, or $13 billion per year in lost wages, lost time at work, medical care, and lost taxes. Fourteen million work days are lost each year by arthritis victims. Every year, $3 billion is spent on medical care for American arthritics. Conventional medicine has so little to offer arthritics that another $400 million annually is spent on quack "cures and remedies" for arthritis. The arthritic is an easy target for the huckster.

There are many different types of arthritis. Arthritis basically involves painful joints stemming from inflammation in the joint region. Osteoarthritis is a degenerative condition of painful and stiff joints (especially after exercise) usually found in the elderly. Rheumatoid arthritis is found commonly in people of all ages, involves an atrophy of the bones, and can cause skeletal deformities. Throughout this chapter we are referring to rheumatoid arthritis.

This disease has monumental proportions: there is no cure, no prevention, and no specific cause. One out of 10 people in the world falls victim to the crippling and painful snare of arthritis. The *Merck Medical Manual* lists over a dozen possible causes for arthritis, including psychological stress (guilt, hate, hurt, rejection, etc.), problems with body chemistry (gout, diabetes, scurvy), infectious organisms, a concussion (fall or injury to that area), allergic reactions, or tumors attacking the joints.[44]

NUTRITION AND ARTHRITIS

The normal bone joint is a marvel of engineering. Two bones are joined by a tough, fibrous protein substance (collagen and elastin) and lubricated by a substance (synovial fluid) that is so slippery that modern chemistry has yet to duplicate its lubricant abilities. Since all bone joints are built from and repaired by dietary nutrients, it seems obvious that diet would influence at least some cases of arthritis. Yet only in the last few years have arthritis groups retracted some of their blanket statements that diet has nothing to do with arthritis. Nutrition can help many arthritics and totally cure a few.

In a well-controlled experiment, a hypoallergenic diet (see chapter on food allergies) produced marked improvements in 75 percent of the arthritis patients studied.[45] Another group of researchers looked at the nutritional status of 50 arthritis patients and 50 healthy controls. While 13 of the arthritis patients were judged to be malnourished, none of the controls had abnormal nutritional levels.[46] Deficiencies of vitamin D, folic acid, and zinc are commonly found in arthritics. Perhaps arthritis, in some instances, is merely some people's way of expressing malnutrition.

Nutrition-related factors in arthritis include:

- *Weight control.* Excess poundage stresses the joints, so losing weight can help some arthritics. (See Chapter 13 for more on this subject.)
- *Allergies.* In some people, the body's immune cells begin to attack its own tissue. When this autoimmune response occurs in the joints, the inflammation of arthritis can result. (See Chapter 8 for more on this subject.)
- *Macronutrient intake.* Some arthritics can be helped with a diet containing less overall fat, saturated animal fat, sugar, meat, and alcohol and with more complex carbohydrates from vegetables and whole grains. This means rigidly adhering to the Core Program. At the very worst, this diet will make the arthritic feel better and more energetic; at the best, it may just be a cure.
- *Specific nutrient intake..* Niacin, pantothenic acid, riboflavin, vitamin A, vitamin B_6, folic acid, vitamin C, bioflavonoids,

magnesium, calcium, zinc, copper, certain amino acids, high-sulfur foods, DMSO, orotic acid, and certain essential fatty acids have all been implicated as having some role in arthritis.

Fats

Fish oil and other special fats provide some of the more exciting work involving nutrition against arthritis. A group of potent body substances called *leukotrienes* cause inflammation of tissue, such as occurs in arthritis. When the diet is high in eicosapentaenoic acid (EPA) and docosahexaenoic acid (DHA), both of which are found primarily in fish oil, there is a marked reduction in leukotrienes produced in the body.[47] Harvard researchers have found that this neat theory applies to human arthritics. Seventeen patients with rheumatoid arthritis were given a diet high in polyunsaturated fats and low in saturated fats plus 10 capsules of EPA daily (totaling 1.8 g of EPA). After 12 weeks, the experimental group reported a noticeable improvement in tender joints and morning stiffness, while the placebo group got worse.[48]

Another special fat is gamma-linolenic acid (GLA), a.k.a *evening primrose oil*. There is some preliminary evidence that GLA may be useful against arthritis.[49] By ensuring a diet higher in plant oils, especially soy, linseed, and safflower oils, you could improve your chances of providing this special dietary fat.

Another use of fat therapy for arthritis is clinically proven but without a well controlled study to support it. Basically, the idea is that arthritics should not drink cold fluids with their meals. If necessary, only hot fluids like herb tea or soup broth should be consumed. The reasoning behind this theory is that cold fluids change the surface tension of fats in the intestines and prevent the proper absorption of the essential fatty acids like linoleic, linolenic, gamma linolenic, EPA, and DHA. Since this therapy offers possible help with no risk, it deserves a try.

Pantothenic Acid

Pantothenic acid has been ignored by some nutritionists because its name implies that it is found "everywhere" and hence is not worth worrying about. The truth is, it is everywhere but in the American diet. Processing wheat removes most of the pantothenic acid from flour. Pantothenic acid is used up more rapidly during high-stress situations, such as are all too common in 20th-century America. Pantothenic acid could be useful in treating certain cases of arthritis.

Arthritics were found to have considerably lower levels of pantothenic acid than healthy controls. When the arthritics were given injections of 50 mg of calcium pantothenate daily (500 percent of the USRDA), blood levels rose to normal, and relief from many symptoms of arthritis was reported. When the injections ceased, the symptoms returned.[50] Results were best in vegetarians, especially those who were given a combination of pantothenic acid injections and royal bee jelly (the richest known source of pantothenic acid). Royal bee jelly also contains a substance called *10-hydroxydec-2-enoic acid*. This substance has been found to have strong antimicrobial properties that may enhance the anti-inflammatory effect that royal bee jelly has against arthritis.[51]

Another small study in 1963 found that oral supplements of pantothenic acid relieved the symptoms of osteoarthritis in some of the subjects tested.[52] For unknown reasons, these data were ignored for the next 17 years until a double-blind study was conducted with oral calcium pantothenate. That study found that pantothenic acid significantly reduced the duration of morning stiffness, degree of disability, and severity of pain in arthritics.[53] Oral doses in this study were 500 mg daily for the first two days, 1,000 mg daily for the next three days, 1,500 mg daily for the next four days, and 2,000 mg daily thereafter. All supplements were taken in divided dosages throughout the day. When supplements of L-cysteine were given along with pantothenic acid, British researchers found a major improvement in patients with both osteoarthritis and rheumatoid arthritis.[54]

The USRDA of pantothenic acid is 10 mg. The discoverer of pantothenic acid, Dr. Roger Williams, considers this level too low. Most Americans get one-third to one-half of the USRDA of pantothenic acid.

Minerals

Zinc is another likely helper in the nutritional treatment of arthritis. Arthritis victims usually have lower-than-normal zinc levels in their blood.[55] In a double-blind study using 24 arthritis patients, zinc supplements provided noticeable improvement in morning stiffness, joint swelling, walking time, and the patients' own impression of their condition.[56] Animal studies show that zinc can inhibit the inflammation process that occurs in arthritis via the release of histamine from mast cells.[57] Mast cells are among the many specialized cells at work in the immune system. This histamine release is a suspected cause in many cases of arthritis.

Copper is a co-worker with zinc in the body. Zinc and copper can compete in some systems and work together in other ways. The diet should provide a 10:1 zinc-to-copper ratio. Arthritis victims often have higher-than-normal copper levels in their arthritic joints. Long ago, this was interpreted to mean that copper may cause arthritis. But now scientists find that the opposite may be true, since copper is involved in anti-inflammatory actions.

Copper bracelets have long been a folk remedy for arthritis, and there may be scientific support for this treatment. Researchers set up a double-blind experiment that provided copper bracelets or similar-looking placebo bracelets to arthritis victims. The osteoarthritis patients whose copper bracelets were replaced with placebo bracelets experienced a significant deterioration in their condition.[58] The researchers found that sweat could dissolve microscopic quantities of copper from the bracelet, which could then be absorbed directly into the skin. Copper may indeed help to reduce bone and tissue swelling, thus relieving certain cases of arthritis.

Superoxide dismutase (SOD) is a potent antioxidant enzyme system in the human body that mops up destructive electron spills. There are various types of SOD, some containing zinc, copper, or molybdenum. When researchers gave injections of zinc-copper SOD (known as Orgotein) directly into human arthritic joints, the symptoms improved.[59]

Manganese is another trace mineral that deserves some attention in the war against arthritis. Manganese is involved in the production of the substance that composes bone ends (mucopolysaccharides). Anecdotally and in a popular book, manganese supplements have improved the symptoms of arthritis.[60] Since the theory is valid, the anecdotal evidence is supportive, and the risks are near zero; it is surprising that no one has scientifically tested the use of manganese supplements against arthritis.

Much of the problem with arthritis is caused by excessive inflammation. Nutrients that can prevent or reverse the unnatural swelling that is found in arthritis would be most welcome in treating the disease. Vitamin E and selenium are two very likely candidates for this job of anti-inflammatory nutrients. A group of 26 girls with juvenile chronic arthritis were found to have selenium levels that were lower than normal.[61] Selenium has definite anti-inflammatory abilities in the human body.[62] Selenium supplements have been approved by the FDA for use in arthritis *on dogs.*[63] Injections of vitamin E and selenium also have been quite successful in treating arthritis conditions in various animals in veterinary practice.[64] Vitamin E has also been used with some success to treat human arthritis.[65]

Protein and Amino Acids

D-phenylalanine (as opposed to the more commonly spoken of L-phenylalanine) supplements helped to reduce the inflammation of arthritis.[66] L-tryptophan is an amino acid that lowered edema and inflammation in rat studies by up to one-third.[67] In the same experiment, researchers found that derivatives of certain amino acids (phenylbutazone, DL-citrulline, DL-leucinamide) were also quite effective in lowering tissue swelling and inflammation.

Beans, eggs, and gelatin are high in the sulfur-bearing amino acids that work toward strengthening the connective tissue in the joints. DMSO (dimethyl sulfoxide) is a naturally occurring organic compound whose by-products are normally present in humans. DMSO has been used with some success to treat human arthritis.[68] It could be the sulfur compound in DMSO that provides the arthritis relief, since sulfur bridges are so important to the strength and integrity of the tough connective tissue that makes up the joints. You should be wary of the purity of DMSO sold in many stores, however, since it often does not meet the exacting standards of the DMSO used in laboratory experiments.

Other Nutrition Factors That May Help Arthritics

Nutrition does indeed relate to arthritis. In many people, optimal nutrition will relieve the symptoms. In some cases, nutrition may cure the condition altogether. Other nutrition factors that have been linked to arthritis include these:

- Vitamin C and aspirin used together were able to reduce the growth of arthritis cells.[69]
- In arthritic patients with low levels of vitamin D (quite common in older adults in America), supplements of vitamin D were able to relieve the symptoms of arthritis.[70]
- A number of physicians have reported excellent results in treating arthritis by using 1,000 mg of niacinamide daily.[71]
- Bioflavonoids not only treat the symptoms of arthritis, but also fortify the joints.[72]

- Some people may temporarily mistake gout for arthritis, since they both cause disabling pain in the joints. Orotic acid (a precursor of the nucleic acids) has been used to treat gout.[73]

DIETARY GUIDELINES
TO PREVENT, TREAT, OR PERHAPS CURE ARTHRITIS

1. Eliminate meat, milk, and wheat for two weeks to see if this improves symptoms. An elimination diet can help many arthritics. (See chapter on food allergies.)

2. A vegetarian regimen can be effective against arthritis.

3. Place special emphasis on beans for their sulfur content.

For Osteoporosis
Calcium   +1,000 mg
Fluoride   +3 mg
Copper   +1.5 mg
Zinc   +15 mg
Magnesium   +500 mg
Iron   +10 mg

Vitamins
Vitamin D   +400 IU (for younger people)
+1,000 IU (for older people)

For Arthritis
Vitamins
  Vitamin A   +10,000 IU
  Vitamin D   +400 IU
  Vitamin E   +200 IU
  Riboflavin +50 mg
  Niacin +400 mg
  Vitamin B_6 +50 mg
  Folic Acid +800 mcg
  Vitamin C   +1,000 mg
  Pantothenic acid   +500 mg/day for first week, adding 500 mg
             more each week until total intake reaches
             2,000 mg/day. If no improvement within 2
             months, slowly reduce the dosage by 500
             mg/day until intake is 50 mg.

Minerals
  Calcium   +800 mg
  Magnesium   +400 mg
  Zinc +15 mg
  Copper +2 mg
  Selenium +200 mcg

Quasi vitamins
  EPA   +2,000 mg
  Royal bee jelly   +200 mg
  Bioflavonoids   +500 mg
  L-tryptophan   +3 g
  D-phenylalanine   +2 g

16
COUNTERING THE EFFECTS OF POLLUTION
Drugs, Tobacco, Alcohol, Radiation, Toxins

There is a good chance that your body is being exposed to poisons on a daily basis. Both voluntarily and involuntarily, Americans are taking in escalating proportions of toxic substances. Any substance that contaminates the normal body chemistry can be considered a pollutant. On the voluntary side, one-third of all adults smoke, and more than half consume liquor regularly. One-third of all *children* and 98 percent of all older adults are on some type of prescription medication. Illicit drug usage is almost beyond estimate. Disregarding pollutants that people *choose* to expose themselves to, even the most careful person is still taking in alarming amounts of air, water, and food pollutants.

The Environmental Protection Agency declared in 1979 that up to 20 percent of all deaths in America are caused by pollutants and environmental hazards.[1] And it's getting worse. Each year, 80–90 *billion* pounds of toxic waste is dumped across America into our 55,000 toxic waste sites, with 90 percent of these toxins disposed of irresponsibly.[2] Including air pollution, there are 600 pounds of toxic waste produced annually for every man, woman and child in America. Urban Americans have 500 times more lead in their bones than the people of 350 years ago.[3] Pesticides, herbicides, certain food additives, smoke, second-hand smoke, alcohol, drugs, radiation, chlorinated water, lead, and other toxins all put a definite limitation on your health and longevity.

Pollution is not new. The Thames River in the 18th century looked more like a thick swamp than a watercourse, since it was the toilet for millions of Londoners. Coal dust and smoke shrouded most big cities in 19th-century Europe with a thick veil of air pollution.

The massive but primitive wastes of yesterday have yielded to the high-tech immortal wastes of today. Whereas feces in the Thames River would eventually degrade, and coal smoke in the air settles to the ground, PCB, asbestos, lead, and various petrochemical derivatives are not biodegradable. Hence, our new pollutants stay in circulation for a very long time. The idea of preserving a balanced ecosystem is gone. It is now a matter of sheer human survival. Millions of people will continue to get cancer, birth defects, and other ailments from Space Age pollution before something is finally done about it. In the meantime, there are several nutrients that are proven defenders against pollutants. This chapter is not intended to stir up paranoia, but rather to instill caution. If you are aware of the obstacles to avoid, then you can reduce your risks. It is the blissfully ignorant person who is more likely to be a victim of 20th-century pollutants.

There are four different efforts you can make to minimize your exposure to environmental pollutants:

1. Minimize or avoid the use of tobacco, drugs, and alcohol.

2. Drink only purified water and rinse your fresh produce in warm water.

3. Seriously lower your intake of high fat animal foods like beef and butter. Many 20th century pollutants are fat soluble and concentrate themselves in animal fat.

4. Take certain nutritional supplements to mitigate the effects of many pollutants.

Healing nutrients can provide a formidable coat of armor to help shield you from the deadly effluvia of 20th-century technology.

DANGEROUS TOXINS

FOOD ADDITIVES

Of the thousands of food additives in use—some FDA approved, others that are "incidental" to agriculture and food processing—some are quite safe, such as the emulsifiers lecithin, gelatin, seaweed, and pectin. Others are questionable, such as the preservatives of BHA and BHT. Still others are risky business, including sodium nitrite, brominated vegetable oils, metabisulfite, and monosodium glutamate (MSG). If you're not interested in learning which additives are safe and which are not, just buy foods without a label. No label means fewer additives. This approach involves considerable home food preparation, but it is possible.

TOBACCO PRODUCTS

Tobacco products have been proven to be so lethal that they should carry a skull and crossbones on their label. Not only does the smoker take risks, but the innocent bystander getting second-hand smoke is also threatened. Nonsmokers in offices, restaurants, planes, and bars are inhaling measurable amounts of tobacco. Children exposed to smoke at home run a 60 percent greater chance of developing cancer. A nonsmoker living with a smoker increases his or her cancer risk by 50 percent. Even smokers living with other smokers run an elevated risk of cancer beyond the risk of their own habit.[4] Actually, sidestream (second-hand) smoke has 300 percent more benzpyrene (a known carcinogen), 600 percent more toluene (the deadly vapors of airplane glue), and 5,000 percent more dimethylnitrosamines (also cancer-causing) than directly inhaled smoke. Second-hand smoke (a.k.a *passive smoking*) is dangerous. Smoking mothers are more likely to deliver premature, defective, or small infants.

DRUGS

Nearly all drugs are found to have some nutrient interaction. Drugs can lower the absorption efficiency, increase the excretion rate, lower the reclamation rate, or just plain use up more of a nutrient. The *Physician's Desk Reference* is filled with the nutritional side effects of various prescription drugs. There is even a professional journal (*Drug-Nutrient Interactions*) that deals exclusively with this subject. As an example, oral contraceptives, which are taken by 50 million women worldwide, create an increased need for vitamin B_6, folacin, and other nutrients. These nutrient interactions can lead to depression and other side effects of poor health. "Recreational" and other illicit drugs are no exception to this drug-nutrient interaction rule.

ALCOHOL

Alcohol is also a drug, but a unique one in that it is more socially acceptable, found on every street corner, and also a nutrient by virtue of its 7 kilocalories per gram. Alcohol causes the loss of many nutrients, including thiamine, zinc, and magnesium. Many heavy drinkers substitute alcoholic beverages for meals, thus creating an even greater chasm between nutrient needs and nutrient intake.[5] One or two drinks daily poses minimal risks for healthy, nonpregnant adults. Yet 33 percent of all drinking adults consume five or more drinks at any given sitting.[6] Excessive alcohol intake becomes a chemical pollutant in the body.

WATER POLLUTION

Water pollution has become a serious issue. The National Cancer Institute has declared that "carcinogens in our water supply pose an unacceptable risk." Chlorine was once added to our water supply to prevent the growth of typhoid and other plague-causing microorganisms. Yet now there is a link between drinking tap water and the development of cancer. When chlorine combines with organic wastes, it forms trihalomethanes, which are known carcinogens.

Agricultural fertilizers run off into rivers and end up in the ground water. These nitrogen compounds join with proteins in the diet to form nitrosamines (known carcinogens) in the stomach. The freeway running down the central valley of California is lined with public drinking fountains that warn against young children and pregnant women consuming the water due to the hazard of cancer-causing nitrosamines.

Chloramines (commonly found in municipal drinking water) are combinations of chlorine and amines. Many municipal water departments have warned people with kidney ailments not to drink their "normal" tap water. Even pet fish will die in most city tap water. If it kills a fish immersed in it, what do you think it is doing to your body? These are only the minor pollutants that are added to drinking water "for your protection." It gets worse.

There are 55,000 chemical dump sites across the nation that are leaking their poisons into the underground drinking water. The city of New Orleans has the dubious distinction of being at the end of the Mississippi River, a favorite "toilet" for the dumping of industrial wastes. Not surprisingly, New Orleans residents have a higher incidence of cancer in the body parts (kidney, bladder, and urinary tract) that are trying to dispose of polluted water.[7] Of the more than 300 chemicals found in the average city drinking water, 22 are known carcinogens.

No one seems to be immune from water pollution. Small towns in Missouri and New England have recently been evacuated due to lethal pollution of underground water supplies. PCB and gasoline, respectively, were the problems in these bucolic rural outposts, where you would think pollution has not tainted the landscape. In the 1950s, General Electric began dumping PCB (polychlorobiphenol), a deadly toxin, into the Hudson River. In two decades, they dumped 1.5 million pounds of PCB. Today, every person on earth and every corner of the world (including the polar ice caps) have detectable levels of PCB. Scientists have yet to determine a safe level of exposure to PCB.

Dioxin is the active ingredient in agent orange, the infamous defoliant used in Vietnam. In 1970, the National Academy of Sciences declared dioxin too dangerous to use in warfare. We then began using dioxin as a herbicide on our own forests. Dow Chemical earns about $12 million annually from the sale of a product that is too dangerous to be used on our enemies in wartime. Dioxin is 100,000 times more teratogenic (likely to cause birth defects) than thalidomide. Much dioxin ends up in our water supply, just one example of the deadly pollutants found there.

On the November 1986 ballot, Californians voted to ban the presence of cancer-causing pollutants in the drinking water supply. That shouldn't be asking too much. Water that is free of carcinogens is something that would normally be assumed by most voters. Yet the governor decided to enforce this law for only 10 percent of the 240 known carcinogens in California drinking water. This perplexing move by the governor was challenged in the state supreme court and overturned in favor of the voters. This just illustrates the ubiquitous and commonly accepted nature of polluted water across America.

The EPA has called water pollution "the most grievous error in judgement we as a nation have ever made." Recently, Congress passed a "superfund" cleanup act to begin purging the water and land of deadly pollutants, but it may be too late. If you still drink normal tap water, you are either uniquely blessed with an isolated pocket of clean water or you are very cavalier about your health. I recommend that people get their own water filtration system or reputable bottled water to drink. Most tap water is okay to wash clothes, dishes, and food, but not for personal consumption.

AIR POLLUTION

The health of 35 million Americans is in immediate jeopardy from air pollution alone. In Los Angeles and New York, you can see the air that you are breathing. This is obviously not good. Ozone from smog can wreak havoc on the lungs. Smog ages cars and houses much faster. In 1883, a granite Egyptian obelisk was placed in New York's Central Park. In the 100 years that the stone has been exposed to New York air, it has lost several inches and experienced more deterioration than the 3,500 years it spent in the Egyptian desert. Imagine what that accelerated oxidation is doing to your body. But air pollution is no longer confined to the big cities. Even some rural communities have hazardous air from nearby industries. Heavy farm equipment spews out a deadly carcinogen (benzpyrene) from its diesel exhaust. One minute of an idling diesel engine produces more carcinogens than you could get from smoking 2,000 cigarettes.[8] Formaldehyde is another by-product of diesel exhaust. Much of these toxins fall on nearby food crops, yet few people recognize this potential hazard.

Most cities lie under a blanket of lead-laden air from leaded gasoline exhaust. Levels of lead that were once thought to be innocuous are now known to be quite harmful and common. Unfortunately, it is the children who get hit hardest by lead pollution. Their active lifestyles and higher metabolic rates bring in more leaded air. Their rapidly growing brains are most vulnerable

to lead toxicity. Many inner-city children with behavioral disturbances or poor learning abilities could be suffering from lead
toxicity.

HERBICIDES AND PESTICIDES

In some regions of the world, pests and insects eat one-third to
one-half of the crops. We don't have that problem in the U.S. due
to potent pesticide sprays. Pesticide sales in America total $4.5
billion per year.[9] However, these sprays are by no means innocuous
once inside the human system. Ask yourself this: If a substance is
lethal enough to kill tenacious weeds and insects, what will it do
to my body? Most foods contain an ever increasing amount of
chemical poisons.[10]

Most pesticides are supposed to be mixed in certain concentrations and ladled out over the crops in certain quantities. Yet many
agricultural workers are either illiterate or uninterested in these
warnings. Migrant workers often use the lids of pesticide containers as family dishes, which illustrates their naive attitude toward
these poisons.

The U.S. Department of Agriculture investigates about 15,000
cases yearly of pesticides poisoning in *city* regions alone. Imagine
the pesticide problem in rural areas where its use is more common.

For over four decades, the potent pesticide EDB (ethylene dibromide) was used on grain crops. In 1983 it was banned in
America because of its cancerous effect on animals. No one will
ever know how many humans were affected by EDB, and it is still
used in other countries that ship their fresh produce to America.

DDT was used for decades in America until Rachel Carson
divulged its insidious effects in her classic book *Silent Spring*.
DDT is now banned for food crop use but is still occasionally used
in forestry. DBCP is another pesticide so lethal that it is now
banned in America. Yet DBCP has been found in 2,450 wells
across America.

In the summer of 1985, watermelon farmers in California had
one-third of their crop (10 million melons) destroyed by state and
federal authorities because the melons contained dangerous levels
of the pesticide aldicarb. Few crops are tested for their levels of
poisons, and even fewer crops are destroyed when their poison

levels exceeds the state and federal standards for "permissible" levels of poisons.

RADIATION

Radiation is found in everything from the sun, to gases emitted from the earth's core (as radon gas), to your dentist's and doctor's X-ray machines, to the nearby nuclear power plant. Radon gas may be the second leading cause of lung cancer, (behind cigarettes) causing between 10,000 and 70,000 cases of fatal lung cancer each year in America alone. In certain regions of this country, radon gas permeates homes that are well sealed (as in the winter) and built into the earth (as with a basement). And there's more:

- Children living near a nuclear processing plant on the north coast of England have a higher rate of leukemia.
- Irradiation of swollen tonsils (a discontinued practice) has been linked to cancer of the thyroid gland.
- Radiation from computer screens has been implicated in raising the incidents of deformed infants when pregnant women work at computer terminals full-time.[11]
- The nuclear disaster in Chernobyl, Russia, in 1986 forewarned the world of the calamitous potential of nuclear power stations. The rate of leukemia and other cancers is expected to rise significantly in the area surrounding Chernobyl.

INDUSTRIAL POLLUTANTS

Industrial pollutants now abound in America. Asbestos, formaldehyde, lead, mercury, PCB, exotic acids, arsenic, and an armada of high-tech garbage has been indiscriminately dumped throughout our country. PCB is both deadly and ubiquitous.[12] It is found in every creature on earth and in every place on earth, even in the polar ice caps. All human milk has predictable amounts of PCB.[13] Health authorities in the Great Lakes region caution against the consumption of more than one locally caught salmon per year, due to the accumulation of PCB in these high-fat fish. Of the 30,000 different chemicals that American industry regularly uses, 1,500 are suspected of causing cancer. Yet the Environmental Protection Agency only regulates the discharge of nine of these chemicals. Industry is free to legally dump the rest anywhere they want.

NUTRITION: A WEAPON AGAINST POLLUTION

What do you have to worry about? Plenty. What can you do about it? Plenty. There are several means by which nutrition can protect you from the ravages of pollution.

- By saturating your body with good substances (such as iodine). This makes it more difficult for your body to take on bad substances (like radioactive iodine).
- By consuming substances that compete with the toxin for absorption sites in the intestines, such as selenium does with lead, arsenic, and mercury.
- By consuming nutrients that bind themselves to the pollutant and carry it out of the system, such as fiber does.
- By consuming nutrients that act like "sacrificial lambs," allowing themselves, rather than healthy body tissue, to be destroyed. Vitamins E, C, and A and the mineral selenium work this way.
- By filling the need for extra nutrients that is created by some pollutants, such as drugs, alcohol, and tobacco. In these cases, it may be the nutritional deficiency that creates the real health hazard.
- By consuming nutrients in doses that give them near "Superman" status. Cysteine, selenium, vitamin A, and niacin seem to act this way.
- By satisfying a nutrient need that exists only in the sick, ailing, polluted body. These "conditionally essential" nutrients, like choline and orotic acid, may become quite therapeutic in protecting some vulnerable people from pollution harm.

Altogether, healing nutrients can provide a substantial shield to protect you from the pollution that we are all exposed to. The malnourished person is much more likely to suffer the effects of pollution than the well-nourished person.The individual nutrients are discussed below.

VITAMIN C

Nitrates and nitrites are food additives used to reduce the risk of botulism poisoning and also to provide a bright red color to otherwise dull-looking meats. But nitrites and nitrates can combine in the stomach with amino acids from protein foods to form nitrosamines, which are known carcinogens.[14] Not only are nitrosamines cancer-causing in themselves, but they also enhance the carcinogenic abilities of certain foods (like overcooked meats) and drinks (such as alcohol).[15] Vitamin C and E both block the formation of nitrosamines in the gastrointestinal tract.[16] When researchers gave 2,000 mg of vitamin C and 400 IU of vitamin E daily to 10 college students, they found that the ascorbic acid alone blocked an average of 81 percent of the nitrosamine formation, and vitamin E blocked 59 percent.

Acetaldehyde is a toxic by-product that results from smoking and drinking. In animal studies, investigators found that supplements of vitamin C, cysteine, and thiamine gave almost complete protection against acetaldehyde toxicity.[17] Smoking binds up considerable amounts of vitamin C.[18] By providing the body with optimal amounts of vitamin C, the smoker can lessen the harm done on the body.

Vitamin C also reduces the harmful effects of radiation.[19] When test animals were given large amounts of vitamin C (equivalent to 3–5 g daily for a human), and then blasted with radiation, the mortality rate was less, and their weight gain was greater when compared to nonsupplemented animals.[20] Vitamin C and E in combination were able to protect another group of test animals substantially from the harmful effects of PCB.[21] Bioflavonoids help to detoxify benzpyrenes, the common cancer-causing substance found in overcooked protein foods.[22]

VITAMIN E AND SELENIUM

Heavy toxic metals, such as lead, mercury, and arsenic, are quite common today. Lead is found in the air (from leaded gasoline exhaust), canned food (leaded seam or plug), lead-base paints eaten by children, leaded ceramic glaze, lead-polluted food and water, and lead/pewter eating utensils. The lead in gasoline can be absorbed through the skin. Lead buildup in the body causes fatigue, lethargy, and a general breakdown of many bodily functions. What were once thought to be safe and acceptable levels of lead in the human body are now known to be both "normal" and hazardous amounts. As much as one-third of all inner-city children suffer mild to severe effects of lead toxicity. Researchers found a direct relationship between fluctuations in the sale of leaded gasoline and the amount of lead in the umbilical cord of newborn babies in that area.[23] Selenium has been found to significantly reduce the absorption and toxicity of these heavy metals.[24]

Cadmium accumulation may cause high blood pressure, among other side effects.[25] Cadmium is found in canned food, tobacco smoke, and industrial pollution. Selenium helps detoxify cadmium from the body.

Mercury is a toxic metal often used in industry. In the 1960s and 1970s, thousands of Japanese infants were born with birth defects from mercury poisoning. Selenium has been shown to reverse the effects of mercury poisoning.[26] It will not cure birth defects from mercury poisoning.

Selenium is involved in the potent detoxifying enzyme in the body, glutathione peroxidase (GSH). Selenium intake is related to GSH production.[27] Scientists found that GSH lowers the toxicity of burned proteins (benzpyrenes), thus lowering the risk for stomach cancer.[28]

Selenium seems to have the ability to lower the risks for virtually all toxins. When animals were given selenium supplements, then exposed to a myriad of pollutants, selenium invariably lowered the cancer rate in the supplemented animals.[29] Other animals were given supplemental selenium and then exposed to the deadly pollutant from tobacco smoke DMBA (dimethylbenzanthracene), with considerably fewer tumors found in the supplemented animals.[30]

In a broad-scoped review, scientists found that selenium levels were closely related to the toxicity of various chemicals and poisons: the lower the selenium levels in the body, the more frequent and severe were the effects of toxins.[31] Selenium/GSH can reduce the toxicity from radiation.[32] When vitamin E and selenium are combined, they have an even greater protective effect against radiation.[33] Selenium supplements in animals are able to blunt the effect of the deadly herbicide paraquat and the potent chemotherapy agent adriamycin.[34] Supplements of coenzyme Q have also been shown to reduce the toxicity of adriamycin on the human heart.[35]

Vitamin E is a potent antioxidant that can protect the blood from the "rusting" effects of air pollution. Vitamin E protects against the effect of various chemical toxins, ozone, and nitrous oxide on the lungs.[36] The enzymes built from selenium and vitamin E are quickly able to repair the damaged DNA to prevent cancer or other harmful effects of pollution.[37]

Selenium and vitamin E are well-established armor plating against the sinister effects of pollutants. Since the ultimate insult of a pollutant to the body is cancer, see Chapter 6 for more information on this subject.

AMINO ACIDS

L-cysteine is a sulfur-bearing amino acid. Researchers at the Argonne Laboratory in Chicago used L-cysteine to significantly reduce the harm done to lab animals by radiation exposure.[38] Cysteine supplements have been found in other experiments at Cornell University to increase the production of GSH, which retards the toxicity of many chemicals.[39] L-methionine is also a sulfur-bearing amino acid that enhances weight gain and reduces mercury concentrations in the tissues of mercury-poisoned animals.[40]

QUASI VITAMINS

Orotic acid is a nonessential nutrient that is a midpoint product in the manufacturing of the nucleic acids DNA and RNA. Supplements of orotic acid have improved the status of both humans and lab animals who were exposed to pollutants.[41]

Orotic acid supplements may be essential for sick, wounded, and poisoned humans. Test animals who were given injections of orotic acid and then exposed to various levels of radiation experienced considerably less damage and more rapid recovery than their unsupplemented peers.[42]

Carnitine is part of the body's shuttle mechanism in burning fats. Scientists at the University of Florida have found that numerous drugs interfere with the body's ability to produce carnitine.[43] Carnitine may be an essential vitamin for people who are exposed to some pollutants or using certain drugs.

VITAMIN A

Vitamin A, especially the plant version beta-carotene, is the most effective free radical sponge yet discovered and thus has its role in preventing the toxicity of pollutants. Beta-carotene supplements equivalent to about 75,000 IU/day for humans were able to cut tumor rates in test animals that were exposed to the carcinogen found in tobacco smoke (DMBA) by 89 percent.[44] Researchers reviewed the history of 308 employees who worked in a Dow Chemical plant in Texas. The higher the intake of beta-carotene, the lower the risk for cancer from either carcinogenic fumes at work or smoking.[45]

Tissue cells that are saturated with beta-carotene and then exposed to radiation, toxins, pollutants, and carcinogenic viruses have a reduced incidence and growth rate of tumors.[46] Various medical procedures, like anesthetics, chemotherapy, and radiation therapy, often deteriorate the immune system of the patient and can worsen his or her overall condition. Vitamin A supplements buffer this immune-suppressive effect[47] and allow the medical treatment to help rather than hinder the patient. Vitamin A supplements also help to restore normal healing in patients undergoing anti-inflammatory drug therapy, including cortisone, aspirin, and others.[48]

B VITAMINS

When niacin is given in large doses (100–1,000 mg daily) it takes on a new role as dilator of blood vessels and general detoxifier. A drug rehabilitation center in Los Angeles claims that niacin supplements have helped to speed recovery to thousands of drug abusers.[49]

Many drugs and some stress stages in life can increase the need for vitamin B_6 by up to 25 times the normal RDA levels.[50]

MINERALS

Zinc is crucial to the manufacture and repair of DNA and RNA. Pollutants often attack RNA and DNA, which then must be rebuilt. Although long-term, high-dose zinc supplements (+100 mg daily for several months) could compete with selenium for sites of absorption and thus actually enhance the toxicity of substances, in most people rational zinc supplements (20–60 mg) would be protective against pollutants. For example:

- Zinc supplements lowered the cancerous effects of toxic chemicals on various lab animals.[51]

- When zinc was combined with vitamin C, both were able to lower the amount of lead absorbed by factory workers.[52]
- Zinc supplements blunt the harmful effects of alcohol on the developing fetus.[53]
- Zinc supplements even prevented birth defects in test animals that were fed the famous teratogenic drug thalidomide.[54]

Copper is another trace mineral that may prevent the cancerous effect of certain pollutants.[55] A copper-salicylate compound was able to inhibit tumors in experimental animals.[56]

Molybdenum supplements protected lab animals from chemical carcinogens.[57] Molybdenum is part of an enzyme system (sulfite oxidase) that neutralizes the many sulfiting food additives found in the American food supply. These sulfites, like metabisulfite, are used extensively in food processing, wine making, and the restaurant industry. Sulfites can cause nausea, diarrhea, asthma, and even death in some individuals.[58] Molybdenum helps to prevent this harm, but much molybdenum is lost in food refining.

Potassium iodide pills are considered standard issue in the case of a nuclear accident. Saturating the body with normal healthy iodide reduces the chance of absorbing radioactive iodide from the atmosphere.

FIBER

Fiber is one of the more staunch bodily defenders against pollution. Animals were fed a variety of questionably safe food additives and/or toxic chemicals. On a low-fiber diet, these substances reduced the health and life span of the animals. Yet, when the animals were fed a high-fiber diet, there seemed to be no harm from these pollutants.[59]

In another study, researchers fed animals small amounts of food additives (2 percent of total diet) containing either red dye number 2, sodium cyclamate (both now banned as carcinogenic), or an emulsifier agent. None of the animals were harmed by these individual food additives. However, when both red dye number 2 and cyclamate were added to the diet, the animals experienced balding scruffy fur, diarrhea, and retarded weight gain. When another group of animals were fed all three food additives at once, they all died within two weeks. Yet when the animals were fed all three additives *plus* a high-fiber diet, all survived seemingly unscathed.[60]

There are compounds called *indoles* found in the cabbage family (cabbage, broccoli, cauliflower, brussels sprouts) that are potent anticancer agents. Fiber has the ability to absorb toxins in the diet and prevent these pollutants from attacking the gastrointestinal tract or being absorbed into the system. Fiber carries pollutants out with the feces, where they belong.

NUTRITIONAL PROTECTION FROM ORAL CONTRACEPTIVES

Birth control pills are now taken by 50 million women world-wide.[61] There are numerous physical, mental, and financial hazards of being continuously pregnant, but there are also certain risks involved in taking birth control pills. Optimal nutrition can minimize this risk. Oral contraceptives (OCs) increase the need for up to a dozen different nutrients,[62] so some experts consider vitamin supplementation to be essential for women taking OCs.[63] OCs seriously increase the need for ascorbic acid,[64] which is a fulcrum for optimal health and longevity.

Many OC users have developed depression due to the increased need for vitamin B_6.[65] And, not surprisingly, B_6 supplements have shown remarkable effectiveness in treating many of the OC users with depression. In one study, 22 depressed women on OC were analyzed, and 11 were found to have clinically abnormal B_6 levels in their blood. In a double-blind test, B_6 supplements cleared up the depression in *all* 11 of these women.[66] Researchers estimate that 80 percent of all OC users have abnormal B_6 metabolism, with 20 percent of users experiencing an absolute B_6 deficiency.

Low riboflavin levels are also commonly found in OC users.[67]

OCs also increase the need for folic acid and B_{12},[68] both of which are crucial to proper fetal development. This is a serious issue in the drug-nutrient interactions that surround oral contraceptives: although all drugs create some degree of nutrient drain, oral contraceptives create a major nutrient drain in women who are both fertile and sexually active. Hence, when they stop taking "the pill," they are both low in nutrients and very likely to get pregnant. This situation does not bode well for either mother or infant-to-be. All women on OCs should take a high-quality, broad-spectrum supplement and allow themselves at least two months after ceasing OC use before attempting to get pregnant.

NUTRITIONAL PROTECTION FROM ALCOHOL

It is the most common drug used in the world today. It is derived from fermenting carbohydrate foods: wine from grapes, beer from barley, rum from molasses, sake from rice, vodka from potatoes. It has been a part of human rituals and diet for at least 8,000 years. Alcohol comprises 10–20 percent of the average drinking adult's energy intake. Some people consume 50 percent or more of their calories from alcohol. In moderation, alcohol seems to have little harmful effect on most healthy adults. However, moderation is not an option for the 6–15 million alcoholics in this country.

Alcohol causes 10 percent of all deaths and up to 50 percent of all birth defects,[69] among other tragedies. Alcohol abuse also causes various nutritional problems. These nutrient deficiencies can cause or worsen the other complications of alcohol abuse. Proper nutrition can dilute the harm done by alcohol. In some cases, optimal nutrition can help return the alcoholic to normal health.

WHAT DOES ALCOHOL DO TO THE BODY?

Most healthy adults can process about 1 ounce of alcohol per hour. Thus a 4-ounce glass of wine, or 12 ounces of beer, or 1 ounce of distilled liquor (all of which contain about 1 ounce of alcohol) when sipped slowly over an hour's time will have minimal impact on the body. Beyond that amount, alcohol must stand in line at the liver and wait to be processed. It is this accumulation of alcohol that can erode health.

Alcohol is a diuretic and can cause considerable loss of body fluid. That fact makes beer drinking on a hot summer's day somewhat ironic. This dehydration of the brain is partly responsible for the pounding headache of a hangover.

Alcohol also lowers blood sugar, which can lead to volatile emotions. Meetings of reformed alcoholics often provide copious quantities of sugared pastries, concentrated coffee with much added sugar, and a fog of tobacco smoke engulfing the room. Each of these agents (caffeine, nicotine, sugar) can cause wild swings in blood glucose levels. Caffeine disturbs blood sugar levels and creates an alcohol craving in some people. Studies with animals show that caffeine intake heightens the desire for alcohol.[70] Stabilizing blood sugar levels through diet and exercise decreases the yearning for drinks in many alcoholics. (See the section on blood glucose in Chapter 10 for more information on how to stabilize blood glucose.)

Alcohol abuse also raises the risk of heart attack (see Chapter 5 for more information on that subject).

Since alcohol must be processed in the liver, alcohol abuse often leads to liver damage. The liver is such a valuable organ that it is probably less expendable than the brain or heart.

Alcohol is a sedative to the central nervous system. The first effect is to dissolve the thin veneer of social inhibitions and make the "happy hour" participant more forward. As alcohol intake continues and infiltrates the brain, speech becomes slurred, movement becomes awkward. The brain can become so saturated with alcohol and sedated that the body just stops breathing and the person dies.

Alcohol abuse seriously retards the absorption efficiency of the intestines and lowers the intake of all nutrients except calories,[71] which compounds the nutritional problems of the alcoholic. Protein-calorie malnutrition (kwashiorkor) is usually envisioned in the context of the poverty belts in Africa, Latin America, and Asia. Yet many American alcoholics have kwashiorkor, which accelerates their downhill health slide.[72]

Although alcohol is higher in calories than either carbohydrates or proteins, many humans do not efficiently process alcohol.[73] Alcohol in the cell furnace is something like a car stuck in the mud: the wheels are turning, and energy is being used, but no work is being done. Recent findings indicate that alcohol may follow biochemical pathways that are unique to alcohol. This may explain why there is such great diversity in human tolerance and desire for alcohol.[74]

Alcohol abuse creates a noteworthy cancer risk, especially in the body parts that are exposed to the alcohol, such as the esophagus and stomach.[75]

Large amounts of alcohol become a vasodilator, thus increasing body heat loss while also impairing the body's ability to adapt to the cold.[76]

Alcohol is not burned up in exercise.[77] Only the liver can render alcohol usable to the body.

Optimal nutrition can mitigate the effects of alcohol. Food

intake is crucial. High-potency vitamins and minerals have been used to quickly rectify poor laboratory blood values in alcoholics.[78] Many specific nutrients can help mollify the damage done by alcohol.

AMINO ACIDS

Ornithine is an amino acid that has been shown to help regenerate healthy liver tissue in animals.[79] Ornithine also helps to stimulate a healthier immune response, which is a serious problem among heavy drinkers.[80]

Cysteine is a sulfur-bearing amino acid that has an unusual capacity to neutralize the damaging aldehydes that occur from smoking, drinking, smog, and fatty diets.[81] When exposed to realistic levels of these aldehydes, 90 percent of the experimental animals died. When protected with supplements of cysteine, thiamine, and ascorbic acid, and then exposed to the toxins, none of the animals died. Cysteine is also a precursor of an important toxin-mopping enzyme (glutathione). When animals were fed diets that were deficient in cysteine and methionine, researchers found lower levels of enzymes that normally protect the body against toxins.[82] Methionine is destroyed by alcohol abuse.[83]

Excessive use of alcohol is known to reduce memory and other mental functions. There are probably many reasons for this. One possibility is the loss of crucial amino acids for thought. Alcoholics with blackout spells have significantly lower levels of tryptophan, which is an important amino acid in making the brain chemical serotonin.[84]

Dr. Roger Williams has found that supplements of glutamine have helped many alcoholics to recover.[85] Glutamine is converted to GABA (gamma-aminobutyric acid), which is one of the most prevalent chemical messengers in the human brain.

VITAMINS AND MINERALS

Thiamine

Alcohol interferes with the absorption of many vitamins.[86] Thiamine deficiency, or beriberi, is very common among alcoholics. Beriberi, literally interpreted from the Indonesian language, means "I cannot, I cannot." Thiamine absorption can be cut in half with alcohol abuse.[87] Not only is thiamine intake cut drastically (because heavy alcohol drinkers eat less), and thiamine absorption reduced (because of its effect on the intestinal wall), but thiamine need goes up considerably since the body eventually burns alcohol as a carbohydrate, a process that demands considerable amounts of thiamine.

Fifty-eight percent of all patients with chronic liver disease were diagnosed with a blatant thiamine deficiency.[88] That number is even higher in alcoholics with cirrhosis of the liver.

Alcoholics often lose the full ability to speak, hear, write, and perform other normal mental functions. This deterioration of the brain is an aphasia known as Wernicke-Korsakoff syndrome. People who abuse alcohol take up such a large portion of health care services that some noted scientists have suggested fortifying alcoholic beverages with thiamine to prevent the dastardly effects of thiamine deficiency that are found in Wernicke-Korsakoff syndrome.[89]

Beriberi of the heart is common in alcoholics and includes symptoms of wide pulse pressure, sweating, warm skin, very warm hands, and excessively rapid heartbeat (tachycardia).[90]

Thiamine is so crucial to the energy metabolism in all cells that thiamine deficiency is often the cause of death in long-term fasting. Thiamine deficiency should be suspected in all heavy drinkers or poor eaters. Most alcoholics are both.

B Vitamins

Vitamin B_{12} absorption is seriously reduced in alcohol abuse.[91] Alcoholics have a difficult time absorbing and activating folacin and B_6.[92] Both of these vitamins are commonly low in the *average* American diet and are even more absent in the drinker. Heavy drinking changes bone marrow cells and serum iron levels;[93] interferes with vitamin D, E, and K metabolism;[94] lowers the absorption efficiency of vitamin A and beta-carotene;[95] reduces B_6 absorption;[96] lowers the absorption of iron and zinc;[97] and lowers the absorption of vitamin C.[98]

Vitamin C

Scurvy is a full-blown vitamin C deficiency and was once thought to be relatively extinct in prosperous America. Scurvy is quite common in alcoholics.[99]

Vitamin A . . . Plus Zinc
In normal people, the enzyme system alcohol dehydrogenase (ADH) is able to activate vitamin A to provide healthy vision. In alcoholics, ADH is so occupied with the processing of alcohol that vitamin A activation is reduced.[100] The result is often night blindness. Researchers found that liver vitamin A levels were well below normal in 45 alcoholics studied, even though their other vitamin A blood values (serum vitamin A, prealbumin, and retinol binding protein) were normal. They suggested that vitamin A supplements be given to heavy drinkers even though deficiency symptoms may not yet be present.[101]

ADH also contains zinc, thus making zinc intake important for the alcoholic. When investigators gave zinc supplements to both healthy subjects and alcoholics at a meal without alcohol, the alcoholics absorbed less of the zinc,[102] which means that alcoholism lowers the zinc absorption mechanism.

Consider the facts: (1) Most Americans are at least marginally low in zinc. (2) Alcoholics absorb even fewer nutrients than normal people. (3) Alcoholics eat fewer nutrients than "normal." (4) Zinc is required to process alcohol. The result is that the alcoholic ends up with a very poor tolerance for alcohol and increased physical damage as the alcohol stays in the system longer due to impaired alcohol-processing ability.[103] Nine of 11 alcoholic patients with liver damage (primary biliary cirrhosis) had poor night vision. Supplements of vitamin A and zinc for one to three months corrected the poor vision to near normal.[104] Zinc supplements alone have also been shown to improve night blindness in alcoholics.[105]

Vitamin E . . . Plus Selenium
In animal studies, vitamin E supplements have markedly reduced the harmful effects of certain toxins on the liver.[106] Selenium levels are low in alcoholics. Low selenium is probably a contributing factor in liver damage from alcoholism.[107]

QUASI VITAMINS AND OTHER NUTRITIONAL HELPERS

Myoinositol is a sugarlike compound that prevents fatty accumulation in the liver of animals.[108] Fatty buildup in the liver is the initial phase of liver disease (such as occurs in alcoholics). Fibrosis and necrosis are the end stages of liver disease.

Choline is another nonessential nutrient that has been proven to reduce fatty infiltration in the liver of alcoholics.[109]

Carnitine is an important fat shuttle mechanism that helps patients with cirrhosis of the liver.[110]

Fructose is a simple sugar found in fruits, honey, and even part of table sugar. When about 60 g, or 2 ounces, of fructose was given to human subjects after alcohol administration, the alcohol cleared the bloodstream 20–30 percent faster than normal.[111]

Researchers have found that coffee oil accelerates the rate of liver recovery in lab animals.[112]

Garlic also protects damaged liver cells.[113]

RNA and DNA supplements are an embattled issue in nutrition. One study found that RNA/DNA helped to speed the rate of liver regeneration in animals.[114] Orotic acid is a precursor of the nucleic acids RNA and DNA and is considered by some experts to be a conditionally essential nutrient for alcoholics and other patients with a damaged liver.[115] Coenzyme Q helps various types of liver ailments, including alcoholic cirrhosis.[116] There is preliminary evidence that gamma-linolenic acid (GLA) can help reduce the cravings for alcohol in some people.[117]

NUTRITIONAL RECOMMENDATIONS FOR PROTECTION FROM POLLUTION

DIETARY GUIDELINES

1. Follow core diet. Consume often: high-fiber plant foods, particularly green vegetables and beans; foods in the cabbage family; and garlic.

2. Minimize intake of: food additives and dyes.

3. Wash fresh produce in warm water before using.

4. Drink only water that is professionally filtered or commercially bottled by reliable suppliers. Most tap water is not safe.

DAILY SUPPLEMENTS TO ADD TO YOUR CORE
PROGRAM

Vitamins
  Vitamin A   +30,000 IU (6,000 RE)
  (beta-carotene)
  Vitamin E   +400 IU
  Thiamine   +50 mg
  Niacin   +100–1,000 mg
  (as niacinamide)
  Vitamin B_6 +50 mg
  Vitamin B_{12} +100 mcg
  Folic Acid   +400 mcg
  Vitamin C   +2,000 mg

Minerals
  Zinc   +20 mg
  Copper   +2 mg
  Selenium   +400 mcg

Quasi vitamins
  L-carnitine   +1,000 mg
  Orotic acid   +200 mg
  L-cysteine   +3,000 mg
  L-methionine   +3,000 mg
  L-ornithine   +3,000 mg

Additional Nutrients for the Alcoholic
  Biotin   +300 mcg
  Coenzyme Q   +60 mg
  Choline   +1,000 mg
  Myoinositol   +2,000 mg
  EPA   +2,000 mg
  GLA   +2,000 mg
  L-glutamine   +6,000 mg
  L-tryptophan   +6,000 mg

17
THE DIGESTIVE SYSTEM

"Part of the secret of success in life is to eat what you like and let the food fight it out inside."

Mark Twain

The study of nutrition basically involves understanding how the raw materials from the diet end up as essential components in the human body. This all begins with digestion. Through a series of mechanical and chemical processes, we are able to consume (and enjoy) an endless array of very different plant and animal material that is rendered into the 50 or so "nutrients" that our body has on its grocery list. A wide variety of problems can arise from this fascinating process called *digestion*.

Cavities, gum disease, heartburn, hiatus hernia, ulcers, hemorrhoids, constipation, and other breakdowns of the digestive tract are among the more common ailments in America. The most common disease in Western society is dental cavities: over 95 percent of us have fillings in our teeth, and eighty percent of older adults in America have no teeth at all.[1] Probably one of the more common complaints of older adults is gastrointestinal upset and constipation. And children with picky appetites jeopardize their own health while often making a war out of dinnertime. Many of these problems can be solved through optimal nutrition.

Other than cancer of the colon, most common problems of the

gastrointestinal tract are more of a nuisance than a life threatening situation. Yet, because of the daily need for food, malfunctions of the gastrointestinal (GI) tract can become the "fingernails scratching on the blackboard of life." People would much rather have their teeth, gums, stomach, intestines, and bowels working properly. Healing nutrients can help to accomplish that goal.

TEETH AND GUMS

Americans consume over 120 pounds of sugar per year per person, and there is a direct relationship between the amount of sugar consumed and the number of decayed, missing, and filled teeth.[2] A prestigious scientist in England says that cavities cannot be produced without sugar in the diet.[3] A Harvard dental researcher has compiled a chart showing the 1,000 percent jump in dental cavities once sugar became a staple in the Western diet.[4] Eighty percent of all dentist's children have no cavities.[5] Hence, we can assume that cavities are quite preventable with proper nutrition and dental care. Cavity incidence would drop off to near zero if we cut sugar consumption to one-fourth of current levels.

But there is more than just sugar in this cavity dilemma. The refining of cereal grains makes them more available to the cavity-producing bacteria in the mouth.[6] Thus, corn on the cob probably won't cause cavities, but corn flakes cereal might. Baked potatoes won't, but potato chips might. Whole wheat won't, but ready-to-eat breakfast cereals might, even without the 65 percent sugar that some of them contain.

Once a hole has been eaten in your teeth by cavity-producing bacteria, the end of that tooth is imminent. The initial cavity must be expanded by the dentist's drill. The metal filling that occupies this void eventually wears out and must be replaced by a larger hole and dental filling. Finally, the cavity can no longer be expanded. The tooth must be replaced by a crown. Root canals and dentures are the next steps in the decline of the teeth. All of this highly uncomfortable, expensive, and unnecessary dental work usually begins with too much sugar in the diet. One of the true obstacles to proper nutrition in the older adult is the lack of teeth. It is difficult to consume normal healthy food regularly when dentures slide and hurt.

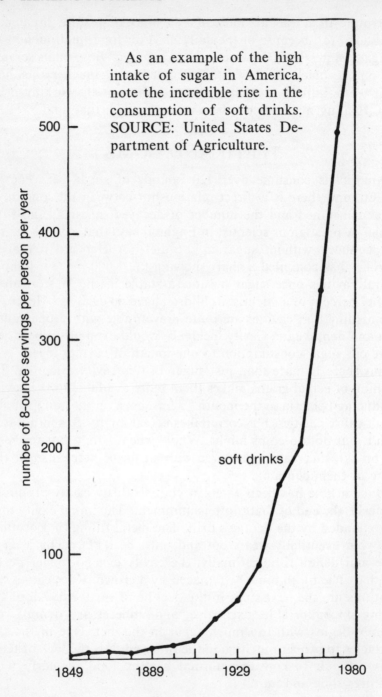

As an example of the high intake of sugar in America, note the incredible rise in the consumption of soft drinks. SOURCE: United States Department of Agriculture.

Sticky, chewy, refined carbohydrates are the favorite fuel for the bacteria that erode tooth enamel and produce a cavity. Yet, if that tooth were formed properly with a thick enamel, compliments of optimal developmental nutrition, a cavity would be less likely to be produced. Fluoride is a primary ingredient in the hardening of teeth. When adequate fluoride is available to developing humans (in pregnancy, lactation, and childhood), the enamel grows thick and strong. In spite of widespread fluoridation of municipal water supplies, the paltry amounts of fluoride used are below effective levels.[7]

Ironically, researchers find that people who had more fillings when they were younger will have fewer fillings as adults.[8] This indicates either an elevation of anticavity immune bodies in the mouth or that these people were strongly motivated to take better care of their teeth.

Another hazard of cavities is the mercury content in tooth fillings. Mercury is a deadly poison. Although mercury fillings are somewhat inert and less lethal than actually swallowing mercury, some sensitive individuals may have health problems from the mercury found in their tooth fillings.

Chewing acid foods (like lemons) or chewable ascorbic acid tablets can disastrously erode tooth enamel.[9] Some chewable vitamin C tablets even contain sugar to further tooth destruction. Yet some mouth problems are symptoms of a vitamin C deficiency. Swollen bleeding gums and weakened tooth foundations can be the early stages of scurvy. In a survey of over 70,000 Americans, 45 percent had noticeable gum disease, and 4 percent had scurvy that was evident from their gums.[10]

Periodontal disease (gum problems) is rampant in America. Some of this stems from a lack of dental care, and some of it results from bacterial infections. High-dose vitamin C supplements were able to prevent gum disease in test animals, even when the offending bacteria strain was injected directly into the animal's mouth.[11]

Coenzyme Q is a quasi vitamin that is effective in treating various types of gum disease.[12]

Topically used folic acid also helps to treat various gum diseases.[13]

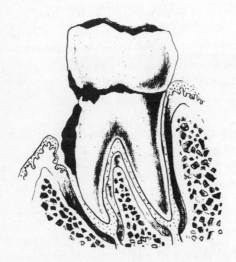
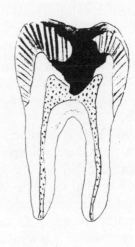

Sugar intake is directly related to cavities. Plaque is a combination of sticky sugar and bacteria. It can eat a hole in the tooth (cavity) or cause gum disease. Bacteria in the mouth use the sugar and give off a strong acid, which dissolves the enamel (outside) of the tooth.

Appetite is a complex interplay of factors, including the emptying rate of the stomach, blood sugar and blood fat levels, mental outlook on food, the hypothalamus in the brain, health of the tongue surface, and other components. A zinc deficiency seriously impairs taste acuity.[14] One-third of all children tested in a study had zinc levels indicative of a chronic zinc deficiency.[15] In a double-blind study with 30 children in Denver, researchers found that supplements of only 5 mg of zinc (half their RDA) markedly improved the children's appetite and calorie intake from food.[16] More than a few children eat poorly because they are zinc-deficient, which then serves to perpetuate their malnutrition. And on the vicious cycle goes. Healing nutrients can interrupt this cycle.

ESOPHAGUS AND STOMACH

The esophagus is the passageway from the mouth to the stomach. A hiatus hernia is a pouch offshoot from the upper stomach/lower esophagus that can catch acid-laden food and be a continuous impediment to enjoying meals. Hiatus hernias are most often caused by overeating or obesity (see Chapter 13 for solutions to that problem). Some people develop pockets of distension in the esophagus from trying to swallow too much food too quickly. Imagine trying to force a golf ball down a garden hose. Distensions and pockets are bound to occur in the garden hose (esophagus) to create great discomfort whenever you eat. Slow down at the dinner table. Eat small bites. Chew them thoroughly and swallow small sections at a time. The hiatus hernia can be a continuous annoyance. But with some rational forethought, most people can avoid it.

Plummer-Vinson syndrome involves a difficulty in swallowing due to a weblike membrane that grows across the upper esophagus. People with this syndrome often develop cancer of the esophagus or stomach. Since iron deficiency is often related to this problem, iron supplementation has practically eliminated it, especially in Sweden, where it was once so prevalent.[17]

The stomach is a large, tough organ situated in the central left region of the viscera. It adds acid to the food, mechanically churns it, absorbs a few items (like water, aspirin, and alcohol), and passes the food mixture on to the small intestines. The strong acid produced by the stomach can eat a hole in your living room carpet or even a hole in your stomach. The result is an ulcer. Ulcers must be quite common, since the most profitable prescription drug sold in America is a medication for ulcers.

Ulcers can be the result of tumultuous emotions. But sometimes ulcers are the product of a poor diet. Here are some nutrition-ulcer links:

- Vitamin E is important in preventing ulcers.[18]
- Vitamin A is important in the formation of the coating (glycoprotein) that protects the stomach from its own acid. High-dose vitamin A (150,000 IU of beta-carotene) supplements accelerate the healing of stomach ulcers in humans.[19]

- Zinc is another nutrient that is crucial to the healing process. Zinc supplements (150 mg daily as zinc sulfate) healed stomach ulcers three times faster than in humans given placebos.[20]
- Patients with stomach (peptic) ulcers had half the serum B_6 levels when compared to intestinal (duodenal) ulcer patients.[21]

Not long ago, the accepted diet for ulcer patients was a high-fat dairy regimen, intended to coat the stomach with fat to allow healing. Yet the high-fat diet also encouraged heart disease. Current recommendations for ulcer healing include small frequent meals (four to six/day), restriction of alcohol (since alcohol stimulates acid production), and moderate intake of fat and protein. Anyone who has overindulged in spicy Mexican or Indian food knows the wrath of an irritated stomach. Yet in a controlled study, chilies did not interfere with the healing of ulcers.[22] Use your own commonsense judgment here. If the food creates "heartburn," then don't eat it.

SMALL INTESTINES

This is where most of the serious business of digestion and absorption occurs.

The appendix is a fingerlike projection extending from the intestines that helps certain animals to digest plant matter that would normally be indigestible. In humans, the appendix is probably useless. However, when the appendix collects bacteria and rotting food, it can swell up, causing appendicitis. The swollen appendix can even burst, which is a life-threatening situation. When researchers analyzed the diets of 135 children with appendicitis and 212 normal children, they found that those who were in the upper 50 percent for fiber intake had a 50 percent reduction in risks for appendicitis.[23] This makes perfect sense. Fiber keeps the food moving through the intestines to prevent poisonous pockets of trapped and stagnant bacteria.

In the 1970s, a trans-Atlantic commercial flight was nearly lost because everyone aboard had eaten food infested with salmonella poisoning. Diarrhea and cramps almost kept the captain from landing the plane. Although the intestinal tract seems nearly invincible, it isn't. Food poisoning comes from bacterially infected foods. *All* foods have some bacteria on them. The bacteria colony just needs a chance to grow. Bacteria multiply exponentially. This means that, under ideal conditions, one bacterium could multiply into a colony of 2 million bacteria in only seven hours.[24] Experts estimate that from 69 million to 275 million cases of food poisoning occur in the United States annually.[25] Statistically, then, each person each year gets at least one case of gastrointestinal upset due to food poisoning. Costs in lost work time and medical expenses from food poisoning run in the billions of dollars per year. Poor sanitation, lack of common sense, and negligent food storage are primarily responsible.

The factors that breed food-borne bacteria are temperature (80–120°F, or 27–49°C), high surface area (as in hamburger, egg salad, liverwurst), time (more than three hours without refrigeration), protein content (meat, chicken, fish, eggs, cheese), and fluid content (dry foods are not easily infested). Through proper sanitation and temperature control of food, you can minimize the risk of food poisoning.

LARGE INTESTINES AND COLON

The large intestines are shorter and fatter than the small intestines and primarily serve to absorb water from the food mixture and to store the feces until they are ready for elimination. Many problems of the digestive system occur in the large intestines and colon. Cancer of the colon is second in prevalence among cancers only to lung cancer (see the chapter on cancer for more on that issue). Diverticulosis is a condition of little ballooned sacs of intestinal membrane that have been forced outward by hardened feces. About 30 percent of Americans over 60 years old have some degree of diverticulosis.[26] These diverticula can produce discomfort, pain, and internal bleeding. Not long ago, diverticulosis was treated with a low-fiber diet. Today, a high-fiber diet has been shown to be much more effective in healing diverticula.[27] Optimal levels of fiber can be a near panacea in maintaining and healing the intestinal tract. Mild increases in fiber intake can significantly improve stool bulk and softness.[28]

Many people and most older adults suffer continuous bouts of constipation. Some tolerate it. Most seek medication. Fiber and fluid intake are the keys to continuous regularity in older adults, according to a 10-week study of nursing home patients.[29] Fiber can improve stool bulk and intestinal transit time to encourage hemorrhoid healing.[30] Fiber is a near miraculous protector of the intestinal tract with benefits to serum lipids, heart, circulation, and other parts of the body.[31] A low-fiber diet increases the risk for hiatus hernia, diverticulosis, and calcified blood clots in the pelvic region (pelvic phleboliths).[32] There were *no* cases of diabetes, hiatus hernia, or coronary thrombosis (blood clots in the heart) and fewer cases of constipation, hemorrhoids, irritable bowel syndrome, appendicitis, and varicose veins among the 75 lifelong vegetarians studied.[33]

Fiber is the main "extra" in a vegetarian diet. Omnivores (meat eaters) consumed 23 g of fiber daily, vegetarians (who also drink milk and eat eggs) consumed 37 g, and vegans (who eat only plant products) consumed an average of 47 g of fiber daily.[34] You don't have to become a vegetarian, but more plant food in the diet would provide limitless health benefits. Since fiber absorbs considerable amounts of water, it is important to increase your fluid intake along with a higher-fiber diet.

Fiber is found almost exclusively in plant food. Fruits, vegetables, whole grains, legumes (beans), and nuts all provide some fiber.[35] The water-soluble fiber found in oats, apples, seaweed, and other foods is particularly valuable. The more refining that is done to a food, the more fiber is probably removed. Long-term cooking, especially high-heat canning, reduces the amount of fiber found in plant foods.[36] Yet there are some plant foods that must be cooked in order to burst the cell wall and be able to derive any nutrients from the food. Potatoes are an example. Raw potatoes provide little more than fluid and fiber. Cooked potatoes provide fluid, fiber, complex carbohydrates, vitamins, minerals, and some protein.

Yogurt and beans are also quite kind to the intestinal tract. Beans provide not only a good source of fiber, but are also able to benefit colonic function.[37] Yogurt contains a bacterial strain called *Lactobacillus acidophilus*, which lowers cholesterol absorption[38] and improves the presence of beneficial bacteria in the intestines.[39] Live yogurt cultures have been scientifically proven to treat diarrhea[40] and constipation and to relieve GI problems associated with long-term antibiotic therapy.[41] Smoking and high sugar intake increase the risks for Crohn's disease and ulcerative colitis.[42]

FLATULENCE

Flatulence (a.k.a *making wind, farting*) is relevant in a nutrition book because food provides the basis for flatus production. Some people have a problem with excessive flatulence, which can cause discomfort or embarrassment.

Gas can be caused by eating too rapidly and swallowing air with the food. This type of gas would be "noisy" but not offensive to the olfactory lobes. Another type of intestinal gas is produced at higher elevations as a result of changes in atmospheric pressure. All other flatus stems from the bacterial fermentation of your food.

Sulfur foods (e.g., eggs, cabbage, broccoli, brussels sprouts, cauliflower, dried apricots, and beans) can produce hydrogen sulfide gas (that rotten egg smell). Most other plant foods provide intestinal bacteria with the raw material to produce methane gas, which is certainly noticeable but not nearly as potent as hydrogen sulfide. Flatus can be so powerful that the human nose can detect concentrations as small as 1 part per 100 million.[43]

A good deal of this book has been spent "selling" you on the merits of a high-fiber diet. Here is one minor drawback of fiber: flatulence. Indigestible food matter (fiber) is quite digestible by certain strains of intestinal bacteria. The bacteria produce methane and other gases that are excreted as flatus. The same gas also allows the feces from a high-fiber diet to float in the toilet. But you can do something about this annoyance. About 30 percent of the population are natural methane makers and have some genetic quirk that predisposes them and their offspring to produce gas.

Because everyone "farts" and many people are offended by it, there is an endless array of drugs that claim to treat the condition. Of all the sophisticated drugs taken for flatulence, the most successful treatment of all is activated charcoal. Activated charcoal is not a drug, needs no prescription, has enormous internal surface area, which apparently binds up the gas, and is harmless. Up to 50 g (nearly 2 ounces) daily has been given to renal dialysis patients for 20 months with no side effects noted.[44] Tablets or bulk powder can be obtained at most drugstores and health food stores. Studies indicate that activated charcoal cuts flatus production by about 75 percent.[45] Five to 10 g of activated charcoal daily should tame even the noisiest and most offensive stomach without major expense or any side effect.

However, for most people, anti-flatus aids are not necessary. By slowly increasing your fiber intake to the recommended 50 g per day, you can minimize flatus production. When some people get enthused about nutrition, they suddenly increase their fiber intake from their customary 10 g daily to the prescribed 50 g. The bacteria in their intestines then run amok, often creating diarrhea and embarrassing quantities of gas. Gradually increasing your fiber intake makes your intestinal bacteria less likely to produce excessive flatus. Also, flatus is most offensive when it is produced from the excreta waiting in the large intestines to be eliminated. Sometimes, merely heeding "nature's call" and defecating can avert any serious problems with flatus.

Foods that are prone toward flatus production, listed in order from most to least, are milk and milk products, onions, beans, celery, carrots, raisins, bananas, apricots, prune juice, pretzels, bagels, wheat germ, brussels sprouts, pastries, potatoes, eggplant, citrus, fruit, apples, bread, meat, fowl, fish, lettuce, cucumbers, broccoli, peppers, avocados, cauliflower, tomatoes, asparagus, zucchini, okra, olives, cantaloupe, grapes, berries, rice, corn chips, potato chips, popcorn, graham crackers, nuts, eggs, nonmilk chocolate, gelatin, fruit ice.

Remember, what produces gas is a very individual matter. Milk creates gas in many people because they are lactose-intolerant. Lacking the enzyme to digest milk, their intestinal bacteria have a field day and produce flatus and distension in abundance. For people who can fully digest milk, it may cause no flatus at all. Through some recorded observations, you can determine which foods are most likely to stoke your flatus machinery. Avoid or minimize them.

Beans are very cheap, tasty, nourishing food. They are also prime offenders in producing flatus. Beans (and various other foods) contain a special type of carbohydrate (oligosaccharides of stachyose and raffinose) that is more quickly digested by bacteria in your intestines than your own digestive enzymes. You can control the flatus production of beans in several ways:

1. Bring beans to a boil for 2 minutes. Then turn off heat and let stand for 1 hour. Drain water. Then cook beans as usual (about 45 minutes in the pressure cooker). This will cut flatus production by 20 percent or more.

2. Sprout the beans. Some of the carbohydrates are changed in form when the bean seeds are allowed to grow. Bean sprouts are also higher in certain vitamins and protein quality. To sprout, add 2 cups of water to 1 cup of beans. Let stand overnight in a glass jar. Next morning, drain water (use a rubber band to secure plastic screen material over the jar opening) and let stand inverted. Both morning and evening for the next 2 days, fill the jar of beans with water, then drain and let stand inverted. The idea is to keep the beans damp but not to allow mold to grow on them. Once the beans have sprouted with about a ¼-inch "tail," steam them for 10 minutes. Bean sprouts can be used as regular beans in recipes or in a cold salad. Sprouting cuts flatulence 40 percent or more.

3. Add certain foods: Yogurt bacteria compete with flatulence-producing bacteria to slow down "wind making." Yogurt cuts flatulence by up to 30 percent. Chicory is a root plant that is often used as a coffee substitute. Chicory has been well documented to be an anti-carminative (flatus stopper).[46] Ginger and garlic can also cut flatus production.

GALLBLADDER, LIVER, AND PANCREAS

The gallbladder is a pear-sized organ lying underneath the liver. The liver produces bile salts for fat digestion. The gallbladder stores and concentrates this bile. Gallstones occur when the duct leading from the gallbladder to the intestines is blocked with concentrated and solidified bile. Gallstones are quite common, and they can be very painful, especially after a high-fat meal in which the gallbladder is attempting to squeeze bile through the blocked duct to the intestines. Gallstones are almost nonexistent in vegetarians, due to their low-fat and high-fiber diet.[47] Gallstones are also very rare in nonobese individuals.[48]

Lecithin is a soaplike food that is derived from soybeans. It can dissolve fats and water-soluble substances at the same time. The food industry capitalizes on this talent by using lecithin as an additive to keep foods from separating out of solution. Dietary lecithin uses its fat-solvent talents to dissolve gallstones in humans.[49] Vitamin C is also involved in processing cholesterol into bile salts. Long-term marginal deficiencies of vitamin C, which are quite common in America, can produce gallstones.[50]

One of the many functions of the liver is to help out in digestion. Hydrogenated dietary fats lower the ability of the liver to alter fats into usable substances.[51] With nearly 60 percent of all fats consumed in America being hydrogenated, this is worthy of concern. Chicory can relieve liver congestion and decrease the vomiting from excess liver bile.[52]

In addition to making insulin for glucose regulation, the pancreas produces some digestive enzymes. Vitamin E supplements have been helpful in relieving the backaches and stomach pains that result from an inflamed pancreas.[53]

DIETARY GUIDELINES

Follow the Core diet, placing special emphasis on high fiber foods. Use Core supplement program (for specific problems, see the text for therapeutic solutions).

18
THE MUSCULAR SYSTEM
Athletic Training

"What a piece of work is man! . . . in form and moving, how express and admirable! in action how like an angel!"

Shakespeare

The human athlete is an amazing creature. No other animal on earth can compete with humans for our combination of speed, strength, endurance, and dexterity. We can thank our muscular system for these diverse talents.

The world-class athletes of the 1980s have created new records of physical achievement, forever pushing back the "limits" of human ability. When Roger Bannister ran the four-minute mile, scientists were quite certain that the human body was incapable of performing such a feat. When Edmund Hillary stood atop Mount Everest, scientist were positive that no human being could live without oxygen at that altitude. Hillary took his mask off to prove them wrong. Recently, a climber made the entire climb up Everest without oxygen. Today's world-class milers could beat yesterday's best mile relay team.

Depending on how athletically endowed you are, your muscular system could compose 40 percent or more of your body weight. Since the muscular system is most valued by active individuals, we will discuss the muscular system and athletes in the same breath throughout this chapter. The nutritional support of the athlete provides some unusual challenges. While the average person is content with normal health, the athlete seeks optimal health in order to excel at his or her event. Optimal health must be supported by optimal nutrition.

You would think that the aesthetically pleasing body of the athlete *must* be well nourished. Not necessarily so. While athletes have higher-than-normal nutrient needs, they often eat the same as or even worse than the normal American. Many athletes are very poorly nourished. They travel much and eat restaurant food often, surrendering control over their food intake. Due to peer pressure and prodigious appetites, they often graze on junk food. Usually their perseverance in training and genetic gifts allow them to perform well in spite of their diet, rather than because of their diet. Thirteen randomly chosen female high school gymnasts were found to be deficient in B_6, folate, iron, calcium, zinc, and magnesium.[1] While 10–25 percent of menstruating women are considered to be anemic, 44 percent of female adolescent runners were found to be anemic.[2]

Active people can eat a succession of pastries and french fries and usually not experience weight problems. Though these foods fill up the stomach and do provide calories, they do not fill up the nutrient stores. Exercise drains the body's blood glucose supplies, which then triggers the appetite mechanism. An insatiable craving for sweets is not uncommon in athletes, as their bodies are trying to replenish the lost glucose. Dancers, wrestlers, jockeys, and other athletes concerned about weight often fast, binge/purge, and take diuretics to lose weight quickly. Young athletes often feel impervious to any damage they might do to their bodies, either on the playing field or from bad eating habits.

So far, we have described a person who is driven indiscriminately toward large amounts of food (especially sweet things), eats in unusual places and on the run, is exposed to inordinate amounts of fan adulation and stress to win, has probably given little consideration to nutrition, and has achieved some success despite this apathy toward nutrition. To truly fulfill your potential, you must pay heed to optimal nutrition. We are talking about milliseconds and inches making the difference between gold, silver, bronze, and "thanks for coming." In the 1984 Winter Olympics, the second-place finisher in the 10-kilometer cross-country skiing event was just three one-hundredths of a second behind the first-place finisher. How would you like it if, after years of intense training and over six miles of arduous skiing, you missed a gold medal by less than the tick of a clock? Each athlete encounters some limiting factor: training, genetic abilities, attitude, or diet. Which is your limiting factor?

THE WEAKEST LINK IN A CHAIN

Nutrition is a weak link in the training of many athletes. Many are gifted with immense natural talent. Many are willing to dedicate thousands of hours of training for their sport. And when the time comes for competition, they often line up next to someone who seems overwhelming. Any gimmick that will provide the athlete with a split-second advantage is welcomed. Of all the vulnerable segments of American society—overweight people, old and decrepit, terminally ill—athletes are the most prone to nutritional quackery.[3] Certain unscrupulous nutritionists and supplement companies feed on this desperate need of athletes to gain an edge over their competition.

Athletes are also somewhat leery of nutrition advice, since they have been deceived by both extremist groups in nutrition:

The ultraconservative nutritionists told athletes that nutrition supplements would do them no good. This statement was based upon some very strange studies. For instance, Dr. Ancel Keys (developer of the infamous "K rations") performed a study in 1943 at the University of Minnesota in which athletes were given supplements of thiamine containing only one-third of the RDA (0.5 mg). Quite obviously, with such infinitesimal amounts, no measurable improvements in athletic performance were noted.[4] Athletes were told that their nutrient needs were no different from those of the average person on the street, except that they needed more calories. Wrong again. Superactive individuals experience a 7- to 20-fold increase in their glucose metabolism with measurable losses in chromium and zinc.[5] Half of all female runners studied were at least borderline iron-deficient.[6] Athletes were told that all of their nutrient needs could be satisfied by "the four food groups." New studies show that the basic four food groups do not even satisfy the nutrient needs of the average sedentary person, much less the vigorous athlete.[7]

On the other end of the spectrum, the ultraliberal nutritionists have been telling athletes that wheat germ oil (containing octacosanol) would improve athletic performance. It probably doesn't. These claims were founded on misinterpreting a scientific paper[8] that spoke of dicobalt octacarbonyl (a catalytic reagent that has nothing to do with wheat germ oil) improving the oxygen-carrying capacity of the muscles.[9] Nutrition formulas that are targeted for bodybuilders claim that their paltry addition of lecithin and choline will "break up fat" to provide a leaner look. That, too, is unlikely. So, you see, athletes are desperate people who have been misled by both liberal and conservative extremists in the nutrition field. They are understandably suspicious and apprehensive at this point. Let us try to clear matters up.

ATHLETES *ARE* DIFFERENT

Essentially, nutrition is important to everyone. But it is crucial to the serious athlete. On a marginal diet, most people still get through the day. Subclinical nutritional deficiencies probably won't prevent you from driving to work, sitting at a desk all day, then watching TV all night. The average person never challenges his or her mental or physical potential and, because of that, may not notice his or her marginal nutrient intake until the cumulative effects arise later in life as some degenerative disease.

It is different for the athlete. The athlete is probing for the upper limits of mental and physical achievement. *Optimal* is the key word here. Anything less than optimal nutrition will produce less than the best athletic performance. To perform at your optimal level of genetic abilities, your diet must also be optimal.

Russian researchers gave vitamin, mineral, and protein supplements to seven male subjects who then underwent a 20-day stress and endurance test. The researchers reported that the "supplements exerted a significant effect on the mental and physical tolerance . . . and that nutritional supplements may become a promising tool in optimizing the health state and performance of men working in unusually demanding circumstances."[10] That obviously applies to women as well.

In order to compete at your highest level, your body must be a product of conscientious nutritional support. With foods as a mainstay and rational supplementation as enhancement, anyone willing to train hard can reach their genetic potential in sports.

NUTRIENT NEEDS OF THE MUSCLES

The muscular system of the body has several distinct nutrient needs:

Energy and the metabolites to "spark" that energy are a critical need. Muscles can burn carbohydrate, fat, or even protein. Carbohydrates are favored in "out of breath" exercises (nonaerobics, such as sprints and weightlifting) since carbohydrates provide a fuel that requires less oxygen in order to be burned. Fats are used by muscles (including the heart) in most endurance events. A small amount of protein is always burned for fuel in humans. In the athlete, the amount of protein burned can become significant. Also, athletes have higher needs for the vitamins (thiamine, niacin, riboflavin, pantothenic acid, biotin) and mineral (chromium) that are required to burn the fuel. Much of the athlete's energy needs are met by burning fats. Carnitine is often found in subsaturation levels in humans and is critical for fat burning.

Oxygen must be delivered via red blood cells. The fuels of fat, protein, and carbohydrate all must eventually be burned in the presence of oxygen. Because of high-volume oxygen intake, blood cells are oxidized more quickly, leaving many athletes anemic. Certain nutrients encourage maximal red blood cell production, while other nutrients protect the blood cells from the destruction caused by above-normal oxygen intake. Building optimal levels of red blood cells should be a key pursuit of athletes involved in distance and aerobic events.

Growth and repair of muscle tissue. Muscles are composed primarily of protein and fluid, with a wide variety of vitamins and minerals involved in making and repairing muscles. Certain nutrients improve the stress adaptability of the muscles to heat, cold, altitude, and other challenges.

Fluid and electrolyte balance. Muscles are dependent on the "electrolyte soup" of water, sodium, potassium, chloride, magnesium, and calcium for proper contraction and relaxation. Deficiency of any of these nutrients or an imbalance can lead to muscle fatigue, cramps, heat stroke, and even death.

The preevent meal. Eating nothing for half a day before an event often leaves the athlete feeling "light" but weak. Yet foods must be chosen carefully for the preevent meal, lest they become a millstone around the athlete's neck for the entire event. What, how much, and when to eat can strongly dictate the athlete's energy levels when competition starts.

ENERGY

While the average sedentary adult may need only 1,200–2,000 kilocalories per day to maintain weight, many athletes need 5,000–10,000. It can be quite a challenge just to eat enough food to avoid losing weight. Carbohydrates are unquestionably the most efficient fuel for the athlete to burn.[11] This means eating a diet high in whole grains, legumes, vegetables, and fruits.

Of the various types of carbohydrates, fructose is the best for the preevent meal.[12] Fructose is found naturally in fruits, some vegetables, corn syrup, and honey. Fructose is passively absorbed, compared to the active absorption of glucose. That difference provides for a more gradual and dependable energy supply during exercise. Anything that is consumed within 45 minutes of the event tends to reduce the endurance of the athlete by lowering the amount of free fatty acids (blood fats) that are available to the muscles.[13] Blood fats normally are a mainstay of fuel throughout endurance events.

Not only does the body need its preferential fuel in the form of carbohydrates, but the body also needs the nutrients to metabolize that fuel. Niacin, thiamine, riboflavin, pantothenic acid, biotin, and chromium are all involved in allowing the body to "burn" its fuel efficiently. Thiamine requirements during intense exercise increase 15-fold.[14] The exhausted athlete shows significantly lower levels of pantothenic acid and thiamine than normal people.[15] Supplements of riboflavin were required to bring blood levels of riboflavin up to normal range in young female joggers.[16] Riboflavin deficiencies are quite common throughout the world, especially among adolescents and poor people.[17] Athletes undergoing intense training have been found to have mild riboflavin deficiencies.[18] When diets high in carbohydrates and marginal in niacin were fed to athletes, they experienced a reduced aerobic capacity and higher lactate levels, probably as a result of the low niacin levels.[19] Lactate, the by-product of burning carbohydrates without sufficient oxygen, produces swollen and sore muscles. Providing the body with optimal levels of the nutrients to burn the carbohydrate food minimizes the levels of lactate that will impair athletic performance.

Caffeine is a mild amphetamine that can stimulate athletic performance. Nine competitive cyclists were tested both with and without caffeine during workouts on stationary bicycles. When the cyclists consumed 330 mg of caffeine (equivalent to about four or five cups of coffee) one hour before exercise, their endurance improved by 20 percent.[20] In a similar follow-up study, investigators found that the caffeine ingestion seems to encourage the body's ability to burn fats, which then extends endurance.[21] Although caffeine may improve alertness, motor control, and endurance, caffeine is also a diuretic. Fluid loss during exercise can be a serious drawback. This could also produce the urge to urinate at the most inopportune moment. Also, caffeine reduces iron absorption, introduces methylxanthines (which are harmful to some people), and alters blood levels of fats and sugars. It would not be a good idea for an athlete to rely on caffeine for performance enhancement.

Energy metabolism is an amazingly complex topic. Nature designed it that way. Because your food energy is released slowly and captured efficiently in a series of small controlled steps, there is also an extensive list of enzymes and by-products, just like descending steps leading from the top of a skyscraper to the ground floor. The final stage of squeezing all the energy out of foodstuffs is called *electron transport*. In this sequence, there is a key juncture called *Coenzyme Q*. CoQ is crucial to energy metabolism,[22] and, since vitamin E protects CoQ from destruction, vitamin E is also important to energy metabolism.[23] Wheat germ oil is the richest natural source of vitamin E, with vegetable oils, mayonnaise, and margarine also containing some vitamin E. Supplements of CoQ have been successful in treating heart disease, indicating that CoQ steps up the efficiency of fat burning.

Most muscles burn some fat. The longer and more intense the event becomes, the greater the amount of fat that will be burned. Therefore, efficiency of fat burning can be very important to athletic performance. Vitamin C is involved in at least three different pathways of maintaining proper levels of fats in the blood. Trained athletes supplemented with 1,000 mg of ascorbic acid daily were able to burn fat more efficiently in both muscle tissue and liver tissue.[24] The scientists in this study noted that vitamin C supplements provided "beneficial effects in both cardiovascular and metabolic parameters during exercise." Ascorbic acid supplements of only 70 mg (slightly more than the RDA) were able to measurably improve aerobic capacity in marginally nourished elementary school boys.[25] In another study, one group of human subjects were given supplements of 2,000 mg of vitamin C daily, while another group received a placebo. Both groups were then tested at high altitudes. The vitamin C group had a 26 percent greater endurance capacity in training at the higher elevations.[26] Vitamin C is also involved in making catecholamines for stress response to cold, heat, and psychological pressure. Test animals who were fed diets high in ascorbic acid had a much better tolerance to the cold.[27]

Carnitine is the shuttle system that gets fat into the cell furnace for use as a fuel. Carnitine supplements improve exercise endurance in animal studies.[28] Carnitine is able to improve the liver's ability to burn fats, which allows the liver to produce more glucose for higher sustained blood sugar levels.[29] Many humans have marginal levels of carnitine in their system, as exhibited by the fact that carnitine supplements often improve human athletic performance.[30] The Italian soccer team were surprising victors in the 1984 World Cup championship. They credited some of their victory to their use of carnitine. Iron is involved in the production of carnitine.[31] The multitudes of iron-deficient athletes may feel fatigue from low carnitine production via their low iron stores.

Arginine is an amino acid that holds great promise for improving athletic performance. Arginine supplements have been shown to prevent nitrogen loss, such as occurs in heavy training. Arginine also encourages the regeneration of ATP, which is the "gold currency" of energy that is found throughout all forms of life.[32]

The average adult body carries about 350 g of glycogen, which is worth 1,400 kilocalories. These glycogen stores are used up after about 90 minutes of intensive exercise.[33] Many distance runners and bikers will attest to "the wall" that they hit when carbohydrate fuel is gone and the cell machinery must switch over to fat burning. You can literally trick your muscles into storing twice the normal amounts of carbohydrate glycogen. "Carb loading," as it is called, consists of thoroughly depleting glycogen stores through intense training and low carbohydrate intake, then restoring the glycogen stores beyond normal levels through a high-carbohydrate diet.

The countdown goes like this: Five days before the event, train intensely. Burn every ounce of glycogen from your muscles. Eat only foods high in protein and fat. This means avoiding grains, vegetables, fruits, and dairy products. Day four is a repeat of day five. You may feel very lethargic by now. Fatigue often sets in because you have depleted blood glucose and glycogen supplies, and these carbohydrates are the favorite fuel of the brain and many muscles. On the third day before the event, work out lightly, thus finishing the depletion phase. Two days before the event, begin the repletion phase. Avoid training and begin eating high-carbohydrate foods. The day before the event is a carbon copy of the previous day. By the day of the event, you should have twice the amount of glycogen stored in your body, through the miracle of enzyme kinetics.[34]

FLUID AND ELECTROLYTE NEEDS

Every year in America, at least five high school football athletes die from dehydration.[35] Many coaches and athletes have developed the dangerous misconception that withholding water during hot workouts will toughen the athletes. It won't. But it may kill them. As the body loses fluid and electrolytes in sweat, exercise ability declines. A high-carbohydrate diet and balanced fluid/electrolyte intake rank number one and number two in priority for simple nutritional suggestions that would markedly improve the performance of many athletes.[36] When eight men were exercised vigorously on a hot summer's day, their muscle magnesium levels dropped by 12 percent after a 5.8 percent loss of body weight from water.[37]

Half of all heat stroke victims have seriously low potassium levels in addition to their dehydration. As muscle potassium levels decline, exercise ability also declines.[38] With only a 1 percent loss of body weight in water, there is a measurable decline in athletic ability.[39] Athletes are advised to drink a solution (tea, juice, water) that contains about a 5 percent sugar concentration every 10–20 minutes in order to avoid a loss of physical abilities.

With the recent renewed interest in amateur sports, there are a number of illustrations of problems that can occur if fluid and electrolyte levels are not maintained. Many athletes just drink large amounts of water, ignoring the electrolytes that are lost in sweat. In a number of marathon events, runners drinking only water have experienced everything from dizziness to grand mal seizures.[40] By drinking only water and not replacing the electrolytes, the athlete dilutes the already imperiled "electrolyte soup." This situation can prevent the nerves (e.g., the brain) and the muscles (e.g., the heart) from working properly. In early stages, this unbalanced electrolyte soup will merely impair athletic ability. Later it affects strength and judgment. If it continues, it may cause death.

As part of regular training, eat foods that are high in magnesium and potassium. This will help to prevent cramps and sore muscles the day after an intense workout. Potassium is found primarily in plant foods. The average American would probably notice an improvement in overall health if he or she doubled potassium intake. Potassium and sodium should be in a two-to-one ratio in the diet. The use of Lite Salt (50 percent potassium) at the dinner table can fortify potassium levels in the body. The average magnesium intake in America is one-half to two-thirds of the RDA. Athletes should try to consume at least 500 mg of magnesium daily from food or supplements.

You can make your own electrolyte replacement beverage to drink during and after workouts. To one quart of clean water, add one teaspoon of Lite Salt (contains large amounts of sodium, potassium, chloride, and smaller amounts of magnesium, calcium, and iodide), one tablespoon of sugar or honey, and some flavoring (mint tea, instant tea, instant orange drink mix) to suit yourself. Mix thoroughly. Regularly drink this concoction or something comparable when you are working out.

MUSCLE GROWTH AND REPAIR

Some athletes want large, sculptured muscles. Some athletes are more concerned about how well their muscles work than about how they look. Muscles are composed primarily of protein and water. Tough connective protein (collagen and elastin) provides a cellular "glue" to keep them durable. Vitamin C helps to build this connective protein. Vitamin B_6 helps to metabolize all proteins. Since muscles are largely protein, a longstanding myth has been that "the more protein you eat, the bigger your muscles will get." Not true. Muscle size depends more upon athletic training and genetic endowment.

Most athletes eat too much protein. Excess protein can stress the kidneys and liver, drain calcium from the bone stores, and even cause weight problems. Even the most active and behemoth athlete needs little more than 100 g of protein daily.[41] Many athletes consume 200–400 g of protein daily. Some protein is used as fuel in exercise. Yet, as the food intake for the athlete increases, so does the protein intake. The Senate Dietary Goals recommend that people consume 12 percent of their calories from protein. When athletes consume 12 percent of their calories from protein, they can easily protect against nitrogen loss in even the most intense athletic training.[42] For instance, athletes who need 4,000 kilocalories to maintain weight would want 12 percent of their calories to come from protein. Twelve percent of 4,000 is 480. Since there are 4 kilocalories/g in protein, this athlete will be getting 120 g of protein daily, which is more than enough for anyone.

Scientists once thought that much nitrogen was lost in sweat, which would therefore increase protein needs during hot weather and serious sweating. Yet the body is able to adjust to heat and significantly conserve the amount of nitrogen that is lost in sweat.

When some athletes decide to take powdered protein supplements, they may be doing themselves more harm than good. Vitamin B_6 is critical to the body's ability to process protein.[43] Higher protein intake without a commensurate rise in B_6 intake could create a B_6 deficiency. Many Americans do not even get RDA levels of B_6. Athletes may need much more than RDA levels of B_6. Animals who were raised on supplements of B_6 had increased muscle stamina.[44] Animals who were reared on oral supplements of B_6 and then exposed to a cold climate ($2°C$, $36°F$ for 20 days) all survived. Of the unsupplemented animals, 69 percent died from the cold.[45] Optimal levels of B_6 probably improve muscle stamina and climate adaptation.

Selenium is a micromineral that helps to build an important protective enzyme system, glutathione peroxidase. The average selenium intake in America is below the minimum recommended level. Selenium deficiencies in animals bring on symptoms that are similar to muscular dystrophy, a condition of gradual weakening of the muscles. Twenty-four muscular dystrophy patients had serum selenium levels that were lower than normal controls. One of these patients was randomly chosen to be given selenium supplements for one year. Considerable improvement in the patient's muscular dystrophy condition was noted.[46] However, in other studies, selenium supplements did not bring major improvement to muscular dystrophy patients.[47] Though few athletes have to worry about muscular dystrophy, it is very likely that a marginal selenium deficiency could bring on mild muscular weakness.

Steroids are potent drugs that are being used by a number of athletes to build muscle bulk. Steroids have some rather dastardly side effects.[48] Liver cancer, impotence, and sterility are some of the risks that steroid users are taking. Some nutrients may offer a safe alternative. Arginine and lysine are two amino acids that are effective in producing marked gains in muscle mass in humans. Taking 1,200 mg each of L-lysine and L-arginine at bedtime on an empty stomach, young male athletes showed measurable improvements in muscle mass after a few weeks of normal intensive training.[49]

Zinc supplements were able to improve muscle stamina in animal studies.[50] Given the common zinc deficiencies in this country, zinc supplements would probably benefit most athletes.

The adrenal glands require large amounts of vitamin C to produce their flow of catecholamines, which are stressor hormones. In exercise, heat, high altitudes, psychological worry, and other situations, the adrenal glands must work overtime to provide catecholamines for the body's stress response. Supplements of vitamin C delay fatigue in the adrenal glands and help to counter the effects of working in high-temperature conditions.[51]

Vitamin E supplements help to relieve common muscle cramps.[52]

By taking 200 mg of magnesium and 600 mg of potassium *after* an intensive workout, the athlete can help to prevent muscle cramps now, tomorrow morning, and at the next contest.

OXYGEN FOR THE BLOOD SUPPLY

In order for the body to burn fuel efficiently, copious supplies of oxygen are needed. Much of athletic training is dedicated to improving the body's ability to bring oxygen to the muscles. Fatigue, lethargy, and irritability are the hallmarks of an anemic person. Half of all runners examined were at least borderline iron-deficient.[53] Although anemia is quite common in young women in America, young female runners are 500 percent more likely to be anemic than their more sedentary counterparts.[54] Iron-deficient animals show a direct corresponding drop in their work capacity.[55] Iron deficiency can also depress growth rate in young animals by up to 82 percent.[56] Iron-deficient animals often show a muscular weakness, even when no anemia is present.[57] Blood iron levels may not be good indicators of the iron that is available to muscles (myoglobin) or the iron available for carnitine synthesis. Often, the muscular impairment from low iron supplies is far beyond what would be expected from mild cases of anemia.[58]

Why are athletes so afflicted with iron shortages? Some iron is lost in sweat, but the amounts are not that significant.[59] However, the abundant oxygen that is brought into the athlete's bloodstream quickly "rusts" the membranes of the red blood cells, causing premature destruction. Also, the continuous pounding action on the feet from running can cause a mechanical crunching of blood cells, which wears them out faster than normal. The antioxidants vitamin E and selenium can slow down the destruction of red blood cells.[60]

Multiple vitamin and mineral supplements (with iron) were effective in improving the running performance and blood indices of borderline malnourished children.[61] Yet iron is not the only important nutrient in the making of red blood cells. Folic acid, B_{12}, B_6, copper, zinc, protein, and iron are all essential for the manufacture of red blood cells. Americans are commonly deficient in folic acid, copper, zinc, iron, and B_6.

PREEVENT MEAL

When Roberto Duran fought "Sugar Ray" Leonard for the world middleweight boxing crown, he stepped into the ring with a belly full of high-fat, high-protein food. Not long afterward, Duran conceded with "No mas [No more]." For centuries, athletes have been preened like prize animals. Raw meat was a favorite preevent meal in certain combat sports. The athletes compared themselves to predatory wild animals, who seem to do quite well on raw meat. What these athletes forgot to notice is that the wild predatory animal is hungry when tracking its prey. After filling up on raw meat, most carnivorous animals find someplace to sleep for a day or so.

The preevent meal should be eaten no less than four hours before the contest. It should be high in simple carbohydrates (especially fructose) and fluid, while being low in fat, fiber, and spices. Many powdered protein diet drinks are available that can neatly satisfy these requirements. In certain distance events, there is a need for athletes to eat something while competing. Soft ripe bananas are a favorite in these situations. They are high in potassium and fructose and easily digestible. The classic preevent meal of steak and eggs is the antithesis of what should be eaten before athletic competition.

OTHER ERGOGENIC NUTRITION FACTORS

When six athletes were given supplements of aspartic acid (3,000 mg), magnesium (500 mg), and potassium (3,500 mg), they were able to increase their exercise capacity by 50 percent.[62] Animals who were supplemented with calcium had improved strength of both skeletal and heart muscles.[63]

Garlic is an impressive agent for energy increase. In animal studies, garlic supplements roughly doubled their endurance capacity.[64]

Ginseng is a root herb that has a 5,000-year old track record, and some enticing scientific data, to prove its value. European scientists have found that ginseng can:

- Improve coordination and reflexes and quicken recovery from physical work done.[65]
- Improve general well-being, reaction abilities, oxygen capacity of the lungs, and sex hormone production.[66]
- Increase the endurance and performance of athletes.[67]
- Enhance work capacity.[68]

NUTRITIONAL RECOMMENDATIONS
DIETARY GUIDELINES

1. Core diet.
2. Moderate use of caffeine may help athletic performance.

DAILY SUPPLEMENTS TO ADD TO YOUR CORE PROGRAM

Vitamins
Vitamin A   +10,000 IU (2,000 RE)
   (beta-carotene)
Vitamin D   +200 IU
Vitamin E   +600 IU
Thiamine   +20 mg
Riboflavin   +20 mg
Niacinamide   +100 mg
Vitamin B_6 +50 mg
Vitamin B_{12} +100 mcg
Folic Acid   +400 mcg
Biotin   +300 mcg
Vitamin C   +2,000 mg
Pantothenic acid   +100 mg

Minerals
Calcium   +800 mg
Potassium   +1,000 mg
Magnesium   +400 mcg
Zinc   +30 mg
Iron   +20 mg (males)
        +30 mg (females)
Copper   +3 mg
Chromium   +400 mcg
Selenium   +200 mcg

Quasi vitamins
L-carnitine   +2,500 mg
EPA   +2,000 mg
Coenzyme Q   +60 mg
L-arginine   +2,000 mg
L-lysine   +2,000 mg
L-aspartic acid   +2,000 mg
Ginseng   +500 mg

19
THE BODY'S PACKAGE
Skin, Nails, Hair

People like to look good. That is perfectly understandable—appearance has much to do with sexual appeal and peer approval, which is also why the cosmetic and hair business is a multibillion-dollar-a-year industry. But physical beauty is more than just external cosmetics; it is related directly to the health of the body. You cannot see the health of someone's blood vessels or pancreas. But you can see that person's skin, hair, and nails, and this exterior package depends on the diet:

- Bumps on the skin can be a symptom of a vitamin A deficiency (hyperfollicular keratosis).
- Cracks at the corner of the mouth (cheilosis) can be a result of low B vitamin intake.
- Excessive bruising can be caused by low zinc, vitamin C, and bioflavonoid intake.

Many nutrient deficiencies show up first in the skin region, since the body considers the skin to be somewhat sacrificial. If the body must make a choice between using a nutrient for survival and using that nutrient to maintain a healthy glowing complexion, the skin

372

will lose out. Many food allergies surface as skin problems: eczema, dermatitis, hives, etc. (see Chapter 8 for more details).

There are precious few motivators to get people to change their lifestyle. Vanity is one. Though the fear of death from cigarettes does not scare many people, the fear of ugliness from smoking (caused by the premature wrinkling of facial skin) is a true motivator. Many people would rather be dead than ugly. You cannot look your best without optimal nutrition. Well-nourished people will make the most of their genetic beauty. Malnourished people will not look their best, in spite of inherited good looks and abundant cosmetic primping.

BEAUTY AND NUTRITION

The skin is the largest organ of the human body. It protects us from the environment and excretes waste products. Your skin, hair, and nails are entirely composed of substances found in your diet.

The skin is often the first place that health care professionals look for signs of malnutrition, because many nutritional deficiencies first manifest themselves as some type of skin problem. Thus, skin problems can often be warning signals that something is going wrong inside your body. Red and scaly skin can mean an allergy or other internal health problem. Scientists at Texas Tech University have found that the symptoms of poor nutrition are very similar to the symptoms of aging of the skin.[1] In many cases, improving the diet and providing certain nutritional supplements can clear up skin conditions. But treating skin ailments with good nutrition goes beyond narcissism. It is often life-saving preventive health.

Attitude, diet, exercise, and physical environment are more influential in the appearance of the skin than external cosmetic approaches. Too much sun, wind, harsh detergents, hair dye, or makeup can age the skin prematurely, in spite of a good diet. Since "you are what you eat" has much truth to it, "you look like what you eat" also has some wisdom. The next time you are in a grocery store, compare the overall appearance of the shopper with the contents of his or her shopping cart. There *is* a link.

People diet because they want to look better. Yet through fasting or weird food intake, they often end up with some deficiency that surfaces as dry, scaly, red, or cracked skin. In trying to look good, these people have forgotten about the importance of nutrition and end up looking bad. Smoking, drinking, drugs, and most marginal American diets can create a nutritional status that allows the person to function but not look his or her best.

FUNCTIONS OF THE SKIN

Your skin is a marvel of design. A section of human skin the size of a postage stamp contains 3 million cells, 3 feet of blood vessels, 12 feet of nerves, 100 sweat glands, 15 oil glands, and 25 nerve ends. Your skin has three layers. The outer layer (epidermis) is all dead cells that have been pushed to the surface by the active middle layer (dermis). Underneath the dermis is the subcutaneous tissue that stores fat to insulate the body from temperature changes. The skin produces various substances that help to fight off infections. The hair provides warmth and also protection from sun and wind. Fingernails and toenails were once valuable for fighting and gripping. They are now relegated to vestige status and serve as "art galleries" for some people.

Much of the skin, hair, and nails is protein. Energy and the corresponding vitamins and minerals are needed to build and repair the skin. A prime constituent of skin is fluid. Oils that are secreted on the skin surface prevent excessive loss of water by evaporation. Oils also act as antibacterial agents. The protective antioxidants vitamins E, A, and C and the mineral selenium are important to the skin. A regular and rich blood flow must constantly bring supplies of nutrients to the area, while also removing waste products. Since the skin cells are among the more rapidly dividing of all body cells, nutrients for new cell growth are critical: zinc, folic acid, B_{12}, vitamin A and others.

NUTRIENTS FOR HEALTHY SKIN, HAIR, AND NAILS

Essentially, if you want to look your best, you must provide your body with an optimal flow of the needed raw materials: nutrients.

FATS

Acne is an infection of a skin pore. Although Americans eat too much fat, we also eat the wrong kind of fats. The results can show up in skin appearance. Acne sufferers have been found to have a deficiency of the essential fatty acid (linoleic acid) in their skin region.[2] When test animals were fed a diet containing 10 percent of the calories from hydrogenated fat (comparable to the typical American diet), the animals developed a deficiency of the essential fatty acid (linoleic acid).[3] Sixty percent of all fats consumed in this country are hydrogenated. Hydrogenation changes a fat just enough so that the body will use it, but the fat does not have the value of normal "cis" fats. Hence, when people get acne from eating the typical American diet, especially chocolate, it may be the hydrogenated fat that is actually causing the problem by creating a deficiency of the essential fatty acid in the skin region. Pet owners have known for centuries that the fat in the diet could improve the animal's coat. What makes humans think that they can eat any type of fat in any quantity and not have it manifested in skin problems?

Eczema is a common skin problem involving red, scaly, inflamed, and sometimes seeping skin regions. Patients with atopic eczema have been found to have problems in fatty acid metabolism. They apparently have low or missing levels of a crucial enzyme for changing certain dietary fats into the desired prostaglandins for skin health.[4] These patients have more cis-linoleic and less gamma-linoleic (GLA) acid in their system than normal. They probably have a defect in the ability to convert the essential fatty acid, linoleic acid, to a more complex fat, GLA. Atopy is an inherited condition found in a large percentage of the population, in which sinus conditions (rhinitis), allergies, and skin problems revolve in and out of these people's lives. Oral doses of GLA were effective in treating many of 99 experimental patients with atopic eczema.[5] Another study (with double-blind, placebo-controlled crossover format) found significant relief in many of 50 eczema patients using GLA.[6] Psoriasis is another skin condition involving red, scaly areas. GLA may also help treat psoriasis.[7]

Infants often develop skin eruptions, diarrhea, or hair loss (acrodermatitis enteropathica) after weaning. In animal studies, GLA supplements given to pregnant and nursing mothers were able to increase the pup's zinc absorption markedly.[8] These scientists propose that weaning produces a sharp drop in both GLA and zinc. Both of these nutrients are involved in skin health. Either GLA, zinc, or both are likely involved in this common problem for infants.

ZINC

Zinc is involved in at least 80 different enzyme systems in the body. Several of these functions involve skin health. Zinc stimulates antibody production for fending off invading organisms in the skin surface. Zinc encourages normal protein metabolism, which is a main function of daily skin growth. And zinc deficiencies are widespread in America. Purpura is a skin condition of subcutaneous bleeding that is common in the older adult. These hemorrhages can be tiny (petechia) or look like large bruises (ecchymoses). Investigators examined 40 patients (aged 65–99) in a hospital geriatric unit. Twenty of these people had significant purpura, and 20 did not. The 20 patients with purpura all had significantly lower zinc levels than the patients without purpura.[9] These authors noted that even the elderly patients without purpura had lower zinc levels than healthy younger patients. Purpura may be an indication of low zinc, which can be more serious than the cosmetic problem of skin bruises.

Acne is found most commonly in adolescents. Although acne is not fatal, many teenagers will tell you otherwise: "I simply died when he saw my zit." Teenage acne is usually caused by temporary hormonal imbalances. Yet bad diet often makes it a worse or longer-lasting condition than it should be. Teens have higher zinc needs (from growth, sexual maturation, and often sexual activity) and lower zinc intake (from copious quantities of "junk food"). Zinc loss is accelerated through sexual activity because sperm and matrix require large amounts of zinc. Carl Pfeiffer, M.D., Ph.D., has found that teens often get acne as a symptom of a marginal zinc deficiency.

Both oral and topical zinc are effective against acne. Topical zinc (when combined with the antibiotic erythromycin) was very effective in healing acne.[10] Other researchers found that oral zinc was as effective against acne as oral antibiotic therapy.[11] In an even larger study of 56 acne patients examined, 27 received a placebo in double-blind fashion, and 29 received 600 mg of zinc sulphate daily. After 12 weeks, none of the placebo patients showed any improvement, while 17 (58 percent) of the zinc-treated patients had marked improvement in their acne.[12] Zinc intake at these dosages should continue only for a few months, since excessive zinc can lower the heart-protective HDLs.

CHROMIUM

Chromium yeast is also effective against acne. In a variety of studies, erratic blood glucose has been tied to acne problems. When nine patients were given 2 teaspoons daily of high-chromium yeast containing 400 mcg of chromium, the improvement in acne was rapid in most subjects.[13]

VITAMIN A

One of the many functions of vitamin A is skin maintenance. Abnormal blood levels of vitamin A may be an accurate indicator of skin problems. Researchers found that serum retinol (which is the blood version of vitamin A) was lower in patients with acne and higher in patients with dry, rough, scaly skin (ichthyosis).[14] Although vitamin A has an excellent track record in treating acne,[15] it can also be toxic in large doses. However, researchers have developed a type of vitamin A that is effective against acne without being toxic.[16] This analog could be toxic to the developing fetus, so pregnant women should be wary of excessive doses of any form of vitamin A.

VITAMIN E AND SELENIUM

Vitamin E and selenium are valuable in treating acne.[17] Researchers selected 42 men with severe acne and 47 women with acne (21 severe, 26 moderate cases). The male acne patients had much lower levels of glutathione peroxidase (GSH), which is a potent protector of the prostaglandins that regulate skin health. GSH levels in women varied, depending whether or not they were using oral contraceptives. Twenty-nine of these patients were selected for selenium and vitamin E therapy. Within six weeks, the 400 mcg of selenium and 20 mg (about 30 IU) of vitamin E helped many of the patients, especially those with low GSH levels and pustular acne.

BIOTIN

Biotin is a B vitamin that is both found in certain foods and produced by intestinal bacteria. Yet biotin deficiencies may be much more common than once thought, say Yale University researchers.[18] In patients on long-term tube feedings without biotin, the early symptoms of deficiency were skin lesions around the eyes, nose, and mouth.[19] Biotin deficiencies are probably quite common in infants and surface as seborrhea, an oily condition of the skin.[20] Biotin (900 mg daily, which is 3,000 times the RDA) was able to cure an inherited cowlick condition (ectodermal dysplasia) and may be useful against some rare types of baldness.[21]

THIAMINE

Thiamine creates a natural insect repellent in human skin. Thiamine therapy (up to 50 mg/day) helps to lower the incidence of insect bites.[22]

NIACIN

In patients with poor diet and/or poor absorption, niacin deficiency can create an unusual sensitivity to the sun. One such patient had no symptoms of pellagra (niacin deficiency), yet was given 200 mg of nicotinic acid (a version of niacin) daily. This quickly cured his reaction to the sun, which involved redness, itching, and blistering.[23]

PABA

Throughout the 1960s, "health faddists" were topically applying ground-up PABA (para-aminobenzoic acid) to help prevent sunburn. PABA is now recognized by the federal government as one of the most effective sunscreens available.[24]

VITAMIN C

Smokers often find their skin, especially the upper lip, wrinkling prematurely from the effects of tobacco. Tobacco binds up huge quantities of vitamin C, which is responsible for maintaining the connective tissue that gives our body a smooth resilience. Two thousand milligrams of vitamin C daily would probably slow down the skin wrinkling but would not stop it.

WATER

Many people have dry rough skin because they do not drink enough water. Five to 10 cups of clean fluids daily will keep the skin looking younger and smoother.

PROTEIN AND OTHER NUTRIENTS

A favorite nutritional "cure" for weak fingernails has been capsules of gelatin. Gelatin is made from animal hooves and hides and hence is collagen, just like your nails. The logic seems to be there, but the results aren't always. Actually, a healthy protein intake will do more to improve nail strength than gelatin capsules will. Vitamin B_6, zinc, copper, GLA, and other nutrients also assist in forming fingernails.

NUTRITIONAL RECOMMENDATIONS

DIETARY GUIDELINES

1. Be aware of possible food allergies and sensitivities that may cause skin problems.

2. Be sure that fat intake is high-quality; that is, restrict intake of saturated animal fat and minimize hydrogenated fat intake. Fats from plant food and fish are preferable.

20
EXCRETION
Kidney Stones, Swollen Prostate, and Urinary Tract Problems

If you compared your bodily fluids to a swimming pool, your kidneys would be the filtration system. It is the job of the kidneys to remove worn-out substances and waste products from the blood while maintaining the proper quantity and consistency of blood. This can be quite a challenge. While the kidneys remove the waste products, they are supposed to retain about 90 percent of the valuable nutrients.

Fluid levels in the body fluctuate throughout the day. This is particularly true for active people in hot, dry climates. The kidneys are supposed to maintain reasonably normal blood pressure and blood volume in spite of the many changes that confront your body. This is no small task. Ask anyone who is on a renal dialysis machine what he or she would pay to get back full function of the kidneys. The answer would probably be "everything I've got."

The most dangerous of all kidney problems is kidney failure. This occurs most often in diabetics. The kidneys are almost totally dependent on blood glucose for energy. Without a dependable supply of fuel, and with the health of tiny capillaries deteriorating, the kidneys often give out in diabetics (see Chapter 14 for more details on the prevention and treatment of diabetes). Infections,

380

concussions, and drug abuse can also kill the kidneys and place the victim indefinitely on a kidney filtration machine (see Chapters 7 and 16 for further information on these subjects).

THE KIDNEYS

KIDNEY STONES

One of the more common problems of the excretory system is kidney stones. These are usually tiny crystals of uric acid (as in gout victims) oxalates or calcium that develop a jagged edge. The body's attempts to excrete these sandlike particles have the effect of dragging a fish hook through the delicate vessels of the excretory system—very, very painful. Kidney stones are probably quite preventable through healing nutrients. Once you get a kidney stone, drugs, surgery, or ultrasonic pounding may be the best therapy.

Years ago, scientists were concerned that calcium supplements may instigate kidney stones, since many kidney stones are composed of calcium. As in many areas of life, the obvious is not always the answer. Actually, kidney stones are more a product of calcium deficiency or imbalance than of calcium excess. Calcium supplements may even prevent kidney stones.[1]

Primitive cultures that eat a diet low in fat and high in magnesium usually have a very low incidence of kidney stones.[2] Soil levels of magnesium in the southeastern United States are lower than normal. This area of the country has become known as the "stone belt" for its prevalence of kidney stones. Magnesium supplements have been quite effective in preventing kidney stones, even in people who have a history of developing this painful condition.[3]

Some people are genetically prone to kidney stones, in spite of a healthy diet and lifestyle. For some of these people, vitamin B_6 therapy (25–600 mg daily) has been amazingly effective at preventing the formation of kidney stones.[4]

Some experts used to recommend against vitamin C supplements on the basis that the oxalate by-products of vitamin C may produce kidney stones. Once again, the obvious is not always the correct answer. In reality, no healthy users of high-dose ascorbic acid have contracted kidney stones. However, the same cannot be said for patients on dialysis machines. Although healthy kidneys can easily remove excess vitamin C, kidney machines cannot do the same. Dialysis patients are prime candidates for kidney stones if they consume too much vitamin C.[5]

SPECIAL FATTY ACIDS AND KIDNEY HEALTH

EPA from fish oil may improve the overall health of the kidneys. A variety of valuable prostaglandins, which help to regulate the kidneys, are readily produced from EPA. During pregnancy, a woman's body adds about 50 percent more to her existing fluid volume. Under this stress, sometimes the kidneys begin mistakenly to dump large amounts of protein into the urine. This condition, proteinuria, can sometimes be prevented or treated with EPA.[6] EPA holds great potential in treating a wide variety of kidney diseases.

RENAL DIALYSIS

More people are being put on artificial kidney machines in America than ever before. Whether more kidneys are failing or medical science is able to keep more marginal people alive, no one knows. Real kidneys are much more efficient than kidney machines. Patients on kidney machines lose much more carnitine than do normal people. Carnitine is probably an essential vitamin for renal dialysis patients.[7] Renal dialysis patients also probably need supplemental vitamin B_6.[8] A version of the B vitamin folic acid (folinic acid) is one of the more effective agents used in treating kidney failure.[9]

Renal dialysis is a life-saving technique for people with kidney failure. Yet these filtration machines remove much of the essential nutrients from the blood. Renal dialysis patients are at great risk for having a variety of malnutritive conditions. For instance, men on renal dialysis often experience impotence due to the zinc that is lost in the kidney filtration process. Zinc supplements were able to restore sexual activity in these men (see Chapter 12 for more details). People using artificial kidney machines should take high-quality, broad-spectrum vitamin-mineral supplements to replenish the nutrients that are lost by the inefficiency of renal dialysis.

SWOLLEN PROSTATE

Another common problem of the excretory system is the inflamed prostate. The prostate is a tiny, doughnut-shaped gland that encircles the urethral tube leading from the bladder through the penis to the outside. The prostate adds certain fluids to sperm. As many men age, the prostate gland can become somewhat of an onerous burden. It swells up and pinches off the urethra, leading to painful urination, urgency followed by no urine, dribbling, and other nonfatal dilemmas. It is interesting to note that many glands of the body swell up when they are deprived of essential nutrients: the thyroid gland swells up when it lacks sufficient iodide, the prostate swells up without adequate zinc, the pancreas swells when lacking vitamin E, and the kidneys become inflamed without adequate EPA. The prostate uses much zinc and is a deposition site for body zinc stores. Zinc is one of the more common deficiencies among Americans, especially as we age. Zinc supplements (150 mg daily for two to four months) reduced the swelling of the prostate gland in many of the men tested.[10] Compared to the expense and pain of prostate surgery, zinc supplementation for prostatitis deserves more use.

URINARY PROBLEMS

URINARY TRACT INFECTIONS

Urinary tract infections are common and uncomfortable and can be dangerous. Urinary tract infections can be caused by the yeast mold organism *Candida albicans*. This is especially common in women (see Chapter 8 for information on how to deal with *Candida* infections).

Normally, a high fluid intake and some acid foods make the urine quite hostile to invading bacteria. Cranberry juice is effective against urinary tract infections for more reasons than just its fluid and acid content. There may be some additional factor in cranberry juice that helps to purge an infection from the urinary tract. Cranberry juice has been used successfully for years to treat urinary tract infections.[11]

CANCER IN THE URINARY TRACT

The abundance of polluted drinking water that is being consumed in this country is causing an increased incidence in cancer of the kidney, bladder, and urethra.[12] These are the regions of the body that are trying to dispose of these toxic substances. With regular fluid intake, the diluted urine helps to flush possible infections from the urinary tract. Yet the water consumed must be relatively pollution-free, or it may cause more harm than good. Quality and quantity of water intake can strongly influence the health of the excretory system. Cancer of the bladder is probably restricted to people who smoke or consume polluted drinking water.

NUTRITIONAL RECOMMENDATIONS
DIETARY GUIDELINES

1. Core diet
2. Core supplements, with the few therapeutic exceptions as noted in the chapter.

21
THE RESPIRATORY SYSTEM
Asthma

You can live weeks without food and days without water. But you can survive only a few minutes without air. All 60 trillion cells in the human body require oxygen. Via an ingenious bellows system of muscles and diaphragm, the lungs bring air into close contact with the blood supply, which then transports oxygen to the body cells.

Several problems can confront this crucial system. Lung cancer and emphysema are common and often fatal conditions and are usually present in people who are exposed to air pollution or tobacco smoke. Certain nutrients can help protect the lungs from these serious conditions (see Chapters 6 and 16 for more details).

The primary cause of death at the turn of the century was tuberculosis and influenza. Both of these conditions are infections of the respiratory system. Thanks to inoculations and improved hygiene, we no longer tremble at the thought of these plagues. Yet pneumonia and influenza still take their toll, especially among older adults (see Chapter 7 to bolster your immune defenses).

Although the brain comprises only 5 percent of the body weight in an adult, it uses up 25 percent of the body's oxygen supply. Hence, the brain (and the behavior and intellect) suffer dramatically when oxygen supply is reduced. This can happen when the red blood cell couriers are in low number, as occurs in anemia (see Chapter 10 for more on that subject).

Also, since the lungs are exposed to a large and continuous oxygen supply, they may "rust" sooner than other body tissues. Of all the bodily functions that deteriorate with age, lung capacity is one of the worst (see Chapter 9 for details on how to slow down oxidation of the lungs).

ASTHMA

One-half million Americans are afflicted with asthma, and food allergies are sometimes the cause.[1] In one study, 107 asthma patients were given 143 different food challenges in a double-blind fashion. Seventy-one percent of the people with a history of food allergies responded with an asthma attack. Fifty-six percent of the people who had no history of food allergies responded with an asthma attack.[2] Asthma and hay fever sufferers are 300 percent more likely to have food sensitivities than the normal healthy person (see Chapter 8 for more on that issue).

Metabisulfite is a food preservative used widely in restaurants, food processing, and wine making. It retards the browning that often occurs on lettuce, potatoes, apples, grapes, and other fresh produce as a result of oxidation. It also may provoke a serious asthma attack in sensitive individuals. Researchers tested 13 asthmatics and 10 healthy controls. Three of the asthmatics had reported a sensitivity to sulfite food additives. The other 10 asthmatics did not consider themselves to be sensitive to sulfites. All 3 of the sensitive people and 4 of the 10 "nonsensitive" asthmatic individuals developed an asthma attack upon double-blind exposure to metabisulfite.[3] None of the 10 healthy controls reacted to metabisulfite. From this small study, we might conclude that roughly half of the 500,000 asthmatics in this country may experience a bronchospasm from exposure to metabisulfite. In some cases, the attack could be fatal. When metabisulfite is used at the level recommended on the label, fresh produce can contain as much as 1 part of metabisulfite per 1,000 parts of food.[4] Since most food additives are found in parts per million or even parts per billion, this metabisulfite concentration is extremely high. A new law specifies that restaurants, wineries, and food manufacturers that use this dangerous food additive must list metabisulfite on the product label.

Asthma may also be linked to a vitamin B_6 problem. Monosodium glutamate (MSG), a flavor enhancer that is popular throughout the developed nations, especially in Oriental food, is no longer used in baby food since it may impair brain development. But people who frequented Chinese restaurants began developing a stiff neck, headache, feverish feeling, burning eyes, and labored breathing. Eventually, the problem was traced to MSG. In large, continuous doses, MSG can cause partial paralysis of the breathing muscles. Researchers at the University of Texas have found that people who develop the "Chinese restaurant syndrome" are low in their levels of vitamin B_6.[5] The same researchers challenged a group of students with MSG. In double-blind fashion, some of the students were given B_6 supplements, and others were given a placebo. When fed MSG-laden foods, none of the students who were protected with B_6 developed upper respiratory distress, while 4 of the unprotected group did develop the condition.[6] Later, using only the students who had reacted to MSG, researchers provided some subjects with B_6 protection and the others with a placebo. Only 1 of the 9 MSG-sensitive individuals who was taking B_6 supplements (50 mg daily) developed any reaction to MSG. MSG apparently has the ability to find a weak link in the metabolism of some people. Vitamin B_6 can protect most people who continue to consume MSG, but MSG should be avoided by infants, and pregnant and lactating women. All other people should minimize MSG intake.

In the above situation, vitamin B_6 supplements prevented the upper respiratory distress from MSG. This gave some clinicians hope that B_6 supplements may help other respiratory conditions. Indeed, B_6 supplements were able to reduce the incidence and severity of childhood asthma attacks.[7] To test this principle further, asthmatics and healthy controls were compared. Seven of the asthma patients showed markedly lower blood levels of vitamin B_6. These seven subjects were then given 100 mg of B_6 daily for 3–10 months. The six healthy controls were given the same amount of B_6 for six weeks. Blood levels of B_6 rose dramatically in the controls, but there was no consistent rise in the levels of B_6 in the blood of the asthmatics. However, the B_6 did reduce the frequency and intensity of asthma attacks.[8] Some cases of asthma may be a symptom of an error in B_6 metabolism, which can be "cured" partially by high-dose supplements of B_6.

Another nutrient that may help the asthmatic is vitamin C. One gram of ascorbic acid daily was able to reduce slightly the sensitivity that asthmatics have to noxious substances in the air.[9] Another study showed that 500 mg of vitamin C taken 90 minutes before exercise was able to reduce bronchial spasms in asthmatics. Overall, vitamin C seems to reduce sensitivity to offensive agents in the air while also preventing serious throat spasms in some asthmatic individuals.[10]

Asthma may also be a symptom of a subclinical deficiency of magnesium. Magnesium sulfate (epsom salts) given intravenously was able to treat asthma attacks quickly and effectively in 10 humans tested.[11] This makes perfect sense. Magnesium is involved in proper muscle relaxation. Asthma may be a violent muscle spasm in the chest and throat region. Most Americans are very low in their magnesium intake, so magnesium supplements would probably provide relief for many asthmatics.

THE NEED FOR OXYGEN

Our bodies are incredibly dependent on a regular supply of oxygen. People with problems in their oxygen delivery system get tired, mean, and listless and have more illnesses. The lungs are one of the most vulnerable parts of the body, since they regularly draw in air from the outside—air that can be laced with infectious organisms and pollutants, air that is, at the very least, a corrosive agent against life. It is ironic that the air we so desperately need is also the cause of our demise in cellular oxidation. Healing nutrients can minimize the health risk from bacteria, viruses, smog, tobacco, and oxygen.

NUTRITIONAL RECOMMENDATIONS TO COMBAT ASTHMA

DIETARY GUIDELINES

1. Avoid MSG and all sulfur-bearing food additives (metabisulfite, sulfur dioxide, etc.).

2. Follow the guidelines in Chapter 8.

DAILY SUPPLEMENTS TO ADD TO YOUR CORE PROGRAM

Vitamin C   +2,000 mg
Vitamin B_6 +100 mg
Magnesium   +400 mg

22
SENSORY ORGANS
Taste, Touch, Smell, Sight, Hearing, Motion

We are intelligent creatures living in a constantly changing environment. Our sense organs allow us to detect these changes in our environment and to imbibe the wild and sweet sensations of life. What magnificent organs these are. We have stereophonic sound detectors (ears) with uncommon sensitivity for hearing music, voices, laughter, and birds. We get stereo vision from wide-angle technicolor "cameras" (eyes), which the sophisticated camera industry is still envious of. We have tactile (touch) responses that are so refined that blind people can "read" the Braille bumps on papers as written language. Our olfactory lobes (smell) in the nasal passages can detect odors as faint as parts per billion in the air. Human noses are still the "instruments" of choice in fields where smell detection is important. Our taste sensors (tongue and nose) detect sour, sweet, salt, and bitter to allow us to seek useful foods, avoid harmful foods, and enjoy eating. Our inner ear provides us with a sense of balance and movement. In the inner ear, fine "sand" particles drift through a fluid medium and are pulled down by gravity to stimulate tiny hair detectors inside of the inner ear. The result is balance so keen that tightrope walkers occasionally "put it all on the line" and walk blindfolded across a dangerous chasm.

Many factors can relate nutrition to the proper functioning of the sense organs. When circulation to the ears and other sense organs is limited, their efficiency begins to diminish. Hence, poor hearing can be a result of circulatory disease (see Chapter 5 for information on how to prevent this tragedy). Cancer, infections, and pollutants could take their toll on the sense organs (see Chapters 6,7, and 16). "Normal" aging can prematurely wear out our sense organs (see Chapter 9 for nutritional tips on how to slow down aging).

Also, be aware of the need for an interdisciplinary approach to health. Exercise improves circulation to these peripheral regions of the body. By protecting the ears from noise, protecting the eyes and skin from the sun, and shielding the mouth from tobacco and pollutants, you can markedly increase your chances of keeping your sense organs functioning well into your 9th or 10th decade of life.

VISION

In spite of the wide availability of vitamin A-rich foods, vitamin A deficiency is still common in the U.S.[1] Vitamin A deficiency is the third most common form of malnutrition in the world, after protein-calorie and iodide deficiencies (goiter). Of the 500,000 new cases of vitamin A deficiency that develop each year in southeast Asia alone, half of these people will go permanently blind. Most of these victims are children. Programs have been instigated in Asia to give semiannual injections of 200,000 IU of vitamin A to children. The result has been an 80 percent drop in serious eye problems (keratomalacia) among children.[2] Twenty percent of all blindness in India is due to vitamin A deficiency.[3]

This malnutrition elsewhere in the world may seem rather distant and irrelevant. It isn't. In a very large study of over 70,000 Americans, one-third of all children under the age of six were found to have low levels of serum vitamin A.[4] One of the first symptoms of low levels of vitamin A is poor visual adaptation to the dark. The longer it takes for the eyes to adjust to darkness, the greater the likelihood of a vitamin A deficiency. Children with poor night vision yet with no clinical signs of vitamin A deficiency were given supplements of vitamin A. In this blind study, the children given placebos took 12 times longer to locate an object in the dark than did the vitamin A-supplemented group.[5] Children have higher needs for vitamin A, since they are rapidly growing, but they often get low intakes of vitamin A. The result can be everything from poor disease resistance to poor vision. Low vitamin A can also lead to low tearing ability, or dry eyes.[6] Researchers found that decreased tearing was related directly to the severity of vitamin A deficiency (xerophthalmia), even in otherwise well-nourished children.

Alcohol abusers also often develop poor night vision (see the section on alcohol in Chapter 16 for more details).

Premature infants may have a limited ability to breathe on their own and are often immersed in an oxygen tent. Born with low levels of vitamin E (an antioxidant) and exposed to rich concentrations of oxygen, the retina of the infant's eyes are often shredded by the excess oxygen in the blood. Blindness in premature infants is quite common. When protected by supplements of vitamin E, these infants suffer far less effects from the destruction of oxygen (see Chapter 11).

Cataracts are a common visual impairment, especially among the elderly. Cataracts may be caused by the cumulative effect of the sun's ultraviolet radiation on the eyes. Eye lenses that were saturated with vitamin E and then exposed to sunlight experienced an 80 percent reduction in the destruction from ultraviolet radiation compared to the nonprotected lenses.[7] These researchers felt that optimal levels of vitamin E might slow cataract formation or prevent them from forming altogether. Recall that a continuous low intake of vitamin E (such as is common among Americans) may lead to premature senility (Alzheimer's disease), early aging, erosion of lung capacity, and visual impairments. The 12 IU of vitamin E daily that the average American consumes is not enough to prevent these common degenerative ailments from occurring. Recent scientific expeditions to the South Pole tell us that 50 percent of the ozone layer that once screened out much of the sun's harmful radiation is now gone.[8] Fluorocarbons from industry, spray cans, and coolants have dissolved the protective ozone layer. Skin cancer and cataracts are expected to increase dramatically in the coming decade due to the erosion of the ozone layer. This makes nutritional protection that much more important.

Patients with cataracts usually have lower-than-normal levels of riboflavin.[9] One of the symptoms of a riboflavin deficiency is cataracts. Riboflavin deficiency is one of the more common malnutritive conditions in America. In studies of 973 schoolchildren in India, a direct link was found between marginal status of the B vitamins and impaired vision. When supplemented with the B vitamins, the children's vision improved markedly.[10]

Diabetics are 25 times more likely to go blind than the average person. Uncontrolled diabetes is a wrecking ball on the eyes. In clinical use, a physician has been able to cut eye problems (diabetic retinopathy) by 80 percent when his antioxidant supplement program is started early enough. Daily intake of vitamin E (800 IU), vitamin C (1,000 mg), vitamin A (10,000 IU), and selenium (500 mcg) has been his time-tested formula for preventing blindness among diabetics.[11] Vitamin E alone has been shown to improve the eye problems (neovascularization) in diabetics and sickle-cell anemia patients.[12]

On an anecdotal level, a college professor reported that he was losing his vision, in spite of a healthy lifestyle. His minor exposure to pollutants from newsprint, photocopies, exhaust fumes, and books were the only possible antagonizing factors. He began taking 500 mg of vitamin C daily, and his eye problems cleared up within a week.[13]

HEARING

In some cases, poor hearing may be related to poor nutrient status. As mentioned in previous Chapters, researchers in China found that regions with low iodide in the diet had an increased incidence of children with hearing problems and that hearing levels and thyroid functions returned to normal after three years of iodide supplementation.[14] And again, this is relevant to Americans because 23–36 percent of Kentucky schoolchildren examined had blatant iodide deficiency in spite of having a seemingly adequate iodide intake.[15]

TASTE AND SMELL

The efficiency of the taste buds is often related directly to zinc intake. Zinc status is marginal at best in the U.S. Anorexics are found to have low zinc levels.[16] Children who are picky eaters often will improve their food intake after taking zinc supplements for a few weeks.[17] Many pica victims with bizarre eating habits have a zinc deficiency.[18] Older adults lose up to 80 percent of their taste buds as they age,[19] with much of this loss due to zinc deficiency.[20]

MOTION AND BALANCE

Motion sickness is a common ailment in humans. There are drugs that can help alleviate some of this problem, but many of them also cause drowsiness. Then there is gingerroot. In a double-blind study at Brigham Young University, a researcher gave Dramamine (a favorite drug to prevent motion sickness), or placebo, or gingerroot to students susceptible to motion sickness. They were then blindfolded and rotated in a tilting chair for up to six minutes. Half of the subjects given ginger could stay for the full six minutes. None of the subjects given placebo or Dramamine could last the full six minutes of movement.[21]

NUTRITIONAL RECOMMENDATIONS
DIETARY GUIDELINES

1. Core diet
2. Core supplements, with the few therapeutic exceptions as noted in the chapter.

CONCLUSION

You have a choice in front of you: continue living the normal American lifestyle and suffer many preventable health problems or follow the guidelines in this book and significantly extend the quality and quantity of your life.

Just as other people cannot live your life for you, they also cannot provide you with health. Only you can do that. Your doctor can't do it. Most physicians wish that their patients would become active partners in averting health catastrophes. Researchers can't do it. In spite of unfathomable money spent and intelligence employed, medical research has precious few "magic bullet" cures for today's diseases. Neither the government nor your insurance company can do it for you. Only you can provide yourself with health. The true healing miracle is what your own body can do for itself when provided with an ideal supply of nutrients, regular challenging exercise, and positive emotions.

You have many things to be grateful for with respect to 20th century health care:

1. You live in a land where food is plentiful. Nutrition knowledge can be somewhat academic and useless in the many starvation-prone areas of the world.

2. Nutrition science has uncovered thousands of ways to fine-tune the body with ideal levels of nutrients, rather than just accepting "survival" nutrition.

3. Modern medicine does have some truly amazing drug and surgery approaches to many emergency health situations.

4. People today are more willing to take charge of their life and use nutrition to improve their overall health. The nutrition-conscious consumer is no longer a freak. There are many others like you. You will find more support than ridicule.

A group of retired Fortune 500 executives were asked: "If you had it to do over again, what would you do differently?" Remember, these are people who have "sipped from the silver cup of life" with abundant money, travel, and prestige. Almost unanimously they had two responses: "I would have spent more time with my family" and "I would have taken better care of my health."

By making a little effort now, you can probably add at least a decade of quality exuberant living to your lifespan. The alternative is to let regrets overwhelm your life later on. You can either make time for wellness, or you will be forced to make time for illness. Take charge of your own life. Pack your own parachute. Use *Healing Nutrients* to find a level of wellness that you never thought possible. Good health to you.

FOR MORE INFORMATION

Dr. Quillin is the author of the *Nutrition Encyclopedia* and *Therapeutic Nutrition*, both of which are full of well-organized and relevant nutrition information. He is also the co-editor of *The Nutrition Times*, a bimonthly newsletter that provides home-study continuing education for physicians, osteopaths, nurses, dieticians, and pharmacists. Please write to Box 336, Fallbrook, CA, 92028 for further information.

ENDNOTES

CHAPTER 1

1. Stini, WA, *Federation Proceedings*, vol. 40, p. 2588, Sept. 1981
2. U.S. Bureau of the Census, *Statistical Abstract of the United States: 1985*, 105th ed., p. 843, Washington, DC, 1984
3. Wagner, MG, *Lancet*, p. 1207, Nov. 27, 1982
4. Hackett, E., *Medical Journal of Australia*, vol. 142, p. 146, Jan. 21, 1985
5. Menzel, P., *Medical Costs, Moral Choices*, Yale University, New Haven, CT, 1985
6. Moramarco, SS, *Los Angeles Times*, Health Supplement, p. 2, Mar. 2, 1986
7. *Los Angeles Times*, Part 1, p. 4, Dec. 7, 1986
8. Braunwald, E., *New England Journal of Medicine*, vol. 309, p. 1181, Nov. 10, 1983
9. Burris, JF, *New England Journal of Medicine*, p. 1350, Nov. 18, 1982
10. Horrobin, DF, *Behavioral and Brain Sciences*, vol. 5, p. 217, June 1982
11. Bailar, JC, et al., *New England Journal of Medicine*, vol. 314, p. 1226, May 8, 1986
12. Roemer, MI, *American Journal of Public Health*, vol. 74, p. 243, Mar. 1984
13. Leaf, A., *New England Journal of Medicine*, vol. 310, p. 718, Mar. 15, 1984

CHAPTER 2

1. O'Dea, K., *Diabetes*, vol. 33, p. 596, June 1984
2. Eaton, S., et al., *New England Journal of Medicine*, vol. 312, p. 283, Jan. 31, 1985
3. Murray, MJ. et al., *American Journal of Clinical Nutrition*, vol. 33, p. 697, Mar.1980
4. Turkel, H., *Journal of Orthomolecular Psychiatry*, vol. 4, no. 2, p. 102, 1975
5. Dipalma, JR, *American Family Physician*, vol. 32, p. 171, Aug. 1985
6. Mazess, RB, et al., *American Journal of Clinical Nutrition*, vol. 42, p. 568, Sept. 1985
7. Schneider, HA, et al., (eds), *Nutritional Support of Medical Practice*, p.26, Harper & Row, Hagerstown, MD, 1977
8. *Journal of American Medical Association*, vol. 231, no. 4, p. 360, Jan. 27, 1975
9. Habibzadeh, N., et al., *British Journal of Nutrition*, vol. 55, p. 23, 1986
10. Wurtman, RJ, et al., *Nutrition and the Brain*, vol. 7, p. 37, 1986
11. Cathcart, RF, *Medical Hypotheses*, vol. 14, p. 423, 1984
12. Styslinger, L., et al., *American Journal of Clinical Nutrition*, vol. 41, p. 21, Jan.1985
13. Harrell, R., et al., *Proceedings of the National Academy of Sciences*, vol. 78, p. 574, Jan. 1981
14. Pauling, L., *American Journal of Psychiatry*, vol. 131, no. 11, p. 1251, Nov. 1974
15. Reed, P., *Nutrition: An Applied Science*, p. 14, West Publishing, St. Paul, MN, 1980
16. Pauling, L., *Science*, vol. 160, p. 265, Apr. 1968
17. Suboticanec, K., et al., *Human Nutrition: Clinical Nutrition*, vol. 40C, p. 421, 1986
18. Ginter, E., *World Review of Nutrition and Dietetics*, vol. 33, p. 104, 1979
19. Bieri, JG, et al., *New England Journal of Medicine*, vol. 65, p. 1063, May, 1983
20. Hegsted, DM, *Nutrition Reviews*, vol. 43, p. 357, Dec. 1985
21. Rimland, B., et al., *American Journal of Psychiatry*, vol. 135, p. 472, 1978
22. Alvarez-Dardet, C., et al., *New England Journal of Medicine*, vol. 312, p. 1521, June 6, 1985
23. Oliver, MF, *Lancet*, p. 1087, May 11, 1985
24. Kanofsky, JD, et al., *New England Journal of Medicine*, p. 173, July 16, 1981
25. Grundy, SM, et al., *Journal of Lipid Research*, vol. 22, p. 24, 1981

26. Banic, S., et al. , *International Journal of Vitamin and Nutrition Research*, supplement, vol. 19, p. 41, 1979

27. Mowrey, DB, *Lancet*, p. 655, Mar. 20, 1982

28. Driskell, JA, et al. , *Nutrition Reports International*, vol. 34, no. 6, p. 1031, Dec. 1986

29. Sandyk, R., et al. , *New England Journal of Medicine*, vol. 314, p. 1257, May 8, 1986

30. Goodwin, JS, et al. , *Journal of American Medical Association*, vol. 251, p. 2387, May 11, 1984

31. King, LS, *Journal of the American Medical Association*, vol. 248, p. 1749, Oct. 8; p. 2329, Nov.12, 1982

32. Bortz, WM, *Journal of American Medical Association*, vol. 248, no. 10, p. 1203, Sept. 10, 1982

33. Taylor, CB, et al. , *Public Health Reports*, vol. 100, no. 2, p. 195, Mar. 1986

34. Welin, L., et al. , *Lancet*, p. 915, Apr. 20, 1985

35. London, RS, et al. , *Obstetrics and Gynecology*, vol. 65, p. 104, Jan. 1985

36. Knaus, WA, et al. , *Annals of Internal Medicine*, vol. 104, no. 3, p. 410, Mar. 1986

37. Kiecolt-Glaser, J., et al. , *Psychosomatic Medicine*, vol. 66, no. 1, p. 7, Jan. 1984

38. *Lancet*, p. 133, July 20, 1985

39. U.S. Department of Health, Education, and Welfare, *Healthy People*, p. 101, U.S. Government Printing Office, 79-55071, Washington, DC, 1979

CHAPTER 3

1. U.S. Bureau of Census, *Statistical Abstract of the United States: 1985*, 105th ed., Washington, DC, 1984, *passim*.

2. Kannel, WB, *Nutrition Today*, p. 2, May 1971

3. Fernandes-Costa FJ, et al. , *American Journal of Clinical Nutrition*, vol. 40, no. 6, p. 1295, Dec. 1984

4. Pollitt, E., et al. , *American Journal of Clinical Nutrition*, vol. 42, p. 348, Aug. 1985

5. Brand, JC, et al. , *American Journal of Clinical Nutrition*, vol. 42, p. 1192, Dec. 1985

6. Reuler, JB, *Journal of the American Dietetic Association*, vol. 253, p. 805, Feb. 8, 1985

7. Reed, P., *Nutrition: An Applied Science*, West Publishing, St. Paul, MN, 1980

8. Hamilton, E., et al. , *Nutrition: Concepts and Controversies*, p. 53, West Publishing, St. Paul, MN, 1985

9. Lowenstein, FW, *Bibliotheca Nutritio et Dieta*, vol. 30, p. 1, 1981

10. Block, G., et al. , *American Journal of Epidemiology*, vol. 122, p. 13, 1985

11. Welsh, SO, et al. , *Food Technology*, p. 70, Jan. 1982

12. Mitchell, H., et al. , *Nutrition in Health and Disease*, 16th ed., p. 18, JB Lippincott Co., Philadelphia, PA, 1976

13. Pearson, JM, et al. , *Journal of the American Dietetic Association*, vol. 86, p. 339, Mar. 1986

14. Schroeder, H., *American Journal of Clinical Nutrition*, vol. 24, p. 562, May 1971

15. Guthrie, HA, et al. , *Journal of Nutrition Education*, vol. 13, p. 46, 1981

16. Morgan, KJ, et al. , *Cereal Foods World*, vol. 30, p. 839, Dec. 1985

17. Ginter, E., *World Review of Nutrition and Dietetics*, vol. 33, p. 104, 1979

18. Gill, GV, et al. , *Journal of Neurology, Neurosurgery, and Psychiatry*, vol. 45, p. 861, 1982

19. Williams RJ, *The Advancement of Nutrition*, p. 13, International Academy of Preventive Medicine, 1982

20. National Institutes of Health, *Journal of the American Medical Association*, vol. 253, p. 2080, Apr. 12, 1985

21. Haglund, K., *Medical News*, p. 3, May 26, 1986

22. National Research Council, *Recommended Dietary Allowances*, p. 1, Academy of Sciences, Washington, DC, 1980

23. Hegsted, DM, *Journal of Nutrition*, vol. 116, p. 478, 1986

24. Lee, CM, et al. , *American Journal of Clinical Nutrition*, vol. 42, p. 226, Aug. 1985

CHAPTER 4

1. Murray, MJ, et al. , *American Journal of Clinical Nutrition*, vol. 33, p. 697, Mar. 1980
2. Randall, E., et al. , *Journal of the American Dietetic Association*, vol. 85, p. 830, July 1985
3. Fabry, P., et al. , *American Journal of Clinical Nutrition*, vol. 23, no. 8, p. 1059, Aug. 1970
4. Metzner, HL, et al. , *American Journal of Clinical Nutrition*, vol. 30, p. 712, May 1977
5. Young, CM, et al. , *Journal of the American Dietetic Association*, vol. 59, p. 474, Nov. 1971
6. Mertz, W., *Journal of the American Dietetic Association*, vol. 84, p. 769, July 1984
7. Guthrie, H., et al., *Journal of Nutrition Education*, vol. 13, p. 46, 1981
8. NutriGuard Research, PO Box 865, Encinitas, CA, 92024; see also Bronson Pharmaceuticals, 4526 Rinetti Lane, La Canada, CA 91011-0628

CHAPTER 5

1. U.S. Bureau of the Census, *Statistical Abstract of the United States, 1985*, 105th ed., Washington, D.C., 1984
2. National Institute of Health, *Journal of American Medical Association*, vol. 253, p. 2080, Apr. 12, 1985
3. Braunwald, E., *New England Journal of Medicine*, vol. 309, p. 1181, Nov. 10, 1983
4. Cherchi, A. et al. , *International Journal of Clinical Pharmacology, Therapy, and Toxicology*, vol. 23, p. 569, 1985
5. Kamikawa, T., et al., *American Journal of Cardiology*, vol. 56, p. 247, 1985
6. Saynor, R., et al., *Atherosclerosis*, vol. 50, p. 3, 1984
7. Norris, PG, ct al., *British Medical Journal*, vol. 293, p. 105, July 1986
8. Paffenbarger, RS, et al., *Journal of American Medical Association*, vol. 252, p. 491, July 27, 1984
9. Kushi, LH, et al., *New England Journal of Medicine*, vol. 312, p. 811, Mar. 28, 1985
10. Fortmann, SP, *American Journal of Clinical Nutrition*, vol. 34, p. 2030, Oct. 1981
11. Hubbard, JD, et al., *New England Journal of Medicine*, vol. 313, p. 52, July 4, 1985
12. Forman, MB, et al., *New England Journal of Medicine*, vol. 313, no. 18, p. 1138, Oct. 31, 1985
13. Robinson, CH, *Fundamentals of Normal Nutrition*, p. 86, Macmillan Publishing, New York, 1978
14. Oh, SY, et al., *American Journal of Clinical Nutrition*, vol. 42, p. 421, Sept. 1985; see also *Nutrition Reviews*, vol. 43, p. 263, Sept. 1985
15. Renaud, S., et al., *American Journal of Clinical Nutrition*, vol. 43, p. 136, Jan. 1986
16. Walker, WJ, *New England Journal of Medicine*, vol. 308, p. 649, Mar. 17, 1983
17. Noppa, H., et al., *American Journal of Epidemiology*, vol. 111, no. 6, p. 682, 1980
18. Puska, P., et al., *Preventive Medicine*, vol. 14, p. 573, Sept. 1985
19. Kritchevsky, D., *Federation Proceedings*, vol. 41, p. 2813, Sept. 1982
20. Smith, EB, *Lancet*, p. 534, Mar. 8, 1980
21. Sgoutas, D., *American Journal of Clinical Nutrition*, vol. 23, no. 8, p. 1111, Aug. 1970
22. Thomassen, MS, et al., *British Journal of Nutrition*, vol. 51, p. 315, May 1984
23. Sohal, PS, et al., *Nutrition Reports International*, vol. 33, no. 1, p. 123, Jan. 1986
24. Potteau, B., et al., *Reproduction, Nutrition, Development*, vol. 23, p. 101, 1983
25. Horrobin, DF, et al., *Lipids*, vol. 18, no. 8, p. 558, 1983
26. Comberg, HU, et al., *Prostaglandins*, vol. 15, p. 193, 1978
27. O'Brien, JR, et al., *Lancet*, p. 995, 1976
28. Hoffman, P., et al., *Prostaglandins, Leukotrienes, and Medicine*, vol. 25, p. 65, 1986
29. Reuter, W., et al., *ZFA (Germany)*, vol. 40, no. 3, p. 171, May 1985
30. Piconneaux, A., et al., *Deutsche Medizinische Wochenschrift*, vol. 44, no. 5, p. 245, 1984

31. Mest, HJ, et al., *Klinische Wochenschrift*, vol. 61, no. 4, p. 187, Feb. 15, 1983
32. Mills, D., et al., *Proceedings of the Society for Experimental Biology and Medicine*, vol. 176, p. 32, 1984
33. Horrobin, D., et al., *Lipids*, vol. 18, p. 558, 1983
34. Sanders, TA, *Proceedings of the Nutrition Society*, vol. 44, p. 391, 1985
35. Sanders, TA, *op. cit.*
36. Kinsella, JE, *Food Technology*, vol. 40, p. 89, Feb. 1986
37. Kromhout, D., et al., *New England Journal of Medicine*, vol. 312, p. 1205, May 9, 1985
38. Fischer, S., et al., *Nature*, vol. 307, p. 165, Jan. 1984
39. Knapp, HR, et al., *New England Journal of Medicine*, vol. 314, p. 937, Apr. 10, 1986
40. Dyerberg, J., *Philosophical Transactions of the Royal Society of London*, vol. 294, p. 373, 1981
41. Lorenz, R., et al., *Circulation*, vol. 67, no. 3, p. 504, Mar. 1983
42. Singer, P., et al., *Prostaglandins, Leukotrienes, and Medicine*, vol. 15, p. 159, 1984
43. Norris, PG, et al., *British Medical Journal*, vol. 293, p. 105, July 1986
44. *Nutrition Reviews*, vol. 43, p. 268, Sept. 1985
45. Phillipson, BE, et al., *New England Journal of Medicine*, vol. 312, p. 1210, May 9, 1985
46. Nestel, PJ, *American Journal of Clinical Nutrition*, vol. 43, p. 752, May 1986
47. Saynor, R., et al., *Atherosclerosis*, vol. 50, p. 3, 1984
48. Culp, BR, et al., *Prostaglandins*, vol. 20, no. 6, p. 1021, Dec. 1980
49. Black, KL, et al., *Stroke*, vol. 15, no. 1, p. 65, 1984
50. Woodcock, B., *British Medical Journal*, vol. 288, p. 592, Feb. 25, 1984; see also Saynor, R., et al., *Atherosclerosis*, vol. 50, p. 3, 1984
51. Saynor, R., *Lancet*, vol. 2, p. 696, Sept. 22, 1984; see also Gunby, P., *Journal of the American Medical Association*, vol. 247, p. 729, Feb. 12, 1982
52. Kinsella, JE, *Food Technology*, vol. 40, p. 89, Feb. 1986
53. *Nutrition Reviews*, vol. 42, p. 189, May 1984
54. Lee, TH, et al., *New England Journal of Medicine*, vol. 312, p. 1217, May 9, 1985
55. *Progress in the Chemistry of Fats and the Other Lipids*, vol. 15, p. 29, 1977
56. Simons, LA, et al., *Australia and New Zealand Journal of Medicine*, vol. 7, p. 262, 1977
57. Saba, P., et al., *Current Therapeutic Research*, vol. 24, no. 3, p. 299, Aug. 1978
58. Hooper, PL, et al., *Journal of American Medical Association*, vol. 244, p. 1960, 1980
59. Freeland-Graves, JH, et al., *American Journal of Clinical Nutrition*, vol. 35, p. 988, 1982
60. Crouse, SF, et al., *Journal of American Medical Association*, vol. 252, p. 785, 1984
61. Southgate, DA, *American Journal of Clinical Nutrition*, vol. 31, p. S107, Oct. 1978
62. Moore, DJ, et al., *Human Nutrition: Clinical Nutrition*, vol. 39C, p. 63, Jan. 1985
63. Kirby, K., et al., *American Journal of Clinical Nutrition*, vol. 34, p. 824, 1981
64. Judd, PA, et al., *British Journal of Nutrition*, vol. 48, p. 451, 1982
65. Penagini, R., et al., *American Journal of Gastroenterology*, vol. 81, no. 2, p. 123, 1986
66. *Food Engineering*, vol. 57, p. 140, Aug. 1985
67. Sharma, RD, et al., *Lipids*, vol. 21, p. 715, 1986
68. Anderson, JW, *Annals of Internal Medicine*, vol. 98, p. 842, 1983
69. Vahouny, GV, *Federation Proceedings*, vol. 41, p. 2801, Sept. 1982
70. Toma, RB, et al., *Food Technology*, vol. 40, p. 111, Feb. 1986
71. Houston, MC, *Archives of Internal Medicine*, vol. 146, p. 179, Jan. 1986
72. Weaver, CM, et al., *Food Technology*, p. 99, Dec. 1986
73. Luger, SW, *New England Journal of Medicine*, vol. 314, p. 1052, Apr. 17, 1986
74. AMA Council, *Journal of American Medical Association*, vol. 249, p. 784, Feb. 11, 1983
75. Witschi, JC, et al., *Journal of the American Dietetic Association*, vol. 85, p. 816, July 1985
76. Wilson, TW, *Lancet*, p. 784, Apr. 5, 1986

77. Beard, TC, et al., *Lancet*, p. 455, Aug. 28, 1982

78. Cullens, M., *Journal of the New Zealand Dietetic Association*, vol. 39, p. 4, Apr. 1985

79. Kromhout, D., et al., *American Journal of Clinical Nutrition*, vol. 41, p. 1299, June 1985

80. Henningsen, NC, et al., *Lancet*, p. 133, Jan.15, 1983

81. Smith, SJ, et al., *Lancet*, p. 362, Feb. 12, 1983

82. Materson, BJ, *Archives of Internal Medicine*, vol. 145, p. 1966, Nov. 1985

83. Kopyt, N., et al., *New England Journal of Medicine*, vol. 313, p. 582, Aug. 29, 1985

84. *Lancet*, p. 1308, June 8, 1985

85. Johnson, NE, et al., *American Journal of Clinical Nutrition*, vol. 42, p. 12, July 1985

86. Sowers, MR, et al., *American Journal of Clinical Nutrition*, vol. 42, p. 135, July 1985

87. Belizan, J., et al., *American Journal of Clinical Nutrition*, vol. 33, p. 2202, 1980

88. *Medical World News*, p. 14, July 14, 1986

89. Marrier, JR, *Reviews of Canadian Biology*, vol. 37, p. 115, 1978

90. Belizan, JM, et al., *Journal of American Medical Association*, vol. 249, p. 1161, Mar. 4, 1983

91. Resnick, LM, et al., *Journal of American College of Cardiology*, vol. 3, p. 616, 1984

92. Altura, BM, et al., *Science*, vol. 223, p. 1315, 1984

93. Dyckner, T., et al., *British Medical Journal*, vol. 286, p. 1847, 1983

94. Johnson, CH, et al., *American Journal of Clinical Nutrition*, vol. 32, p. 967, 1979

95. Altura, B., et al., *Science*, vol. 221, p. 376, July 22, 1983

96. Fassler, CA, et al., *Archives of Internal Medicine*, vol. 145, p. 1604, Sept. 1985

97. Iseri, *Western Journal of Medicine*, vol. 138, p. 823, 1983

98. Specter, M., et al., *Circulation*, vol. 52, p. 1001, 1975

99. Altura, BM, *Medical Hypotheses*, vol. 5, p. 843, 1979

100. McGuire, R., *Medical News*, p. 7, Nov. 24, 1986

101. Lee, CM, et al., *Annals of Clinical and Laboratory Science*, vol. 14, p. 151, 1984

102. Anderson, RA, et al., *American Journal of Clinical Nutrition*, vol. 36, p. 1184, Dec. 1982

103. Schroeder, HA, *Journal of Nutrition*, vol. 88, p. 439, 1966

104. Kumpulainen, J., et al., *Journal of Agricultural and Food Chemistry*, vol. 27, p. 490, 1979

105. Mertz, W., *Federation Proceedings*, vol. 41, p. 2807, Sept. 1982

106. Newman, HA, et al., *Clinical Chemistry*, vol. 24, p. 541, 1978

107. Pyorala, K., *Diabetes Care*, vol. 2, p. 131, 1979

108. Offenbacher, EG, et al., *Diabetes*, vol. 29, p. 919, 1980

109. Abraham, AS, et al., *American Journal of Clinical Nutrition*, vol. 33, p. 2294, Nov. 1980

110. Elwood, JC, et al., *Journal of American College of Nutrition*, vol. 1, p. 263, 1982

111. Simonoff, M., *Cardiovascular Research*, vol. 18, p. 591, 1984

112. Mertz, W., in *Present Knowledge in Nutrition*, p. 373, Nutrition Foundation, New York, 1973

113. Saner, G., *Chromium in Nutrition and Disease*, p. 129, Alan R. Liss, Inc., New York, 1980

114. *Nutrition Reviews*, vol. 38, p. 25, 1980

115. Bremer, J., *Physiological Reviews*, vol. 63, no. 4, p. 1420, Oct. 1983

116. Rebouche, CJ, *Mayo Clinic Proceedings*, vol. 58, no. 8, p. 533, Aug. 1983

117. Borum, PR, *Annual Reviews of Nutrition*, vol. 3, p. 233, 1983

118. Garzya, G., et al., *International Journal on Tissue Reactions*, vol. 11, p. 175, 1980

119. Cherchi, A., et al., *International Journal of Clinical Pharmacology, Therapy and Toxicology*, vol. 23, p. 569, 1985

120. Folts, J., et al., *American Journal of Cardiology*, vol. 41, p. 1209, 1978; see also Suzuki, Y., et al., *Advances in Myocardiology*, vol 4, p. 549, 1983

121. Brooks, H., et al., *Journal of Clinical Pharmacology*, vol. 17, p. 561, 1977

122. Lacour, B., et al., *Lancet*, vol. 2, p. 763, Oct. 11, 1980

123. Pola, P., et al., *Current Therapeutic Research*, vol, 27, p. 208, 1980
124. Thomsen, J., et al., *American Journal of Cardiology*, vol. 43, p. 300, 1979
125. Schiavoni, G., et al., *Clinical Therapeutics*, vol. 96, p. 263, 1981
126. Makarova, VG, *Farmakologiia I Toksikologiia*, vol. 48, p. 57, Mar. 1985; see also Iimura, O., et al., *Advances in Myocardiology*, vol. 6, p. 437, 1985
127. Beetens, JR, et al., *Archives Internationales de Pharmacodynamie et de Therapie*, vol. 259, p. 300, 1982
128. Ginter, E., *World Reviews of Nutrition and Dietetics*, vol. 33, p. 104, 1979
129. Haglund, K., *Medical News*, p. 3, May 26, 1986
130. Garry, PJ, et al., *American Journal of Clinical Nutrition*, vol. 36, p. 332, Aug. 1982
131. Adam, K., *American Journal of Clinical Nutrition*, vol. 34, p. 1712, Sept. 1981
132. Yoskioka, M. et al., *International Journal for Vitamin and Nutrition Research*, vol. 54, p. 343, 1984
133. Cordova, C., et al., *Atherosclerosis*, vol. 41, p. 15, 1982
134. Sarji, E., et al., *Thrombosis Research*, vol. 15, p. 639, 1979
135. Horsey, J., et al., *Journal of Human Nutrition*, vol. 35, p. 53, Feb. 1981
136. Verlangieri, AJ, et al., *Blood Vessels*, vol. 14, p. 157, 1977
137. Bordia, AK, *Atherosclerosis*, vol. 35, p. 181, 1980
138. *Lancet*, p. 907, Oct. 20, 1984
139. Spittle, C., *Lancet ii*, p. 199, 1973
140. Havsteen, B., *Biochemical Pharmacology*, vol. 32, p. 1141, 1983
141. Jones, E., et al., *IRCS Medical Science*, vol. 12, p. 320, 1984
142. Marshall, M., *Fortschrittle der Medizin*, vol. 102, no. 29, p. 772, Aug. 16, 1984
143. Rathi, A., et al., *Acta Vitaminologica et Enzymologica*, vol. 5, no. 4, p. 255, 1983
144. McEwan, AJ, et al., *British Medical Journal*, vol. 2, p. 138, 1971
145. Johnson, EF, *American Journal of Pharmacology*, vol. 118, p. 164, 1946
146. Griffith, JQ, et al., *Rutin and Related Flavonoids*, Mack Publishing, Easton, PA, 1955
147. Rhead, WJ, et al., *Nutrition Reviews*, vol. 29, p. 262, 1971
148. Tsao, CS, et al., *International Journal for Vitamin and Nutrition Research*, vol. 54, p. 245, 1984
149. White, JD, *New England Journal of Medicine*, vol. 304, p. 1491, June 11, 1981
150. Pru, C., et al., *Nephron*, vol. 39, p. 112, 1985
151. Guang-lu, X., et al., *Nutrition Research*, sup. 1, p. 187, 1985
152. Salonen, JT, et al., *Lancet*, p. 175, July 24, 1982
153. Moore, JA, et al., *Clinical Chemistry*, vol. 30, no. 7, p. 1171, 1984
154. Shamberger, RJ, et al., *Trace Substances and Environmental Health*, vol. 9, p. 15, 1975
155. Stead, NW, et al., *American Journal of Clinical Nutrition*, vol. 39, p. 677, 1984
156. Schiavon, R., et al., *Thrombosis Research*, vol. 34, p. 389, Jun. 1984
157. Doni, MG, et al., *Haemostasis*, vol. 13, p. 248, 1983
158. Masukawa, T., et al., *Experientia*, vol 39, p. 5, 1983
159. Frost, DV, et al., *Annals of Pharmacology*, vol. 18, p. 259, 1975
160. Nikolaev, SM, et al., *Farmakologiia I Toksikologiia*, vol. 39, p. 571, 1976
161. Bieri, J., et al., *New England Journal of Medicine*, vol. 308, no. 18, p. 1063, May 5, 1983
162. FitzGerald, GA, et al., *Annals of New York Academy of Science*, vol. 393, p. 209, 1982
163. Steiner, M., *Thrombosis and Haemostasis*, vol. 49, no. 2, p. 73, 1983
164. FitzGerald, GA, et al., *Annals of New York Academy of Sciences*, vol. 393, p. 209, 1982
165. Barboriak, JJ, *American Journal of Clinical Pathology*, vol. 77, p. 371, Mar. 1982
166. Gaby, AR, et al., *Journal of American Medical Association*, vol. 248, p. 1066, Sept. 3, 1982
167. Kanofsky, J., et al., *New England Journal of Medicine*, p. 173, July 16, 1981
168. Haegar, K., *American Journal of Clinical Nutrition*, vol. 27, p. 1179, 1974
169. Ayres, JR, et al., *Southern Medical Journal*, vol. 67, no. 11, p. 1308, Nov. 1974
170. Yang, G., et al., *American Journal of Clinical Nutrition*, vol. 37, p. 872, May 1983

171. Levander, O., et al., *American Journal of Clinical Nutrition*, vol. 34, p. 2662, Dec. 1981

172. Palmer, I., et al., *Journal of Food Science*, vol. 47, p. 1595, 1982

173. Wei-Han, Y., *Japanese Circulation Journal*, vol. 46, 1201, Nov. 1982

174. Bordia, A., *American Journal of Clinical Nutrition*, vol. 34, p. 2100, Oct. 1981

175. Rashid, A., et al., *Journal of the Pakistan Medical Association*, vol. 35, p. 357, Dec. 1985

176. Lau, BH, et al., *Nutrition Research*, vol. 3, p. 119, 1983

177. Visudhiphan, S., et al., *American Journal of Clinical Nutrition*, vol. 35, p. 1452, June 1982

178. Kumar, N., et al., *British Medical Journal*, vol. 288, p. 1803, June 1984

179. *Nutrition Reviews*, vol. 44, no. 1, p. 20, Jan. 1986

180. Nagabhushan, M., et al., *Nutrition and Cancer*, vol. 8, p. 201, 1986

181. Giri, J., et al., *Indian Journal of Nutrition and Dietetics*, vol. 21, p. 433, Dec. 1984

182. Gupta, AK, et al., *IRCS Medical Science*, vol. 14, p. 212, 1986

183. Gilliland, S., et al., *Applied and Environmental Microbiology*, vol. 49, no. 2, p. 377, Feb. 1985; see also Hepner, G., et al., *American Journal of Clinical Nutrition*, vol. 32, p. 19, Jan. 1979

184. Willett, W., et al., *New England Journal of Medicine*, p. 1159, Nov. 13, 1980

185. Blackwelder, WC, et al., *American Journal of Medicine*, vol. 68, p. 164, Feb. 1980

186. Nestel, PJ, et al., *Metabolism* vol. 29, no. 2, p. 101, Feb. 1980

187. Greenspon, AJ, et al., *Annals of Internal Medicine*, vol. 98, p. 135, Feb. 1983

188. Gruchow, HW, et al., *Journal of American Medical Association*, vol. 253, p. 1567, Mar. 15, 1985

189. Malhotra, H., et al., *Lancet ii*, p. 584, Sept. 14, 1985

190. Read, M., et al., *Journal of American Dietetic Association*, vol. 82, p. 401, Apr. 1983

191. Gordon, T., et al., *Archives of Internal Medicine*, vol. 146, p. 262, Feb. 1986

192. Donahue, RP, et al., *Journal of American Medical Association*, vol. 255, p. 2311, May 2, 1986

193. Camargo, CA, et al., *Journal of American Medical Association*, vol. 253, p. 2854, May 17, 1985

194. Story, JA, *Federation Proceedings*, vol. 41, p. 2797, Sept. 1982

195. Karlstrom, B., et al., *Human Nutrition: Clinical Nutrition*, vol. 39C, p. 289, July 1985

196. Mertz, W., *Federation Proceedings*, vol. 41, p. 2807, Sept. 1982

197. Tilson, MD, *Archives of Surgery*, vol. 117, p. 1212, 1982

198. Meydani, SN, et al., *Journal of Nutrition*, vol. 112, p. 1098, 1982

199. Pachotikarn, C., et al., *Nutrition Reports International*, vol. 32, p. 373, Aug. 1985

200. Festa, MD, et al., *American Journal of Clinical Nutrition*, vol. 41, p. 285, Feb. 1985

201. Mertz, W., *Science*, vol. 213, p. 1332, Sept. 1981

202. Sullivan, JL, *Lancet*, p. 1293, June 13, 1981

203. Levander, OA, *Federation Proceedings*, vol. 36, no. 5, p. 1683, Apr. 1977; see also Glauser, SC, et al., *Lancet i*, p. 717, 1976

204. Hooper, PL, et al., *International Journal for Vitamin and Nutrition Research*, vol. 53, p. 412, 1983

205. *Journal of American Medical Association*, vol. 231, p. 360, Jan. 27, 1975

206. McGregor, L., et al., *Atherosclerosis*, vol. 38, p. 129, 1980

207. Kane, JP, et al., *New England Journal of Medicine*, vol. 304, p. 251, 1981

208. Grundy, SM, et al., *Journal of Lipid Research*, vol. 88, p. 53, 1978

209. *Lancet*, p. 1299, June 13, 1981

210. Olson, RE, *Vitamins and Hormones*, vol. 40, p. 1, 1983

211. *Resident and Staff Physician*, vol. 29, p. 102, 1983

212. Folkers, K., et al., *Journal of Molecular Medicine*, vol. 2, p. 431, 1977

213. Yamagami, T., et al., *Research Communications in Chemical Pathology and Pharmacology*, vol. 14, p. 721, 1976

214. Angelucci, L., et al., *Nature*, vol. 181, p. 911, 1958

215. McCarty, M., *Medical Hypothesis*, vol. 7, p. 515, 1981

216. Rastopchin, IP, *Zhurnal Nevropatologii I Psikhiatrii Imeni S.S. Korsakova*, vol. 84, no. 7, p. 1020, 1984

217. Nagorna-Stasiak, B., et al., *Polskie Archiwum Weterynaryjne*, vol. 23, no. 4, p. 63, 1983

218. Sullivan, W., *Australian and New Zealand Journal of Medicine*, vol. 3, p. 417, 1973

219. Bailey, B., in *Recent Developments in Cardiac Muscle Pharmacology*, Shibata, H. et al., (eds), Igaku-Shoin, Tokyo, 1982

220. McCarty, M., *Medical Hypothesis*, vol. 7, p. 515, 1981

221. Nakazawa, K., et al., *Journal of International Medical Research*, vol. 6, no. 3, p. 217, 1978

222. *Lancet ii*, p. 1283, Dec. 7, 1985

223. Kark, JD, et al., *British Medical Journal*, vol. 291, p. 699, Sept. 14, 1985

224. Williams, PT, et al., *Journal of American Medical Association*, vol. 253, p. 1407, Mar. 8, 1985

225. Knapp, JA, et al., *American Journal of Epidemiology*, vol. 22, p. 1, July 1985

226. Rosenberg, L., et al., *American Journal of Epidemiology*, vol. 111, p. 675, 1980

227. Carroll, KK, *Federation Proceedings*, vol. 41, p. 2792, Sept. 1982

228. Rouse, IL, et al., *Lancet*, p. 5, Jan. 1, 1983

229. Sved, AF, et al., *Proceedings of National Academy of Sciences*, vol. 76, p. 3511, 1979

230. Tanaka, O., et al., *Fortschritte Der Chemie Organischer Naturstoffe*, vol. 46, p. 1, 1984: see also Quiroga, H., *Orientacion Medica*, vol. 31, no. 1281, p. 201, 1982

231. Young, CM, et al., *Journal of the American Dietetic Association*, vol. 59, p. 473, Nov. 1971; see also Fabry, P., et al., *American Journal of Clinical Nutrition*, vol. 23, no. 8, p. 1059, Aug. 1970

CHAPTER 6

1. Bailar, JC, et al., *New England Journal of Medicine*, vol. 314, p. 1226, May 8, 1986

2. U.S. Bureau of the Census, *Statistical Abstract of the United States: 1985*, 105th edition, p. 74, Washington, DC, 1984

3. Lourau, J. et al., *Experientia*, vol. 6, p. 25, 1950

4. Spector, L., et al., *Proceedings of the Society for Experimental Biology and Medicine*, vol. 100, p. 405, 1959

5. Walford, R., *Maximum Life Span*, WW Norton, New York, 1983

6. Ames, B., *Science*, vol. 221, p. 1256, 1983

7. National Research Council, *Diet, Nutrition and Cancer*, p. 13-20. National Academy Press, Washington, DC, 1982

8. Blair, A., et al., *Journal of the National Cancer Institute*, vol. 78, no. 1, p. 191, Jan. 1987

9. Brody, J., *Jane Brody's Nutrition Book*, p. 227, WW Norton, New York, 1983

10. Sandler, DP, et al., *Lancet*, p. 312, Feb. 9, 1985

11. *Lancet*, p. 133, July 20, 1985

12. Locke, S., et al., *Foundations of Psychoneuroimmunology*, Aldine Publishers, New York, 1985

13. Yoneyama, T., et al., *Japanese Journal of Cancer Research*, vol. 77, p. 625, July 1986

14. Maugh, TH, *Science*, vol. 217, p. 36, July 1982

15. Sugimura, T., *Science*, vol. 233, p. 312, July 1986

16. Ames, BN, *Science*, vol. 221, p. 1256, Sept. 1983

17. Willett, WC, et al., *New England Journal of Medicine*, vol. 310, p. 633, Mar. 8-15, 1984

18. Watson, RR, et al., *Journal of the American Dietetic Association*, vol. 86, p. 505, Apr. 1986

19. Lawrence, W., *Cancer*, vol. 43, p. 2020, 1979

20. Orr, J., et al., *Gynecologic Oncology*, vol. 17, p. 257, 1984

21. Clark, LC, et al., *Journal of Nutrition*, vol. 116, p. 170, 1986

22. Schrauzer, GN, *Vitamins, Nutrition, and Cancer*, p. 240, 1984

23. Salonen, J., et al., *British Medical Journal*, vol. 290, p. 417, 1985
24. Schrauzer, GN, et al., *Japanese Journal of Cancer Research*, vol. 76, p. 374, May 1985
25. Wald, NJ, et al., *British Journal of Cancer*, vol. 49, p. 321, 1984
26. Stahelin, HB, et al., *Journal of the National Cancer Institute*, vol. 73, p. 1463, Dec. 1984
27. Burton, GW, et al., *Lancet*, p. 327, Aug. 7, 1982
28. Sparnins, VL, et al., *Journal of the National Cancer Institute*, vol. 66, p. 769, 1981
29. Masukawa, T., et al., *Biochemical Pharmacology*, vol. 33, no. 16, p. 2635, 1984
30. Combs, GF, et al., *BioScience*, vol. 27, no. 7, p. 467, 1977
31. Schrauzer, GN, et al., *Bioinorganic Chemistry*, vol. 7, p. 23, 1977
32. McConnell, KP, et al., *Journal of Surgical Oncology*, vol. 18, p. 67, 1980
33. Willett, JC, et al., *Lancet*, p. 130, 1983
34. Salonen, JT, et al., *American Journal of Epidemiology*, vol. 120, p. 342, 1984
35. Wagner, DA, et al., *Cancer Research*, vol. 45, p. 6519, Dec. 1985
36. Trickler, D., et al., *Journal of the National Cancer Institute*, vol. 78, p. 165, Jan. 1987
37. van Rensburg, SJ, et al., *Nutrition and Cancer*, vol. 8, p. 163, 1986
38. McCarty, MF, *Medical Hypotheses*, vol. 14, p. 213, 1984
39. Salonen, JT, et al., *British Medical Journal*, vol. 290, p. 417, Feb. 1985
40. Van Vleet, JF, et al., *American Journal of Veterinary Research*, vol. 39, p. 997, 1978
41. Prasad, KN, et al., *Proceedings of the Society for Experimental Biology and Medicine*, vol. 164, p. 158, 1980
42. Ip, C., *Cancer Research*, vol. 41, p. 4386, 1981
43. Lawson, T., et al., *Chemico-Biological Interactions*, vol. 45, p. 95, 1983
44. Milner, JA, et al., *Cancer Research*, vol. 41, p. 1652, 1981
45. Watrach, AM, et al., *Cancer Letters*, vol. 25, p. 41, 1984
46. Spallholz, JE, *Advances in Experimental Medicine and Biology*, vol. 135, p. 43, 1981
47. *Journal of American Medical Association*, vol. 244, no. 10, p. 1077, Sept. 5, 1980
48. London, R., et al., *Cancer Research*, vol. 41, p. 3811, 1981
49. Horvath, P., et al., *Cancer Research*, vol. 43, p. 5335, 1983
50. Palmer, J., et al., *Journal of the American Dietetic Association*, vol. 82, p. 511, 1983
51. Levander, OA, et al., *American Journal of Clinical Nutrition*, vol. 34, p. 2662, Dec. 1981
52. Levander, OA, et al., *American Journal of Clinical Nutrition*, vol. 39, p. 809, May 1984
53. Clark, LC, et al., *Journal of Nutrition*, vol. 116, p. 170, Jan. 1986
54. Yang, G., et al., *American Journal of Clinical Nutrition*, vol. 37, p. 872, 1983
55. *Nutrition Reviews*, vol. 34, p. 347, 1976
56. Yang, G., et al., *American Journal of Clinical Nutrition*, vol. 37, p. 872, May 1983
57. Kumpulainen, J., et al., *American Journal of Clinical Nutrition*, vol. 42, p. 829, Nov. 1985
58. Luo, X., et al., *American Journal of Clinical Nutrition*, vol. 42, p. 439, Sept. 1985
59. Mason, AC, et al., *Journal of Nutrition*, vol. 116, p. 1883, 1986
60. Palmer, IS, et al., *Journal of Food Science*, vol. 47, p. 1595, 1982
61. Burkitt, L., *Lancet*, p. 1229, 1969
62. Graf, E., et al., *Cancer*, vol. 56, p. 717, Aug 1985
63. Kromhout, D., et al., *Lancet*, p. 518, Sept. 4, 1982
64. *Science*, vol. 221, p. 1256, 1983
65. National Research Council, *Diet, Nutrition, and Cancer*, National Academy Press, Washington, DC, 1982, *passim*.
66. Ershoff, B., *American Journal of Clinical Nutrition*, vol. 27, p. 1395, 1974
67. Howie, BJ, et al., *American Journal of Clinical Nutrition*, vol. 42, p. 127, July 1985
68. Zile, MH, et al., *Proceedings of the Society for Experimental Biology and Medicine*, vol. 172, p. 139, 1983
69. Peto, R., et al., *Nature*, vol. 290, p. 201, Mar. 1981

70. Skekelle, RB, et al., *Lancet*, p. 1185, 1981
71. Samet, JM, et al., *American Review of Respiratory Disease*, vol. 131, p. 198, 1985
72. Ziegler, RG, et al., *Journal of the National Cancer Institute*, vol. 73, p. 1429, Dec. 1984
73. La Vecchia, CL, et al., *International Journal of Cancer*, vol. 34, p. 319, 1984
74. Orr, JW, et al., *American Journal of Obstetrics and Gynecology*, vol. 151, p. 632, Mar. 1985
75. Stehr, PA, et al., *American Journal of Epidemiology*, vol. 121, p. 65, Jan. 1985
76. Stich, HF, et al., *Lancet*, p. 1204, 1984
77. Basu, TK, et al., *European Journal of Cancer and Clinical Oncology*, vol. 18, p. 339, 1982
78. Kark, JD, et al., *Journal of the National Cancer Institute*, vol. 66, p. 7, Jan. 1981
79. Mahmoud, LA, et al., *International Journal of Cancer*, vol. 30, p. 143, 1982
80. Stahelin, HB, et al., *Journal of the National Cancer Institute*, vol. 73, p. 1463, Dec. 1984
81. Modan, B., et al., *International Journal of Cancer*, vol. 28, p. 421, 1981
82. Magnus, K., (ed.), *Trends in Cancer Incidence*, Hemisphere Publishing Corp., Washington, DC, 1982
83. Peto, R., *Cancer Surveys*, vol. 2, p. 327, 1983
84. Micksche, M., et al., *Oncology*, vol. 34, p. 234, 1977
85. Bollag, W., et al., *Acta Dermato-Venereologica*, vol. 55, supp. 74, p. 163, 1975
86. Gunby, P., *Journal of the American Medical Association*, vol. 247, p. 1799, Apr. 2, 1982
87. *Nutrition Reviews*, vol. 43, p. 240, Aug. 1985
88. *Lancet*, p. 28, July 3, 1982
89. Goodman, DS, *New England Journal of Medicine*, vol. 310, p. 1023, Apr. 1984
90. Vakil, DV, et al., *Nutrition Research*, vol. 5, p. 911, 1985
91. Ragavan, VV, et al., *American Journal of the Medical Sciences*, vol. 283, p. 161, May 1982
92. Wald, NJ, et al., *Cancer Letters*, vol. 29, p. 203, 1985
93. Bieri, J., et al., *American Journal of Clinical Nutrition*, vol. 34, p. 289, Feb. 1981
94. Dahl, H., et al., *Acta Pathologica Microbiologica Scandinavia*, vol. 84, p. 280, 1976
95. Wagner, DA, et al., *Cancer Research*, vol. 45, p. 6519, Dec. 1985
96. Wassertheil-Smoller, B., et al., *American Journal of Epidemiology*, vol. 114, p. 714, 1981
97. Orr, JW, et al., *American Journal of Obstetrics and Gynecology*, vol. 151, p. 632, Mar. 1985
98. Kolonel, LN, et al., *American Journal of Clinical Nutrition*, vol. 34, p. 2478, 1981
99. Stahelin, HB, et al., *Journal of the National Cancer Institute*, vol. 73, p. 1463, Dec. 1984
100. *Nutrition Reviews*, vol. 43, p. 146, May 1985
101. Cameron, E., et al., *Proceedings of the National Academy of Sciences*, vol. 75, p. 4538, Sept. 1978
102. *Nutrition Reviews*, vol. 44, p. 28, Jan. 1986
103. Anthony, HM, et al., *British Journal of Cancer*, vol. 46, p. 354, 1982
104. Yung, S., et al., *Journal of Pharmaceutical Sciences*, vol. 71, p. 282, Mar. 1982
105. Molnar, J., et al., *Neoplasma*, vol. 28, p. 11, 1981
106. Carroll, KK, *Cancer Research*, vol. 35, p. 3374, 1975
107. Willett, WC, et al., *New England Journal of Medicine*, vol. 310, p. 633, Mar. 8–15, 1984
108. Bristol, JB, et al., *British Medical Journal*, vol. 291, p. 1467, Nov. 23, 1985
109. Snowdon, DA, *Journal of the American Medical Association*, vol. 254, p. 356, July, 1985
110. Rose, DP, et al., *Journal of the American Medical Association*, vol. 254, p. 2553, Nov. 1985
111. Shirley, RL, et al., *Journal of the American Medical Association*, vol. 225, p. 259, Jan. 1986

112. National Academy of Sciences, *Diet, Nutrition, and Cancer*, p. 13-20, National Academy Press, Washington, DC, 1982

113. Lam, CW, et al., *Archives of Toxicology*, vol. 58, p. 67, 1985

114. Armstrong, B., et al., *International Journal of Cancer*, vol. 15, p. 617, 1975

115. Lubin, F., et al., *American Journal of Epidemiology*, vol. 122, p. 579, Oct. 1985

116. Bird, RP, et al., *Nutrition and Cancer*, vol. 8, p. 93, 1986

117. Tisdale, MJ, *Experimental Cell Biology*, vol. 51, p. 250, 1983

118. Karmali, RA, et al., *Journal of the National Cancer Institute*, vol. 73, no. 2, p. 457, Aug. 1984

119. van der Merwe, CF, *South African Medical Journal*, vol. 65, p. 712, May 1984

120. Garland, C., et al., *Lancet*, p. 307, Feb. 9, 1985

121. Lipkin, M., et al., *New England Journal of Medicine*, vol. 313, p. 1381, Nov. 1985

122. Lin, HJ, et al., *Nutrition Reports International*, vol. 15, p. 635, 1977

123. Davies, IJ, et al., *Journal of Clinical Pathology*, vol. 21, p. 363, 1968

124. Habib, FK, *Journal of Steroid Chemistry*, vol. 9, p. 403, 1978

125. Duncan, JR, et al., *Journal of the National Cancer Institute*, vol. 55, p. 195, 1975

126. van Rensburg, SJ, *Journal of the National Cancer Institute*, vol. 67, p. 243, Aug. 1981

127. *Journal of Parenteral and Enteral Nutrition*, vol. 4, p. 561, 1980

128. Schrauzer, G., et al., *Bioinorganic Chemistry*, vol. 7, p. 23, 1977

129. Yang, CS, *Cancer Research*, vol. 40, p. 2633, 1980

130. Ames, BN, et al., *Proceedings of the National Academy of Sciences*, vol. 78, p. 6858, 1981

131. Luo, X., et al., *Federation Proceedings*, vol. 46, p. 928, 1981

132. Thompson, H., et al., *Carcinogenesis*, vol. 5, p. 849, 1984

133. Fields, M., et al., *Nutrition Reports International*, vol. 34, no. 6, p. 1071, Dec. 1986

134. Kensler, RA, et al., *Science*, vol. 221, p. 75, 1983

135. Oberley, LW, et al., *Cancer Research*, vol. 39, p. 1141, 1979

136. Webber, MM, *Nutrition Research*, vol. 6, p. 35, 1986

137. Boing, H., et al., *Nutrition and Cancer*, vol. 7, p. 121, 1985

138. Nader, CJ, et al., *Nutrition Reports International*, vol. 23, p. 113, Jan. 1981

139. van der Westhuyzen, J., *Nutrition and Cancer*, vol. 7, p. 179, 1985

140. Edes, RS, et al., *Proceedings of the Society for Experimental Biology and Medicine*, vol. 162, p. 71, 1979

141. Oeriu, S., et al., *Journal of Gerontology*, vol. 20, p. 417, 1965

142. Tas, E., et al., *Mechanisms of Ageing and Development*, vol. 12, p. 65, 1980

143. Milner, JA, et al., *Journal of Nutrition*, vol. 109, p. 489, 1979

144. Tayek, J., et al., *Clinical Research*, vol. 33, p. 72A, 1985

145. Pollack, ES, et al., *New England Journal of Medicine*, vol. 310, p. 617, Mar. 1984

146. Minton, J., et al., *Nutrition Action*, vol. 135, no. 1, p. 157, 1979

147. Rosenberg, L., et al., *American Journal of Epidemiology*, vol. 122, p. 391, Sept. 1985

148. Ishihara, S., *Journal of Vitaminology*, vol. 15, p. 305, 1969

149. Butterworth, CE, et al., *American Journal of Clinical Nutrition*, vol. 35, p. 73, Jan. 1982

150. Rivlin, RS, *Cancer Research*, vol. 33, p. 1977, 1973

151. Disorbo, RL, et al., *Nutrition and Cancer*, vol. 5, p. 10, 1983

152. De Simone, C., et al., *Nutrition Reports International*, vol. 33, p. 419, Mar. 1986

153. *Nutrition Reviews*, vol. 42, p. 374, Nov. 1984

154. Lourau, R., et al., *Experientia*, vol. 6, p. 25, 1950

155. Spector, H., et al., *Proceedings of the Society for Experimental Biology and Medicine*, vol. 100, p. 405, 1959

156. Hamilton, EM, et al., *Nutrition: Concepts and Controversies*, p. 452, West Publishing, St. Paul, MN, 1985

157. Lathia, D., et al., *Nutrition and Cancer*, vol. 1, no. 2, p. 19, 1979

158. Lai, L., et al., *Nutrition and Cancer*, vol. 1, p. 27, 1978

159. Colkitz, GA, et al., *American Journal of Clinical Nutrition*, vol. 41, p. 32, Jan. 1985

160. Yamamoto, I., et al., *Cancer Letters*, vol. 26, p. 241, Apr. 1985
161. Lau, BH, et al., *Nutrition Research*, vol. 3, p. 119, 1983
162. McCarty, MF, *Medical Hypotheses*, vol. 7, p. 591, 1981
163. Weaver, RG, et al., *Second Annual Research Convocation Exhibit Synopses*, no. 20, Portland, Nov. 1983
164. Tanaka, O., et al., *Fortschritte der Chemie Organischer Naturstoffe*, vol. 46, p. 1, 1984
165. Moertel, CG, et al., *New England Journal of Medicine*, vol. 306, p. 201, Jan. 1982
166. Frank, B., *Nucleic Acid and Anti-Oxidant Therapy of Aging and Degeneration*, Rainstone Publishing, New York, 1977
167. Odens, RR, *Journal of the American Geriatrics Society*, vol. 21, p. 450, 1973
168. Rigby, PG, *Cancer Research*, vol. 31, p. 4., Jan. 1971
169. Lacoue, L., et al., *Lancet*, p. 161, July 26, 1980
170. Michelson, RA, et al., *Superoxide and Superoxide Dismutases*, p. 496, Academic Press, New York, 1977
171. Lam, LK, et al., *Cancer Research*, vol. 42, p. 1193, Apr. 1982
172. Gold, E., et al., *Cancer*, vol. 55, p. 460, 1985
173. Bristol, JB, et al., *British Medical Journal*, vol. 291, p. 1467, Nov. 1985
174. Ames, BN, *Science*, vol. 221, p. 1256, 1983
175. Oterdoom, HJ, *Lancet*, p. 330, Aug. 3, 1985
176. Wayne, IG, et al., *Science*, vol. 213, p. 909, 1981
177. Linsell, CA, *Carcinogenic Risks: Strategies for Intervention*, Davis, C., et al., (eds.), Lyon Publisher, World Health Organization, International Agency for Research on Cancer, 1974

CHAPTER 7

1. Locke, S., et al., (eds.), *Foundations of Psychoneuroimmunology*, Aldine Publishers, New York, 1985, *passim*.
2. Ishigami, T., *American Review of Tuberculosis*, vol. 2, p. 470, 1918
3. *Lancet*, p. 133, July 20, 1985
4. Chandra, S., et al., *Progress in Food and Nutrition Science*, vol. 10, p. 1, 1986
5. Puri, S., et al., *Pediatric Clinics of North America*. vol. 32, p. 499, Apr. 1985
6. *Nutrition Reviews*, vol.43, p. 305, Oct. 1985
7. Chandra, RK, et al., *British Medical Journal*, vol. 291, p. 705, Sept. 1985
8. Butterworth, CE, *Nutrition Today*, p. 4, Mar. 1974
9. Jensen, JE, et al., *Journal of Bone and Joint Surgery*, vol. 64A, p. 1263, Dec. 1982
10. *Lancet*, p. 1491, June 29, 1985
11. Bienia, R., et al., *Journal of the American Geriatrics Society*, vol. 30, p. 433, July 1982
12. Smale, BF, et al., *Cancer*, vol. 47, p. 2375, May 1981
13. Wright, RA, et al., *Nutritional Assessment, passim.*, Blackwell, Boston, 1984
14. Carruthers, R., *Drugs*, vol. 6, p. 164, 1973; see also Pories, WJ, et al., Lancet, vol. i, p. 1069, 1969
15. *Nutrition Reviews*, vol. 40, p. 72, Mar. 1982
16. Moser, PB, et al., *Nutrition Research*, vol. 5, p. 253, 1985
17. Chandra, RK, *Journal of the American Medical Association*, vol. 252, p. 1443, Sept. 1984
18. Duchateau, J., et al., *American Journal of Medicine*, vol. 70, p. 1001, May, 1981
19. Pories, WJ, et al., *Annals of Surgery*, vol. 165, no. 3, p. 432, 1967
20. Frommer, JA, *Medical Journal of Australia*, vol. 2, p. 793, 1975
21. Eby, GA, et al., *Antimicrobial Agents and Chemotherapy*, vol. 25, p. 20, 1984
22. Bjorksten, B., et al., *Acta Paediatrica Scandinavica*, vol. 69, p. 183, 1980
23. Hoogenraad, T., et al., *Lancet*, vol. ii, p. 1262, 1978
24. Weiner, RG, *Journal of the American Medical Association*, vol. 252, p. 1409, Sept. 1984
25. Jain, VK, et al., *Nutrition Research*, vol. 4, p. 537, 1984
26. Moseson, M., *Nutrition Research*, vol. 6, p. 729, 1986

27. Moore, JA, et al., *Clinical Chemistry*, vol. 30, no. 7, p. 1171, 1984
28. Spallholz, JE, *Advances in Experimental Medical Biology*, vol. 135, p. 43, 1981
29. Greeder, GA, et al., *Science*, vol. 209, p. 825, 1980
30. Desowitz, R., *Infection and Immunity*, vol. 27, p. 87, 1980
31. *Physiological Reviews*, vol. 60, p. 188, 1980
32. Malkovsky, M., et al., *Proceedings of the National Academy of Sciences*, vol. 80, p. 6322, 1983
33. Gerber, LE, et al., *Journal of Nutrition*, vol. 112, p. 1555, 1982
34. Hunt, TK, *American Journal of Surgery*, vol. 125, p. 12, 1973
35. Seifter, E., et al., *Annals of Surgery*, vol. 194, no. 1, p. 42, July 1981
36. Chernov, MS, et al., *Journal of Trauma*, vol. 12, p. 831, 1972
37. Patty, I., et al., *Lancet*, vol. ii, p. 876, 1982
38. Barton, GM, et al., *International Journal of Vitamin and Nutrition Research*, vol. 42, p. 524, 1972
39. Ringsdorf, WM, et al., *Oral Surgery*, vol. 53, p. 231, Mar. 1982
40. Schorah, CJ, et al., *American Journal of Clinical Nutrition*, vol. 34, p. 871, May 1981
41. Taylor, TV, et al., *Lancet*, vol. ii, p. 544, 1974
42. Afifi, AM, et al, *British Journal of Dermatology*, vol. 92, p. 339, 1975
43. Spittle, C., *Lancet*, vol. ii, p. 199, 1973
44. Fraser, RC, et al., *American Journal of Clinical Nutrition*, vol. 33, p. 839, 1980
45. Anderson, R., et al., *American Journal of Clinical Nutrition*, vol. 33, p. 71, 1980
46. Anderson, TW, *Nutrition Today*, vol. 12, p. 6, 1977; see also Pauling, L., *Medical Tribune*, p. 18, Mar. 24, 1976
47. Carr, AB, et al., *Acta Geneticae Medicae et Gemellologiae*, vol. 30, p. 249, 1981
48. Terezhalmy, GT, et al., *Oral Surgery*, vol. 45, p. 56, 1978
49. Cathcart, RF, *Medical Hypotheses*, vol. 7, p. 1359, 1981
50. Kuodell, RG, et al., *American Journal of Clinical Nutrition*, vol. 34, p. 20, 1981
51. Banic, S., et al., *International Journal of Vitamin and Nutrition Research*, supplement, vol. 19, p. 41, 1979
52. Banic, S., *Nature*, vol. 258, p. 153, 1975
53. Kennes, B., et al., *Gerontology*, vol. 29, p. 305, 1983
54. Cathcart, RF, *Medical Hypotheses*, vol. 14, p. 423, 1984
55. Jones, E., et al., *IRCS Medical Science*, vol. 12, p. 320, 1984
56. Shub, T., et al., *Antiobiotiki*, vol. 26, p. 268, 1981
57. Miller, D., et al., *Proceedings of the National Academy of Sciences*, vol. 78, p. 3605, 1981
58. Cheraskin, E., *Journal of the American Medical Association*, vol. 254, p. 2894, Nov. 1985
59. Chandra, RK, et al., *Nutrition Research*, vol. 2, p. 223, 1982
60. Walsh, DE, et al., *Journal of Antimicrobial Chemotherapy*, vol. 12, p. 489, 1983
61. Tsen, CC, et al., *Journal of Food Science*, vol. 42, p. 1370, 1977
62. Meydani, M., et al., *Drug-Nutrient Interactions*, vol. 2, p. 217, 1984
63. Barbul, A., et al., *Surgery*, vol. 90, p. 244, 1981
64. Barbul, A., et al., *Surgery Forum*, vol. 28, p. 101, 1977
65. Visek, WJ, *Journal of Nutrition*, vol. 116, p. 36, Jan. 1986
66. Barbul, A., et al., *Federation Proceedings*, vol. 37, p. 264, Apr. 1978
67. Gaull, GE, *Journal of the American College of Nutrition*, vol. 5, p. 121, 1986
68. *Journal of Clinical Nutrition*, vol. 35, p. 442, 1982
69. Prohaska, JR, et al., *Science*, vol. 213, p. 559, 1981
70. Newberne, PM, et al., *British Journal of Experimental Pathology*, vol. 51, no. 3, p. 229, 1970
71. Soskel, NT, et al., *American Review of Respiratory Disease*, vol. 126, p. 316, 1982
72. Nockels, CF, *Federation Proceedings*, vol. 38, p. 2134, 1979
73. Prasad, JS, *American Journal of Clinical Nutrition*, vol. 33, p. 606, 1980
74. Machtey, I., et al., *Journal of the American Geriatrics Society*, vol. 26, p. 328, 1978
75. Baker, J., *Plastic and Reconstructive Surgery*, vol. 68, no. 5, p. 696, Nov. 1981
76. Lundin, E., et al., *Plastic and Reconstructive Surgery*, vol. 69, p. 1029, June 1982

77. Saperstein, H., et al., *Archives of Dermatology*, vol. 120, p. 906, July 1984
78. Kanofsky, JD, et al., *New England Journal of Medicine*, p. 173, July 16, 1981
79. *American Journal of Clinical Nutrition*, vol. 35, p. 418, supp. , Feb. 1982
80. Talbot, MC, et al., *American Journal of Clinical Nutrition*, vol. 46, p. 659, Oct. 1982; see also Casciato, D., et al., *Nephron*, vol. 38, no. 1, p. 9, Sept. 1984
81. Barton-Wright, L., et al., *Martindale-The Extra Pharmacopeia*, p. 1752, The Pharmaceutical Press, London, 1982
82. Aprahamian, M., et al., *American Journal of Clinical Nutrition*, vol. 41, p. 578, Mar. 1985
83. Nardi, GL, et al., *Surgical Gynecology and Obstetrics*, vol. 112, p. 526, 1961
84. Ralli, EP, et al., *Vitamins and Hormones*, vol. 11, p. 133, 1953
85. Kathman, JV, et al., *Nutrition Research*, vol. 4, p. 245, 1984
86. Walsh, J., et al., *Annals of Nutrition and Metabolism*, vol. 25, p. 178, 1981
87. Barlow, GB, et al., *Clinica Chimica Acta*, vol. 29, p. 355, 1970
88. Vogel, R., *Journal of Oral Medicine*, vol. 33, p. 20, 1978
89. Elmer, G., *Nurse Practitioner*, p. 40, Sept. 1981
90. Dutta, P., et al., *Lancet*, p. 1040, Nov.9, 1985
91. Bordier, P., et al., *Journal of Clinical Endocrinology*, vol. 46, p. 284, Feb. 1978
92. Bliznakov, E., *Mechanisms of Aging and Development*, vol. 7, p. 189, 1978
93. Wilkinson, E., et al., *Research Communications in Chemical Pathology and Pharmacology*, vol. 12, p. 111, 1975
94. Simon, LN, et al., *Cancer Treatment Reports*, vol. 62, p. 1963, 1978
95. Bohles, H., et al., *Journal of Parenteral and Enteral Nutrition*, vol. 8, p. 9, 1983
96. *Journal of the American Medical Association*, vol. 248, p. 1369, Sept. 1982
97. Gregori, B., et al., *Acta Bio-Medica de L., Ateneo Parmense*, vol. 56, p. 23, 1985
98. Ngumbi, PM, et al., *East African Medical Journal*, vol. 61, p. 372, May 1984
99. Foxman, B., et al., *American Journal of Public Health*, vol. 75, p. 1314, Nov. 1985
100. Lau, BH, et al., *Nutrition Research*, vol. 3, p. 119, 1983
101. Tanaka, O., et al., *Fortschritte der Chemie Organischer Naaturstoffe*, vol. 46, p. 1, 1984
102. Sinai, Y., et al, *Infection and Immunology*, vol. 9, p. 781, May 1974
103. Prickett, JD, et al., *Immunology*, vol. 46, p. 819, 1982
104. Hamilton, D., *Bulletin of the History of Medicine*, vol. 56, p. 30, 1980

CHAPTER 8

1. Forman, MB, et al., *New England Journal of Medicine*, vol. 313, no. 18, p. 1138, Oct. 1985
2. Dobersen, MJ, et al., *New England Journal of Medicine*, vol. 303, no. 26, p. 1493, Dec. 1980
3. Stefanini, GF, et al., *Lancet*, vol. i, p. 207, Jan.25, 1986
4. Darlington, LG, et al., *Lancet*, vol. i, p. 236, Feb.1, 1986
5. Cant, AJ, *Human Nutrition: Applied Nutrition*, vol. 39A, p. 277, Aug. 1985
6. Gunderson, CH, *American Family Physician*, vol. 33, p. 137, Jan. 1986
7. Stefanini, GF., et al., *op.cit.*
8. Darlington, LG, et al., *op.cit.*
9. Winter, R., *Food Additives*, p. 4, Crown Books, New York, 1984
10. Willett, W., et al., *New England Journal of Medicine*, vol. 310, p. 633, Mar. 1984
11. Breneman, J., *Basics of Food Allergy*, CC Thomas, Springfield, IL 1984, *passim.*
12. Fontana, VJ, et al., in *Modern Nutrition in Health and Disease*, p. 924, Goodhard, RS, et al., (eds.), Lea & Febiger, Philadelphia, 1976
13. Taylor, B., et al., *Lancet*, vol. ii, p. 1255, 1984
14. Rudin, DO, *Biological Psychiatry*, vol. 16, p. 489, 1981
15. Nasr, S., et al., *Journal of Affective Disorders*, vol. 3, p. 291, 1981
16. Jakobsson, I., et al., *Pediatrics*, vol. 71, p. 268, 1983
17. Chandra, RK, *Acta Paediatrica Scandinavica*, vol. 68, p. 691, 1979
18. Cant, A., *Human Nutrition: Applied Nutrition*, vol. 38A, p. 455, Dec. 1984
19. Crayton, JW, *Food Technology*, p. 153, Jan. 1986

20. Ayres, S., et al., *Cutis*, vol. 21, p. 321, Mar,1978
21. Crayton, JW, *op.cit.*
22. Bennett, J., et al., *Drug Research*, vol. 31, p. 433, 1981
23. Strasser, T., et al., *Proceedings of the National Academy of Sciences*, vol. 82, p. 1540, Mar. 1985
24. Lee, TH, et al., *Clinical Allergy*, vol. 16, p. 89, 1986
25. *Veterinarian Medicine and Small Animal Clinician*, vol. 61, p. 986, 1966
26. Long, P., et al., *Nutrition: An Inquiry into the Issues*, p. 389, Prentice-Hall, Englewood Cliffs, NJ, 1983
27. Truswell, AW, *British Medical Journal*, vol. 291, p. 951, Oct. 1985
28 Ershoff, BH, *Journal of Food Science*, vol. 41, p. 949, 1976
29. Koepke, J., et al., *Annals of Allergy*, vol. 54, no. 3, p. 213, Mar. 1985
30. Folkers, K., et al., *Hoppe-Seylers Zeitschrift Fur Physiologische Chemie*, vol. 365, p. 405, Mar. 1984
31. Wurtman, RJ, *Lancet*, p. 1060, Nov. 9, 1985
32. Bodey, G., et al., *Candidiasis*, Raven Press, New York, 1985, *passim.*
33. *Lancet*, p. 662, Mar. 20, 1982; see also Egger, J., et al., *Lancet*, p. 540, Mar. 9, 1985
34. Bolsen, B., *Journal of the American Medical Association*, vol. 247, p. 948, Feb. 1982
35. Swain, A., et al., *Lancet*, p. 41, July 6, 1985
36. Swain, A., et al., *op.cit.*
37. Ross, DM, et al., *Hyperactivity*, p. 3, John Wiley & Sons, New York, 1982

CHAPTER 9

1. Hayflick, L., *Federation Proceedings*, vol. 38, p. 1847, 1979
2. Guthrie, H., *Introductory Nutrition*, 5th ed., p. 506, CV Mosby, St. Louis, MO, 1983
3. Ross Laboratories, *Aging and Nutrition*, Ross Laboratories, 1979, *passim.*
4. Schneider, EL, et al., *New England Journal of Medicine*, vol. 312, p. 1159, May 2, 1985
5. Sempos, CT, et al., *Journal of the American Dietetic Association*, vol. 81, p. 35, July 1982
6. Horrobin, DF, *Behavioral and Brain Sciences*, vol. 5, p. 217, June 1982
7. Hendler, S., *The Complete Guide to Anti-aging Nutrients*, p. 23, Simon & Schuster, New York, 1985
8. Fisher, S., et al., *American Journal of Clinical Nutrition*, vol. 31, p. 667, 1978
9. Geissler, C., et al., *American Journal of Clinical Nutrition*, vol. 39, p. 478, Mar. 1984
10. Walford, R., *Maximum Life Span*, WW Norton, New York, 1983
11. Winick, M., *Modern Medicine*, p. 69, Feb. 15, 1978
12. Bortz, WM, *Journal of the American Medical Association*, vol. 248, no. 10, p. 1203, Sept. 10, 1982
13. Neldner, KH, *Geriatrics*, vol. 39, p. 69, Feb. 1984
14. Brin, H., *Postgraduate Medicine*, vol. 63, no. 3, p. 155, Mar. 1978
15. Garry, P., et al., *American Journal of Clinical Nutrition*, vol. 36, p. 319, Aug. 1982
16. Sempos, C., et al., *Journal of the American Medical Association*, vol. 81, p. 35, July 1982
17. Norton, L., et al., *Journal of Gerontology*, vol. 39, p. 592, 1984
18. Exton-Smith, A., *Proceedings of the Royal Society of Medicine*, vol. 70, p. 615, 1977
19. Reuler, JB, et al., *Journal of the American Medical Association*, vol. 253, p. 805, Feb. 8, 1985
20. Cheraskin, E., *Journal of the American Medical Association*, vol. 254, p. 2894, Nov. 1985
21. Addis, GM, et al., *Medical Laboratory Sciences*, vol. 42, p. 90, 1985
22. Walsh, J., et al., *Annals of Nutrition and Metabolism*, vol. 25, p. 178, 1981
23. Hutton, C., et al., *Journal of the American Dietetic Association*, vol. 82, p. 148, Feb. 1983
24. Lee, C., et al., *Annals of Clinical and Laboratory Science*, vol. 14, p. 151, 1984
25. Addis, GM, et al., *Medical Laboratory Sciences*, vol. 42, p. 90, 1985

26. Hofmann, L., (ed.), *The Great American Nutrition Hassle*, p. 89, Mayfield Publishers, Palo Alto, CA, 1978

27. Henkin, J., *Annals of Internal Medicine*, vol. 99, p. 227, 1983

28. Fanelli, MT, et al., *Journal of the American Dietetic Association*, vol. 85, p. 1570, Dec. 1985

29. Schneider, EL, et al., *New England Journal of Medicine*, vol. 314, p. 157, Jan. 16, 1986

30. Munro, HN, *Hospital Practice*, p. 143, Aug. 1982

31. Lee, CM, et al., *American Journal of Clinical Nutrition*, vol. 42, p. 226, Aug. 1985

32. Guilland, J., et al., *International Journal of Vitamin and Nutrition Research*, vol. 54, p. 185, 1984

33. Elmer, G., *Nurse Practitioner*, p. 40, Nov. 1981

34. Deacon, R., et al., *Scandinavian Journal of Haematology*, vol. 28, no. 4, p. 289, 1982

35. Samson, D., et al., *British Journal of Haematology*, vol. 35, p. 217, Feb. 1977

36. Kobrosielski-Vergona, K., *Age*, vol. 10, p. 11, 1987

37. Lazarov, J., *Experimental Gerontology*, vol. 12, p. 75, 1977

38. McIntosh, E., *American Journal of Public Health*, vol. 72, p. 1412, Dec. 1982

39. McKenna, M., et al., *Irish Medical Journal*, vol. 74, no. 11, p. 336, Nov. 1981

40. Weisman, Y., et al., *Israel Journal of Medical Science*, vol. 17, p. 19, Jan. 1981

41. Bass, L., *American Journal of Nursing*, p. 254, Feb. 1977

42. Gersovitz, M., et al., *American Journal of Clinical Nutrition*, vol. 35, p. 6, Jan. 1982

43. O'Hanlon, P., et al., *American Journal of Clinical Nutrition*, vol. 31, p. 1257, July 1978

44. Maiani, G., et al., *Annals of Human Biology*, vol. 11, p. 476, 1984

45. Wechsler, H., et al., *New England Journal of Medicine*, vol. 308, p. 97, Jan. 13, 1983

46. *Lancet*, p. 423, Feb. 22, 1986

47. Hancock, MR, et al., *British Journal of Psychiatry*, vol. 147, p. 404, 1985

48. Newton, HM, et al., *American Journal of Clinical Nutrition*, vol. 42, p. 656, Oct. 1985

49. Ratfy, AK, et al., *IRCS Medical Science*, vol. 14, p. 815, 1986

50. Cerklewski, FL, et al., *Journal of Nutrition*, vol. 116, p. 618, 1986

51. Burns, A., et al., *Lancet*, p. 805, Apr. 5, 1986

52. Meydani, M., et al., *Nutrition Research*, vol. 5, p. 1227, 1985

53. Weder, B., et al., *Neurology*, vol. 34, p. 1561, Dec. 1984

54. Roach, ES, et al., *American Family Physician*, vol. 25, p. 111, Jan. 1982

55. Blundell, EL, et al., *Journal of Clinical Pathology*, vol. 38, p. 1179, 1985

56. Craig, GM, *op. cit.* et al., *British Journal of Nutrition*, vol. 54, p. 613, 1985

57. Goggans, FC, *American Journal of Psychiatry*, vol. 141, p. 300, Feb. 1984

58. Older, MWJ, et al., *Age and Aging*, vol. 11, p. 101, 1982

59. Chandra, RK, et al., *Nutrition Research*, vol. 2, p. 223, 1982

60. Chandra, RK, et al., *British Medical Journal*, vol. 291, p. 705, Sept. 1985

61. Paterson, PG, et al., *Journal of the American Dietetic Association*, vol. 85, p. 186, Feb. 1985

62. Duchateau, J., et al., *American Journal of Medicine*, vol. 70, p. 1001, 1981

63. Haboubi, NY, et al., *Journal of Clinical Pathology*, vol. 38, p. 1189, 1985

64. Schorah, CH, et al., *American Journal of Clinical Nutrition*, vol. 34, p. 871, May 1981

65. Schorah, CJ, et al., *Lancet*, p. 403, Feb. 24, 1979

66. Kennes, B., et al., *Gerontology*, vol. 29, p. 305, 1983

67. Aprahamian, M., et al., *American Journal of Clinical Nutrition*, vol. 41, p. 578, 1985; see also *Practitioner*, vol. 224, p. 208, 1980

68. Walsh, JH, et al., *Annals of Nutrition and Metabolism*, vol. 25, p. 178, 1981; see also Bhat, KS, *Nutrition Reports International*, vol. 36, no. 3, p. 685, Sept. 1987

69. Shalka, HW, et al., *American Journal of Clinical Nutrition*, vol. 34, p. 861, May 1981

70. Elmer, G., *Nurse Practitioner*, p. 40, Sept. 1981

71. Varma, S., et al., *Photochemistry and Photobiology*, vol. 36, no. 6, p. 623, Dec. 1982

72. Weindruch, R., et al., *Journal of Nutrition*, vol. 116, p. 641, 1986

73. Firbas, JH, *Age*, vol. 9, p. 25, 1986

74. Schneider, EL, et al., *New England Journal of Medicine*, vol. 312, no. 18, p. 1159, May 1985

75. Wartanowicz, M., et al., *Annals of Nutrition and Metabolism*, vol. 28, p. 186, 1984

76. Vatassery, G., et al., *Journal of the American College of Nutrition*, vol. 2, no. 4, p. 369, 1983

77. Dauber, J., et al., *Survey on Synthesis of Pathology Research*, vol. 3, no. 1, p. 83, 1984

78. McCarty, MF, *Medical Hypotheses*, vol. 13, p. 77, 1984

79. Tappel, A., et al., *Journal of Gerontology*, vol. 28, no. 4, p. 415, Oct. 1973

80. Weitzman, B., *Immunology*, vol. 128, p. 2770, 1982

81. Mahmud, SA, et al., *Hamdard*, vol. 27, p. 166, Jan. 1984

82. Szent-Gyorgyi, A., *New York Academy of Science*, vol. 61, p. 732, 1955

83. Havsteen, B., *Biochemical Pharmacology*, vol. 32, p. 1141, 1983

84. Jones, E., et al., *IRCS Medical Science*, vol. 12, p. 320, 1984

85. Kastenbaum, R., *Journal of Nutrition for the Elderly*, vol. 4, p. 15, Spring 1985

86. Barboriak, JJ, et al., *Journal of the American Dietetic Association*, vol. 72, p. 493, May 1978

87. Tanaka, O., et al., *Fortschritte Der Chemie Organischer Naturstoffe*, vol. 46, p. 1, 1984

88. Hayes, KC, *Nutrition Reviews*, vol. 43, no. 3, p. 65, Mar. 1985

89. Pasantes-Morales, H., et al., *Journal of Neuroscience Research*, vol. 11, p. 303, 1984

90. Huxtable, R., et al., *Progress in Clinical Biological Research*, vol. 125, p. 5, 1983

CHAPTER 10

1. Brown, R., case study presented at a medical conference at the University of Virginia Medical School, Sept. 1986

2. Seaker, M., *East West Journal*, vol. 12, p. 26, July 1982

3. The Surgeon General, *Healthy People: The Surgeon General's Report on Health Promotion and Disease Prevention*, DHEW, p. 68, pub. #79-55071 and 79-55071A, Washington, DC, 1979

4. Ross, DM, et al., *Hyperactivity*, p. 3, John Wiley & Sons, New York, 1982

5. Schauss, A., *Diet, Crime, and Delinquency*, p. vi, Parker House, Berkeley, CA, 1981

6. Franklin, J., *Molecules of the Mind*, Athenium Press, 1986

7. *Nutrition and Mental Health: Hearings Before the Select Committee on Nutrition and Human Needs of the United States Senate*, p. 70, Parker House, Berkeley, CA, 1980

8. Taylor, CB, et al., *Public Health Reports*, vol. 100, no. 2, p. 195, Apr. 1985

9. Schauss, A., *op.cit.*, *passim*.

10. Bolton, R., *Ethnology*, vol. 12, p. 227, July 1973

11. Freedland, RA, et al., *A Biochemical Approach to Nutrition*, John Wiley & Sons, New York, 1977, *passim*.

12. Hale, F., *Biological Psychiatry*, vol. 17, p. 125, 1982

13. Nelson, RL, *Mayo Clinic Proceedings*, vol. 60, p. 844, Dec. 1985

14. The United States Senate Select Committee on Nutrition and Human Needs, *Nutrition and Mental Health*, p. 70, Parker House, Berkeley, CA, 1980

15. Piziak, VK, *Medical Times*, vol. 114, p. 119, June 1986

16. Pollitt, E., et al., *American Journal of Clinical Nutrition*, vol. 42, p. 348, Aug. 1985

17. Lester, ML, et al., *Nutrition and Behavior*, vol. 1, p. 3, 1982

18. Fields, M., et al., *Nutrition Reports International*, vol. 34, no. 6, p. 1071, Dec. 1986

19. Salway, R., et al., *Lancet*, p. 1282, 1978

20. Clements, CA, et al., *American Journal of Clinical Nutrition*, vol. 33, p. 1954, 1980

21. Borum, PR, et al., *Journal of the American College of Nutrition*, vol. 5, p. 177, 1986

22. Sato, Y., et al., *International Journal of Sports Medicine*, vol. 7, p. 307, 1986

23. Grobin, D., *Journal of the American Geriatric Society*, vol. 23, p. 31, Jan. 1975

24. Anderson, RA, et al., *American Journal of Clinical Nutrition*, vol. 36, p. 1184, Dec. 1982

25. Anderson, RA, et al., *Federation Proceedings*, vol. 43, p. 471, 1984

26. Older, MW, et al., *Age and Ageing*, vol. 11, p. 101, 1982

27. Botez, MI, et al., *Journal of Neurology and Neurosurgical Psychiatry*, vol. 45, p. 731, Aug. 1982

28. Plaitakis, A., et al., *Neurology*, vol. 28, p. 691, July 1978

29. Walsh, J., et al., *Annals of Nutrition and Metabolism*, vol. 25, p. 178, 1981

30. Kathman, J., et al., *Nutrition Research*, vol. 4, p. 245, 1984

31. Vir, SC, et al., *International Journal of Vitamin and Nutrition Research*, vol. 47, p. 336, 1977

32. Buzina, R., et al., *International Journal of Vitamin and Nutrition Research*, vol. 49, p. 136, 1979

33. Galler, J., (ed.) *Nutrition and Behavior*, Plenum Press, New York, 1984, *passim.*

34. Leibel, RL, *Journal of the American Dietetic Association*, vol. 71, p. 398, Oct. 1977

35. Oski, FA, et al., *Journal of Pediatrics*, vol. 92, p. 21, 1978

36. Oski, FA, *Pediatric Clinics of North America*, vol. 32, p. 493, Apr. 1985

37. Oski, FA, et al., *Pediatrics*, vol. 71, p. 877, June 1983

38. Voors, AW, et al., *Public Health Reports*, vol. 96, p. 45, Jan. 1981

39. Pastides, H., *Yale Journal of Biology and Medicine*, vol. 54, p. 265, 1981

40. Seoane, NA, et al., *Journal of the Canadian Dietetic Association*, vol. 46, p. 298, Nov. 1985

41. Nickerson, HJ, et al., *American Journal of Diseases of Children*, vol. 139, p. 1115, Nov. 1985

42. Handing, A., et al., *Acta Medica Scandinavica*, vol. 209, p. 315, 1981

43. Brune, M., et al., *American Journal of Clinical Nutrition*, vol,43, p. 438, Mar. 1986

44. Horwitt, MK, et al., *American Journal of Clinical Nutrition*, vol. 12, p. 99, Feb. 1963

45. Soemantri, AG, et al., *American Journal of Clinical Nutrition*, vol. 42, p. 1221, Dec. 1985

46. Pollitt, E., et al., *American Journal of Clincial Nutrition*, vol. 43, p. 555, Apr. 1986

47. Natta, C., et al., *American Journal of Clinical Nutrition*, vol. 33, p. 968, 1980; see also Giardini, O., et al., *New England Journal of Medicine*, vol. 305, p. 644, 1981

48. Ono, K., *Nephron*, vol. 40, p. 440, 1985

49. Hodges, RE, et al., *American Journal of Clinical Nutrition*, vol. 31, p. 876, May 1978

50. Majia, L., et al., *American Journal of Clinical Nutrition*, vol. 30, p. 1175, July 1977

51. Seshadri, S., et al., *Human Nutrition: Applied Nutrition*, vol. 39A, p. 151, Apr. 1985

52. *American Journal of Obstetrics and Gynecology*, vol. 83, p. 1269, 1962

53. Beutler, R., *Modern Nutrition in Health and Disease*, p. 324, Lea & Febiger, Philadelphia, 1980

54. Nadiger, HA, et al., *British Journal of Nutrition*, vol. 43, p. 45, 1980

55. Samson, D., et al., *British Journal of Haematology*, vol. 35, p. 217, Feb. 1977

56. Breskin, MW, et al., *Journal of the American Dietetic Association*, vol. 85, p. 49, Jan. 1985

57. *Nutrition Reviews*, vol. 43, p. 220, July 1985

58. Rhew, TH, et al., *Journal of Nutrition*, vol. 116, p. 2263, 1986

59. Daeschner, CW, et al., *Journal of Pediatrics*, vol. 98, p. 778, May 1981

60. Frizzell, RT, et al., *Journal of the American Medical Association*, vol. 255, p. 772, Feb. 1986

61. Kott, E., et al., *European Neurology*, vol. 24, p. 221, 1985

62. Beard, TC, et al., *Lancet*, p. 455, Aug. 1982

63. Fonseca, V., et al., *British Medical Journal*, vol. 291, p. 1680, Dec. 1985

64. Altura, BM, *Magnesium*, vol. 4, no. 4, p. 169, 1985

65. Johnson, ES, et al., *British Medical Journal*, vol. 291, p. 569, Aug. 1985

66. Massey, LK, et al., *Nutrition Research*, vol. 5, p. 1281, 1985

67. Lenhert, H., et al., *Brain Research*, vol. 303, p. 215, 1984

68. Gelenberg, AJ, et al., *American Journal of Psychiatry*, vol. 137, p. 622, 1980

69. *Advances in Neurology*, vol. 5, p. 235, 1974

70. Pfeiffer, C., *Zinc and Other Micro-nutrients*, Keats, New Canaan, CT, 1978

71. Kunin, RA, *Mega-Nutrition*, New American Library, New York, 1981,

72. Budd, K., in *Advances in Pain Research and Therapy*, Bonica, J., et al., (eds), p. 305, Raven Press, New York, 1983

73. *Pain*, vol. 8, p. 231, 1980
74. Sandyk, R., et al., *New England Journal of Medicine*, vol. 314, p. 1257, May 1986
75. Yogman, MW, et al., *American Journal of Clinical Nutrition*, vol. 42, p. 352, Aug. 1985
76. Fitten, LJ, et al., *Journal of the American Geriatric Society*, vol. 33, p. 294, Apr. 1985
77. Hartmann, E., et al., *Journal of Nervous and Mental Disorders*, vol. 167, p. 497, 1979
78. Seltzer, S., et al., *Pain*, vol. 13, p. 385, 1982
79. Leiberman, HR, et al., *American Journal of Clinical Nutrition*, vol. 42, p. 366, Aug. 1985
80. Thomson, J., et al., *Psychological Medicine*, vol. 12, p. 741, 1982
81. Cho-chung, YS, et al., *European Journal of Biochemistry*, vol. 3, p. 401, 1968
82. Mohler, H., et al., *Nature*, p. 563, Apr. 1979
83. Driskell, JA, et al., *Journal of the American Dietetic Association*, vol. 85, p. 46, Jan. 1985
84. Adams, P., et al., *Lancet*, p. 897, Apr. 1973
85. Tkacz, C., et al., *Journal of Orthomolecular Psychiatry*, vol. 10, p. 119, 1981
86. Ellis, J., et al., *Research Communications in Chemical Pathology and Pharmacology*, vol. 33, p. 331, Aug. 1981
87. Driskell, JA, et al., *Nutrition Reports International*, vol. 34, no. 6, p. 1031, Dec. 1986
88. Folkers, K., et al., *Hoppe-Seylers Zeitschrift Fur Physiologische Chemie*, vol. 365, p. 405, Mar. 1984
89. Martineau, J., et al., *Biological Psychiatry*, vol. 20, p. 467, 1985
90. Bartus, R., et al., *Science*, vol. 209, p. 301, 1980
91. Peters, B., et al., *Annals of Neurology*, vol. 6, p. 219, Sept. 1979
92. Signoret, J., et al., *Lancet*, p. 837, Oct.14, 1978
93. Gelenberg, A., et al., *American Journal of Psychiatry*, vol. 136, p. 772, June 1979
94. Wood, J., et. al., *Federation Proceedings*, vol. 41, p. 3015, Dec. 1982
95. Wurtman, RJ, *Scientific American*, p. 50, Apr. 1982
96. Kastenbaum, R., *Journal of Nutrition for the Elderly*, vol. 4, p. 15, Spring, 1985
97. Wong, PT, *Annals of the Academy of Medicine, Singapore*, vol. 14, p. 147, Jan1985
98. Williams, RJ, *Nutrition Against Disease*, p. 164, Bantam Books, New York, 1971
99. Pauling, L., *Science*, p. 265, Apr. 19, 1968
100. Newton, HM, et al., *American Journal of clinical Nutrition*, vol. 42, p. 656, Oct. 1985
101. Snyder, SH, *Scientific American*, vol. 236, p. 44, Mar. 1977
102. Bhathena, SJ, et al., *American Journal of Clinical Nutrition*, vol. 43, p. 42, Jan. 1986
103. Waller, DA, et al., *American Journal of Clinical Nutrition*, vol. 44, p. 20, July 1986
104. Jonas, JM, et al., *Lancet*, p. 390, Feb.1, 1986
105. Hayes, KC, *Nutrition Reviews*, vol. 43, p. 65, Mar. 1985
106. Durelli, L., et al., *Clinical Neuropharmacology*, vol. 6, p. 37, Mar. 1983
107. Barbeau, A., et al., *Life Sciences*, vol. 17, p. 669, Sept 1975
108. *Journal of the American Medical Association*, vol. 248, p. 1369, Sept. 1982
109. Rudolph, R., et al., *Chronic Problem Wounds*, Little, Brown, and co., Boston, 1983
110. Paintz, M., et al., *Pharmazie*, vol. 34, p. 839, 1979
111. Sasajima, M., et al., *Folia Pharmacologica Japonica*, vol. 74, p. 897, 1978
112. Hippchen, LF, (ed.), *Ecologic-Biochemical Approaches to Treatment of Delinquents and Criminals*, p. 6, Van Nostrand Reinhold, New York, 1978
113. Goodman, RA, et al., *American Journal of Public Health*, vol. 76, p. 144, Feb. 1986
114. Gunderson, CH, *American Family Physician*, vol. 33, p. 137, Jan. 1986
115. Jones, RJ, et al., *Lancet*, p. 720, Oct.3, 1981
116. Rudin, DO, *Biological Psychiatry*, vol. 16, p. 837, 1981
117. Lieberman, HR, et al., *Food Technology*, vol. 40, p. 139, Jan. 1986
118. Cant, AJ, *Human Nutrition: Applied Nutrition*, vol. 39A, p. 277, Aug. 1985
119. Rabinowitz, M., *Lancet*, p. 63, Jan.1, 1983

120. Nelson, H., *Los Angeles Times*, part 1, p. 3. Apr.23, 1987
121. Roberts, HJ, *New England Journal of Medicine*, vol. 304, p. 423, Feb. 1981
122. Wheater, RH, *Journal of the American Medical Association*, vol. 253, p. 2288, Apr. 1985
123. Wurtman, RJ, *Lancet*, p. 1060, Nov. 1985
124. *Journal of the American Medical Association*, vol. 254, p. 400, July 1985
125. Lindebaum, J., et al., *Nature*, vol. 224, p. 806, Nov. 1969
126. Martinez, FA, et al., *Journal of Neurological Science*, vol. 48, p. 315, Dec. 1980
127. Baker, H., et al., *Journal of the American Geriatric Society*, vol. 26, p. 218, 1978
128. Botez, MI, et al., in *Folic Acid in Neurology, Psychiatry, and Internal Medicine*, p. 401, Raven Press, New York, 1979
129. *New Scientist*, p. 619, June 1981
130. Wells, TE, et al., *American Journal of Medical Genetics*, vol. 23, p. 291, 1986
131. Harrell, RF, et al., *Proceedings of the National Academy of Sciences*, vol. 78, p. 574, Jan. 1981
132. Sandstead, HH, *American Journal of Clinical Nutrition*, vol. 43, p. 293, Feb. 1986
133. O'Sullivan, H., *Australian and New Zealand Journal of Medicine*, vol. 3, p. 417, 1973
134. Pauling, L., *Science*, vol. 160, p. 265, Apr. 1968
135. Choudhry, M., et al., *Indian Journal of Nutrition and Dietetics*, vol. 21, p. 1, Jan. 1984
136. Kehoe, AB, et al., *American Anthropologist*, vol. 83, p. 549, 1981

CHAPTER 11

1. Robinson, CH, *Fundamentals of Normal Nutrition*, p. 286, MacMillan, New York, 1978
2. Barrett, DE, et al., *American Journal of Clinical Nutrition*, vol. 42, p. 102, July 1985
3. McLester, JS, *Handbook of Nutrition*, American Medical Association, UOL 14S, no. 16, 1951
4. Sandstead, HH, *American Journal of Clinical Nutrition*, vol. 43, p. 293, Feb. 1986
5. Connolly, KJ, et al., *Lancet*, p. 1149, Dec. 1979
6. Ziporyn, T., *Journal of the American Medical Association*, vol. 253, p. 1846, Apr. 1985
7. Vobecky, JS, et al., *International Journal for Vitamin and Nutrition Research*, vol. 55, p. 205, 1985
8. Listernick, R., et al., *American Journal of Diseases of Children*, vol. 139, p. 1157, Nov. 1985
9. Crawford, JD, *New England Journal of Medicine*, vol. 305, p. 163, July 1981
10. Hunt, IF, et al., *American Journal of Clinical Nutrition*, vol. 40, p. 508, Sept. 1984
11. Kadam, SS, et al., *Indian Journal of Nutrition and Dietetics*, vol. 21, p. 69, Feb. 1984
12. Habibzadeh, N., et al., *British Journal of Nutrition*, vol. 55, p. 23, 1986
13. Guthrie, HA, *Introductory Nutrition*, p. 417, CV Mosby, St. Louis, 1983
14. Leader, A., et al., *Canadian Medical Association Journal*, vol. 125, p. 545, Sept. 1981
15. Dorner, G., et al., *Experimental Clinical Endocrinology*, vol. 84, p. 129, 1984
16. Choudhry, M., et al., *Indian Journal of Nutrition and Dietetics*, vol. 21, p. 1, Jan. 1984
17. Dostalova, L., *Developmental Pharmacology and Therapeutics*, vol. 4, sup. 1, p. 45, 1982
18. Baker, H., et al., *American Journal of Clinical Nutrition*, vol. 28, p. 56, Jan. 1975
19. Sayetta, RB, *American Family Physician*, vol. 33, p. 181, May 1986
20. Guthrie, H., *Introductory Nutrition*, 5th ed., ch.16, CV Mosby, St. Louis, 1983
21. Zamenhof, S., et al., *Biology of the Neonate*, vol. 32, p. 205, 1977
22. *Science*, vol. 160, p. 322, 1968
23. Korhs, MB, et al., *American Journal of Clinical Nutrition*, vol. 32, p. 1206, 1979
24. Rosso, P., *American Journal of Clinical Nutrition*, vol. 41, p. 644, Mar. 1985
25. Drunin, JV, et al., *Lancet*, p. 823, Oct.12, 1985

26. Michael, HN, et al., *British Medical Bulletin*, vol. 37, p. 31, 1981
27. Meadows, NJ, et al., *Lancet*, p. 1135, Nov.21, 1981
28. Park, JH, et al., *Journal of Nutrition*, vol. 116, p. 610, 1986
29. Mukherjee, MD, et al., *American Journal of Clinical Nutrition*, vol. 40, p. 496, Sept. 1984
30. Eckhert, CD, et al., *Journal of Nutrition*, vol. 107, p. 855, 1977
31. Cherry, FF, et al., *American Journal of Clinical Nutrition*, vol. 34, p. 2367, Nov. 1981
32. Hunt, IF, et al., *American Journal of Clinical Nutrition*, vol. 40, p. 508, Sept. 1984
33. Mutch, PB, et al., *Journal of Nutrition*, vol. 104, p. 828, 1974
34. Meiners, CR, et al., *American Journal of Clinical Nutrition*, vol. 30, p. 879, 1977
35. Collipp, PJ, et al., *Annals of Nutrition and Metabolism*, vol. 26, p. 287, 1982
36. Hambridge, KM, et al., *American Journal of Clinical Nutrition*, vol. 29, p. 734, 1976
37. Butrimovitz, GP, et al., *American Journal of Clinical Nutrition*, vol. 31, p. 1409, 1978
38. Milne, DB, et al., *American Journal of Clinical Nutrition*, vol. 39, p. 535, 1984
39. Breskin, MW, et al., *American Journal of Clinical Nutrition*, vol. 38, p. 943, Dec. 1983
40. Mukherjee, MD, et al., *op.cit.*
41. Krebs, NF, et al., *American Journal of Clinical Nutrition*, vol. 41, p. 560, Mar. 1985
42. Halmesmaki, E., et al., *British Medical Journal*, vol. 291, p. 1470, Nov. 1985
43. *Nutrition Reviews*, vol. 40, p. 43, Feb. 1982
44. Yip, R., et al., *American Journal of Clinical Nutrition*, vol. 42, p. 683, Oct. 1985
45. Taper, LJ, et al., *American Journal of Clinical Nutrition*, vol. 41, p. 1184, June 1985
46. Courtney Moore, ME, et al., *Journal of Pediatrics*, vol. 105, p. 600, Oct. 1984
47. Crouse, SF, et al., *Journal of the American Medical Association*, vol. 252, p. 785, Aug. 1983
48. Gipoulox, JD, et al., *Roux's Archives of Developmental Biology*, vol. 195, p. 193, 1986
49. Breskin, M., et al., *American Journal of Clinical Nutrition*, vol. 38, p. 943, Dec. 1983
50. Sandstead, HH, *Nutrition Reviews*, vol. 43, p. 129, May 1985
51. Welsh, SO, et al., *Food Technology*, p. 70, Jan. 1982
52. Moser, PB, et al., *Journal of the American Dietetic Association*, vol. 84, p. 42, Jan. 1984
53. *Nutrition Reviews*, vol. 44, p. 181, May 1986
54. Goodman, LS, et al., *The Pharmacological Basis of Therapeutics*, p. 1344, MacMillan, New York, 1977
55. Surgeon General, *Healthy People*, p. 26, U.S. Department of Health, Education, and Welfare, Washington, DC, 1979
56. Smithells, RW, *Pediatrics*, vol. 69, p. 498, Apr. 1982
57. Rhoads, GG, et al., *American Journal of Epidemiology*, vol. 120, p. 803, Dec. 1984
58. Laurence, KM, *Pediatrics*, vol. 70, p. 648, Oct. 1982
59. Tchernia, G., et al., *Developmental Pharmacology and Therapeutics 4*, sup. 1, p. 58, 1982
60. *Lancet*, p. 1412, Dec.18, 1982
61. Smithells, RW, et al., *Lancet*, p. 339, Feb. 1980
62. Laurence, KM, et al., *British Medical Journal*, vol. 282, p. 1509, May 1981
63. *Nature*, vol. 299, p. 198, Sept. 1982; vol. 300, p. 102, Nov. 1982; vol. 300, p. 302, Nov. 1982
64. *Lancet*, p. 1308, June 1984
65. Rhoads, GG, et al., *op.cit.*
66. Deacon, R., et al., *Scandinavian Journal of Haematology*, vol. 28, p. 289, Apr. 1982
67. Tolarova, M., *Lancet*, p. 217, July 1982
68. Blot, I., et al., *Gynecology and Obstetrics Investigations*, vol. 12, p. 294, 1981
69. Bates, CJ, et al., *Human Nutrition: Clinical Nutrition*, vol. 40C, p. 3, 1986
70. Colman, N., et al., *American Journal of Clinical Nutrition*, vol. 27, p. 339, Apr. 1974
71. Borschel, MW, et al., *American Journal of Clinical Nutrition*, vol. 43, p. 7, Jan. 1986

72. Reynolds, R., et al., *Journal of the American Dietetic Association*, vol. 84, p. 1339, 1984

73. Styslinger, L., et al., *American Journal of Clinical Nutrition*, vol. 41, p. 21, Jan. 1985

74. Borschel, MW, et al., *American Journal of Clinical Nutrition*, vol. 43, p. 7, Jan. 1986

75. Atkins, JN, *American Reviews of Respiratory Disease*, vol. 126, p. 714, 1982

76. *British Medical Journal*, vol. 2, p. 13, 1975

77. Garry, PJ (ed.), *Human Nutrition: Clinical and Biochemical Aspects*, p. 219, American Association for Clinical Chemistry, Washington, DC, 1981

78. Temesvari, P., et al., *Acta Pediatrica Scandinavica*, vol. 72, p. 525, 1983

79. Reinken, L., et al., *International Journal of Vitamin and Nutrition Research*, vol. 48, p. 341, 1978

80. Bhagavan, HN, *International Journal of Vitamin Research*, vol. 39, p. 235, 1969

81. Wighton, MC, et al., *Medical Journal of Australia*, vol. 14, p. 1, July 1979

82. *Lancet*, p. 682, Mar. 1983

83. Jones, KI, et al., *Lancet*, p. 999, Nov. 1973

84. Little, RE, et al., *American Journal of Epidemiology*, vol. 123, p. 270, 1986

85. Weiner, L., et al., *Clinical Nutrition*, vol. 4, p. 10, Feb. 1985

86. Lecos, C., *FDA Consumer*, p. 6, Oct. 1980

87. Brody, J., *Jane Brody's Nutrition Book*, p. 241, WW Norton, New York, 1981

88. Linn, S., et al., *New England Journal of Medicine*, vol. 306, p. 141, 1982

89. Hughes, RN, et al., *Life Sciences*, vol. 38, p. 861, 1986

90. Villar, J., et al., *International Journal of Gynecology and Obstetrics*, vol. 21, p. 271, 1983

91. Belizan, J., et al., *American Journal of Clinical Nutrition*, vol. 33, p. 2202, 1980

92. Belizan, J., et al., *American Journal of Obstetrics and Gynecology*, vol. 146, p. 175, 1983

93. Altura, BM, et al., *Science*, vol. 221, p. 376, July 1983

94. Elliot, J., *American Journal of Obstetrics and Gynecology*, vol. 147, p. 277, Oct. 1983

95. Oski, FA, *Pediatric Clinics of North America*, vol. 32, p. 493, Apr. 1985

96. Oski, FA, et al., *Pediatrics*, vol. 71, p. 877, June 1983

97. Walter, J., et al., *Journal of Pediatrics*, vol. 102, p. 519, 1983

98. Wallenberg, HC, et al., *Journal of Perinatal Medicine*, vol. 12, p. 7, 1984

99. Oski, FA, *op.cit.*

100. Connolly, KJ, et al., *op.cit.*

101. Yan-You, W., et al., *Lancet*, p. 518, Sept. 1985

102. Ziporyn, T., *op.cit.*

103. Bruhn, JC, et al., *Journal of Food Protection*, vol. 48, p. 397, May 1985

104. Kumpulainen, J., et al., *American Journal of Clinical Nutrition*, vol. 42, p. 829, Nov. 1985

105. Cockburn, F., et al., *British Medical Journal*, p. 11, July 5, 1980

106. Greer, FR, et al., *Journal of Pediatrics*, vol. 98, p. 696, May 1981

107. Curtis, JA, et al., *Canadian Medical Association Journal*, vol. 128, p. 150, Jan. 1983

108. Elidrissy, AT, et al., *Calcified Tissue International*, vol. 36, p. 266, 1984

109. Haworth, JC, et al., *Canadian Medical Association Journal*, vol. 134, p. 237, Feb. 1986

110. Goodman, DS, *New England Journal of Medicine*, vol. 310, p. 1023, Apr. 1984

111. Hustead, VA, et al., *Journal of Pediatrics*, vol. 105, p. 610, 1984

112. Hutchings, DE, et al., *Developmental Psychobiology*, vol. 7, p. 225, 1974

113. Lennep, EV, et al., *Prenatal Diagnosis*, vol. 5, p. 35, 1985

114. Stirling, HF, et al., *Lancet*, p. 1089, May 1986

115. Schearer, MJ, et al., *Lancet*, p. 460, Aug. 1982

116. Dunn, PM, *Lancet*, p. 770, Oct. 1982

117. Merkel, R., *American Journal of Obstetrics and Gynecology*, p. 416, Aug. 1952

118. Salmenpera, L., *American Journal of Clinical Nutrition*, vol. 40, p. 150, Nov. 1984

119. *Nutrition Reviews*, vol. 29, p. 260, 1971

120. Ongari, MA, et al., *American Journal of Obstetrics and Gynecology*, vol. 149, p. 455, 1984

121. Kornfeld, J., *Medical News*, p. 14, Apr.28, 1980

122. Harris, WS, et al., *American Journal of Clinical Nutrition*, vol. 40, p. 780, Oct. 1984

123. O'Brien, PM, et al., in *Clinical Uses of Essential Fatty Acids*, p. 163, Eden Press, Montreal, 1982

124. Lewis, P., *British Journal of Hospital Medicine*, p. 393, Oct. 1982

125. Stumpf, DA, et al., *Neurology*, vol. 35, p. 1041, July 1985

126. Hahn, P., et al., *Federation Proceedings*, vol. 44, p. 2369, Apr. 1985

127. Borum, PR, et al., *Journal of the American College of Nutrition*, vol. 5, p. 177, 1986

128. Hittner, HM, et al., *New England Journal of Medicine*, vol. 305, p. 1365, Dec. 1981

129. Speer, ME, et al., *Pediatrics*, vol. 74, p. 1107, Dec. 1984

130. Bell, EF, et al., *Pediatrics*, vol. 63, p. 830, 1979

131. Jagadeesan, V., et al., *Nutrition Reports International*, vol. 23, p. 135, Jan. 1981

132. Shiono, PH, et al., *Journal of the American Medical Association*, vol. 255, p. 82, Jan. 1986

133. Sexton, M., et al., *Journal of the American Medical Association*, vol. 251, p. 911, Feb. 1984

134. Istoel, WJ, et al., *British Heart Journal*, vol. 48, p. 493, 1982

135. Ericson, A., et al., *American Journal of Obstetrics and Gynecology*, vol. 135, p. 348, 1979

136. Linn, S., et al., *New England Journal of Medicine*, vol. 306, p. 141, Jan. 1982

137. Caster, WO, et al., *International Journal for Vitamin and Nutrition Research*, vol. 54, p. 371, 1984

138. Brown, JE, et al., *American Journal of Clinical Nutrition*, vol. 43, p. 414, Mar. 1986

139. Eisa, OA, et al., *British Journal of Nutrition*, vol. 54, p. 593, 1985

140. Habicht, JP, et al., *American Journal of Epidemiology*, vol. 123, p. 279, Feb. 1986

141. Schneider, MH, et al., in *Contemporary Developments in Nutrition*, p. 481, CV Mosby, St. Louis, MO, 1980

142. Barness, L., in *Nutritional Support of Medical Practice*, Schneider, H., et al., (eds.), p. 441, Harper & Row, Hagerstown, MD, 1977

143. Forman, MR, et al., *American Journal of Clinical Nutrition*, vol. 42, p. 864, Nov. 1985

144. Whitehead, R., *Lancet*, p. 167, Jan. 1983

145. Huang, L., et al., *Nutrition Research*, vol. 4, p. 977, 1984

146. *Nutrition Reviews*, vol. 41, p. 80, Mar. 1983

147. Nelson, GH, et al., *Journal of the American Medical Association*, vol. 253, p. 1880, Apr. 1985

148. Monti, JC, et al., *Experientia*, vol. 42, p. 39. 1986

149. Kintzel, H., et al., *Acta Pediatrica Scandinavica*, vol. 60, p. 1, 1971

150. Freundlich, M., et al., *Lancet*, p. 527, Sept. 1985

151. Zeisel, SH, et al., *Journal of Nutrition*, vol. 116, p. 50, Jan. 1986

152. Hayes, KC, *Nutrition Reviews*, vol. 43, p. 65, Mar. 1985

153. Gaull, GE, *Journal of the American College of Nutrition*, vol. 5, p. 121, 1985

154. Ahn, CH, et al., *American Journal of Clinical Nutrition*, vol. 33, p. 183, Feb. 1980

155. Sims, LS, *Journal of the American Dietetic Association*, vol. 73, p. 139, Aug. 1978

156. Borschel, MW, et al., *American Journal of Clinical Nutrition*, vol. 43, p. 7, Jan. 1986

157. Ronnholm, KA, *American Journal of Clinical Nutrition*, vol. 43, p. 1, Jan. 1986

158. Varra, MV, et al., *American Journal of Clinical Nutrition*, vol. 43, p. 495, Apr. 1986

159. Sneed, SM, et al., *American Journal of Clinical Nutrition*, vol. 34, p. 1338, July 1981

160. Cant, AJ, *Human Nutrition: Applied Nutrition*, vol. 39A, p. 277, Aug. 1985

161. Marx, CM, et al., *American Journal of Obstetrics and Gynecology*, vol. 152, p. 668, July 1985

CHAPTER 12

1. Virag, R., et al., *Lancet*, p. 183, Jan.26, 1985
2. Antoniou, LD, et al., *Lancet*, p. 895, Oct.29, 1977
3. Sudesh, K., et al., *Annals of Internal Medicine*, vol. 97, p. 357, 1982
4. *Nutrition Today*, Mar. 1981
5. Hartoma, G., et al., *Lancet*, vol. 2, p. 1125, 1977
6. Wanger, PA, et al., *Human Nutrition: Clinical Nutrition*, vol. 39C, p. 459, Nov. 1985
7. Schachter, A., et al., *Journal of Urology*, vol. 110, p. 311, Sept. 1973
8. *Medical News*, vol. 249, no. 20, p. 2747, May 27, 1983
9. Kohengkull, S., et al., *Fertility and Sterility*, vol. 23, p. 1333, 1977
10. Kabir, M., et al., *Food and Nutrition Bulletin*, vol. 6, p. 40, Sept. 1984
11. Kemmann, E., et al., *Journal of the American Medical Association*, vol. 249, p. 926, Feb. 1983
12. Seymour, L., et al., *American Journal of Obstetrics and Gynecology*, p. 890, Dec. 1981
13. Abraham, GE, et al., *Infertility*, vol. 2, p. 315, 1980
14. Stage, S., *Female Complaints: Lydia Pinkham and the Business of Women's Medicine*, WW Norton, New York, 1979
15. Labrum, AH, *Journal of Reproductive Medicine*, vol. 28, no. 7, p. 438, July 1983
16. Cowan, LD, et al., *American Journal of Epidemiology*, vol. 114, p. 209, 1981
17. Reid, R., et al., *Clinical Obstetrics and Gynecology*, vol. 26, no. 3, p. 710, Sept. 1983
18. Hargrove, JT, et al., *Journal of Reproductive Medicine*, vol. 28, p. 435, July 1983
19. Rossignol, AM, *American Journal of Public Health*, vol. 75, p. 1335, Nov. 1985
20. Minton, JP, et al., *Surgery*, vol. 86, p. 105, 1979
21. London, RS, et al., *Journal of the American College of Nutrition*, vol. 3, p. 351, 1984
22. London, RS, et al., *Journal of the American College of Nutrition*, vol. 3, p. 351, 1984
23. Abraham, GE, et al., *Infertility*, vol. 3, p. 155, 1980
24. Snider, BL, et al., *Archives of Dermatology*, vol. 110, p. 130, 1974
25. Schaumberg, H., et al., *New England Journal of Medicine*, vol. 309, p. 445, 1983
26. Morton, JH, et al., *American Journal of Obstetrics and Gynecology*, vol. 65, p. 1182, 1953
27. Dennefors, BL, et al., *Journal of Clinical Endocrinology and Metabolism*, vol. 55, p. 102, 1982
28. Hill, PB, et al., *American Journal of Clinical Nutrition*, vol. 43, p. 37, Jan. 1986
29. Horrobin, DH, *Journal of Reproductive Medicine*, vol. 28, p. 465, July 1983
30. Frankel, TL, et al., *British Journal of Nutrition*, vol. 39, p. 227, 1978
31. Oelkers, W., et al., *Journal of Clinical Endocrinology and Metabolism*, vol. 43, p. 1036, 1976
32. Lee, CM, et al., *Annals of Clinical and Laboratory Science*, vol. 14, p. 51, 1984
33. Kishimoto, H., et al., *Yokohama Medical Bulletin*, vol. 27, p. 89, 1976
34. Goei, GS, et al., *Journal of Reproductive Medicine*, vol. 28, p. 527, Aug. 1983
35. Belfer, ML, et al., *Archives of General Psychiatry*, vol. 25, p. 540, 1971
36. Rubinow, DE, et al., *American Journal of Psychiatry*, vol. 141, p. 163, Feb. 1984

CHAPTER 13

1. Mayer, J., in *Modern Nutrition in Health and Disease*, Goodhart & Shils (eds.), Lea & Febiger, Philadelphia, 1973
2. *Lancet*, p. 1223, May 29, 1982
3. Tullis, F., et al., in *Nutritional Support of Medical Practice*, Schneider, H., et al., (eds.), p. 392, Harper & Row, Hagerstown, MD, 1977
4. Stunkard, AJ, et al., *New England Journal of Medicine*, vol. 314, p. 193, Jan.23, 1986
5. Drabman, RS, et al, *Journal of Nutrition Education*, vol. 9, no. 2, p. 80, Apr. 1977
6. Owen, OE, et al., *American Journal of Clinical Nutrition*, vol. 44, p. 1, July 1986
7. Braitman, LE, et al., *Journal of Chronic Diseases*, vol. 38, p. 727, 1985
8. Michael, HN, et al., *British Medical Bulletin*, vol. 37, p. 31, 1981
9. Garrow, JS, et al., *Lancet*, p. 670, Mar.23, 1985

10. Ashley, DV, et al., *American Journal of Clinical Nutrition*,vol. 42, p. 1240, Dec. 1985
11. Anderson, GH, *American Journal of Clinical Nutrition*, vol. 44, p. 158, July 1986
12. Jonas, JM, et al., *Lancet*, p. 390, Feb.1, 1986
13. Van Itallie, TB, *New England Journal of Medicine*, vol. 314, p. 239, Jan.23, 1986
14. Klesges, RC, et al., *International Journal of Eating Disorders*, vol. 5, no. 2, p. 335, 1986
15. Garn, SM, et al., *Ecology of Food and Nutrition*, vol. 10, p. 237, 1981
16. Dietz, WH, et al., *Pediatrics*, vol. 75, p. 807, May 1985
17. Hallfrisch, J., et al., *Nutrition Research*, vol. 2, p. 263, 1982
18. Duggan, JP, et al., *Science*, vol. 231, p. 609, Jan. 1986
19. Salmon, DM, et al., *International Journal of Obesity*, vol. 9, p. 443, 1985
20. Acheson, KJ, et al., *American Journal of Physiology*, vol. 246, p. 62, 1984
21. Lin, P., et al., *Journal of Nutrition*, vol. 109, p. 1143, 1979
22. Taber, LA, et al., *Journal of the American Dietetic Association*, vol. 76, p. 21, Jan. 1980
23. Morley, JE, et al., *American Journal of Clinical Nutrition*, vol. 34, no. 8, p. 1489, 1981
24. Allen, DW, et al., *Medical Journal of Australia*, vol. 2, p. 434, 1977; see also Bjorntorp, P., *Clinics in Endocrinology and Metabolism*, vol. 5, no. 2, p. 431, July 1976
25. Stuart, RB, et al., *Journal of the American Dietetic Association*, vol. 75, p. 258, Sept. 1979
26. O'Hara, WJ, et al., *Journal of Applied Physiology*, vol. 46, no. 5, p. 872, 1979
27. Vallerrand, AL, et al., *Diabetes*, vol. 35, p. 329, Mar. 1986
28. Acheson, KJ, et al., *Metabolism*, vol. 31, no. 12, p. 1234, Dec. 1982
29. Gibbs, J., et al., *American Journal of Physiology*, vol. 230, no. 1, p. 15, Jan. 1976
30. Schwartz, RS, et al., *Metabolism*, vol. 34, p. 285, Mar. 1985
31. King, RF, et al., *American Journal of Clinical Nutrition*, vol. 42, p. 177, Aug. 1985
32. Chomard, P., et al., *Human Nutrition: Clinical Nutrition*, vol. 39C, p. 371, Sept. 1985
33. Taber, LA, et al., *Journal of the American Dietetic Association*, vol. 76, p. 21, Jan. 1980
34. Ozelci, A., et al., *Journal of Nutrition*, vol. 108, p. 1724, 1978
35. Leveille, GA, et al., *Nutrition Today*, p. 4, Nov. 1974
36. Hunt, JN, et al., *Gastroenterology*, vol. 89, p. 1326, Dec. 1985
37. Metzner, HL, et al., *American Journal of Clinical Nutrition*, vol. 30, p. 712, May 1977
38. Clausen, JD, et al., *Journal of the American Dietetic Association*, vol. 77, p. 249, Sept. 1980
39. Yang, MU, et al., *Journal of Clinical Investigation*, vol. 58, p. 722, Sept. 1976
40. Duncan, KH, et al., *American Journal of Clinical Nutrition*, vol. 37, p. 763, May 1983
41. *Nutrition Reviews*, vol. 38, p. 25, 1980
42. Leibovitz, B., *Carnitine: The Vitamin B-T Phenomenon*, p. 107, Dell Publishers, New York, 1984
43. Maebashi, M., et al., *Lancet*, p. 805, 1978
44. McCarty, MF, *Medical Hypotheses*, vol. 8, p. 269, 1982
45. Ferguson, J., in *Lipoplasty*, Hetter, G. (ed.), p. 49, Little, Brown, & Co., Boston, MA, 1984
46. Sayetta, RB, *American Family Physician*, vol. 33, no. 5, p. 181, May 1986
47. Miller, TM, et al., *Journal of the American Dietetic Association*, vol. 77, p. 561, Nov. 1980
48. Bryce-Smith, D., et al., *Lancet*, p. 350, Aug.11, 1984
49. Bakan, R., *Lancet*, p. 874, Oct.13, 1984
50. Krebs, N., et al., *American Journal of Diseases of Children*, vol. 138, p. 270, Mar. 1984
51. Sayetta, RB, *op.cit.*
52. Hutton, CW, et al., *Journal of the American Dietetic Association*, vol. 82, p. 148, Feb. 1983
53. Humphrey, LL, *International Journal of Eating Disorders*, vol. 5, no. 2, p. 223, 1986
54. Waller, DA, et al., *American Journal of Clinical Nutrition*, vol. 44, p. 20, July 1986

55. Bhathena, SJ, et al, *American Journal of Clinical Nutrition*, vol. 43, p. 42, Jan. 1986

CHAPTER 14

1. Krall, L., (ed.), *Joslin Diabetes Manual*, 11th ed., Lea & Febiger, Philadelphia,1978, *passim.*
2, O'Dea, K., *Diabetes*, vol. 33, p. 596, June 1984
3. Henry, RR, et al., *Diabetes*, vol. 35, p. 155, Feb. 1986
4. Bialkowska, M., et al., *Materia Medica Polona*, vol. 3, no. 32, p. 244, 1977
5. Dobersen, MJ, et al., *New England Journal of Medicine*, vol. 303, p. 1493, 1980
6. Dorner, G., et al., *Experimental Clinical Endocrinology*, vol. 84, no. 2, p. 129, Oct. 1984
7. Norkins, AL, *Scientific American*, vol. 241, p. 62, Nov. 1979
8. Cox, DJ, et al., *Journal of the American Medical Association*, vol. 253, p. 1558, Mar. 1985
9. Mertz, W., in *Chromium in Nutrition and Metabolism*, Shapcott, D., et al., (eds.), p. 1, Elsevier, Amsterdam, 1979
10. Anderson, RA, et al., *American Journal of Clinical Nutrition*, vol. 41, p. 1177, June 1985
11. Kumpulainen, JT, et al., *Agriculture and Food Chemistry*, vol. 27, p. 490, 1979
12. Offenbacher, EG, et al., *Diabetes*, vol. 29, p. 919, 1980; see also Check, WA, *Journal of the American Medical Association*, vol. 247, p. 3046, 1982
13. Elwood, JC, et al., *Journal of the American College of Nutrition*, vol. 1, p. 263, 1982
14. Mossop, RT, *Central African Journal of Medicine*, vol. 29, p. 80, 1983
15. Elias, AN, et al., *General Pharmacology*, vol. 15, p. 535, 1984
16. Rabinowitz, MB, et al., *Diabetes Care*, vol. 6, p. 319, July 1983
17. *Journal of Clinical Investigation*, vol. 71, no. 1523, p. 1581, 1983
18. Mertz, W., in *Present Knowledge in Nutrition*, p. 373, The Nutrition Foundation, Washington, DC, 1976
19. Bierman, EL, *American Journal of Clinical Nutrition*, vol. 441, p. 1113, May 1985
20. Kiehm, J., et al., *American Journal of Clinical Nutrition*, vol. 29, p. 895, 1976
21. Snowdon, DA, et al., *American Journal of Public Health*, vol. 75, p. 507, May 1985
22. Toma, RB, et al., *Food Technology*, vol. 40, p. 118, Feb. 1986
23. Viswanathan, M., et al., *Diabetologia Croatica*, vol. 13, p. 163, Nov. 1984
24. Pavlovic, M., et al., *Diabetologia Croatica*, vol. 13, p. 199, Nov. 1984
25. Jenkins, DJ, et al., *American Journal of Clinical Nutrition*, vol. 34, p. 362, Mar. 1981
26. Jenkins, DJ, et al., *American Journal of Clinical Nutrition*, vol. 35, p. 1339, June 1982
27. Jenkins, DJ, et al., *American Journal of Clinical Nutrition*, vol. 43, p. 516, Apr. 1986
28. Hallfrisch, J., et al., *Journal of Nutrition*, vol. 109, p. 1909, 1979
29. Reiser, S., et al., *American Journal of Clinical Nutrition*, vol. 43, p. 151, Jan. 1986
30. Anderson, JW, *Medical Times*, vol. 108, p. 41, May 1980
31. Jenkins, DJ, et al., *Lancet*, vol. ii, p. 779, 1977
32. Osilesi, O., et al., *American Journal of Clinical Nutrition*, vol. 42, p. 597, Oct. 1985
33. McIvor, ME, et al., *Diabetes Care*, vol. 8, p. 274, May 1985
34. Holt, S., et al., *Lancet*, p. 636, Mar.24, 1979
35. Moore, DJ, et al., *Human Nutrition: Clinical Nutrition*, vol. 39C, p. 63, Jan. 1985
36. *Nutrition Reviews*, vol. 44, p. 232, July 1986
37. Maebashi, M., et al., *Lancet*, vol. ii, p. 805, 1978
38. *Metabolism*, vol. 33, p. 358, Apr. 1984
39. Bierenbaum, M., et al., *Nutrition Reports International*, vol. 31, p. 1171, June 1985
40. Gilbert, V., et al., *Hormone and Metabolic Research*, vol. 15, p. 320, 1983
41. Pritchard, KA, et al., *Diabetes*, vol. 35, p. 278, Mar. 1986
42. Seifter, E., et al., *Annals of Surgery*, vol. 194, p. 42, 1981
43. Ginter, E., et al., *International Journal of Vitamin and Nutrition Research*, vol. 48, p. 368, 1978
44. *Lancet*, p. 788, Apr.10, 1976

45. Brown, RR, et al., *Journal of Clinical Investigation*, vol. 40, p. 617, 1961; see also *Lancet*, vol. i., p. 897, 1973
46. Dubuc, A., *Journal of Medicine Bordeaux*, vol. 138, p. 881, 1961
47. *British Medical Journal*, vol. 2, p. 13, 1975
48. Roth, HP, et al., *Biological Trace Element Research*, vol. 3, p. 13, 1981
49. Kinlaw, B., et al., *American Journal of Medicine*, vol. 75, p. 273, 1983
50. Winegrad, AI, et al., *New England Journal of Medicine*, vol. 308, p. 152, 1983
51. Salway, B., *Lancet*, vol. ii, p. 1282, 1980
52. Clements, A., et al., *American Journal of Clinical Nutrition*, vol. 33, p. 1954, 1980
53. *The Vitamins*, vol. 3, 2nd ed., Academic Press, New York, 1971
54. Singer, P., et al., *Biomed Bioc*, vol. 43, p. S438, 1984
55. Klein, C., *Munchener Medizinische Wochenschrift*, vol. 117, p. 957, 1975
56. Kinoshito, J., *Journal of the American Medical Association*, vol. 246, p. 257, 1981
57. Shigeta, Y., et al., *Journal of Vitaminology*, vol. 12, p. 293, 1966
58. Visek, WJ, *Journal of Nutrition*, vol. 116, p. 36, Jan. 1986
59. Brekhman, I., et al., *Drug Research*, vol. 25, p. 539, 1975
60. Sharma, RD, *Nutrition Research*, vol. 6, p. 1353, 1986
61. Young, CM, et al., *Journal of the American Dietetic Association*, vol. 59, p. 473, Nov. 1971
62. Connor, H., et al., *Human Nutrition: Applied Nutrition*, vol. 39A, p. 393, Dec. 1986
63. Galbo, H., et al., *Journal of Applied Physiology*, vol. 40, p. 855, June 1976

CHAPTER 15

1. Davies, R., et al., *American Family Physician*, vol. 32, p. 107, Nov. 1985
2. Boyce, W., et al., *Lancet*, p. 150, Jan. 19, 1985
3. Fisher, S., et al., *American Journal of Clinical Nutrition*, vol. 31, p. 667, 1978
4. Lee, CJ, et al., *American Journal of Clinical Nutrition*, vol. 34, p. 819, May 1981
5. Haspels, AA, et al., *Maturitas*, vol. 1, p. 15, June 1978
6. *Journal of the American Medical Association*, vol. 252, p. 799, Aug. 1984
7. Schnitzler, C., et al., *South African Medical Journal*, vol. 66, no. 19, p. 730, Nov. 1984
8. Schwartz, R., et al., *American Journal of Clinical Nutrition*, vol. 26, p. 519, May 1973
9. Linkswiler, HM, et al., *Federation Proceedings*, vol. 40, p. 2429, July 1981
10. Boyce, BF, et al., *Lancet*, p. 1009, Nov.6, 1982
11. Recker, R., *New England Journal of Medicine*, vol. 313, p. 70, July 1985
12. Garrison, R., et al., *The Nutrition Desk Reference*, p. 59, Keats Publishing, New Canaan, CT, 1985
13. Lutz, J., et al, *The American Journal of Clinical Nutrition*, vol. 44, p. 99, July 1986
14. Simeon, O., et al., *Lancet*, p. 432, Aug.24, 1985
15. Strause, LG, et al., *Journal of Nutrition*, vol. 116, p. 98, 1986
16. Raisz, LG, *Journal of the American Geriatrics Society*, vol. 30, p. 127, Feb. 1982
17. *Lancet*, p. 423, Aug. 21, 1982
18. Korcok, M., *Journal of the American Medical Association*, vol. 247, p. 1106, Feb. 1982
19. Rambaut, PC, et al., *Lancet*, p. 1050, Nov. 9, 1985
20. *Lancet*, p. 1370, June 15, 1985
21. Albanese, AA, et al., *American Family Physician*, vol. 18, no. 4, p. 162, Oct. 1978
22. Albanese, AA, et al., *Nutrition Reports International*, vol. 33, no. 6, p. 879, June 1986
23. Draper, HH, et al., *Federation Proceedings*, vol. 40, p. 2434, July 1981
24. Hamilton, E., et al., *Nutrition: Concepts and Controversies*, p. 53, West Publishing, St. Paul, MN, 1985
25. Sandler, RB, et al., *American Journal of Clinical Nutrition*, vol. 42, p. 270, Aug. 1985
26. Zikaras, MB, *Journal of Health Promotion*, vol. 2, p. 9, Spring, 1985
27. Roberts, HJ, *New England Journal of Medicine*, vol. 304, p. 423, Feb. 1981

424 HEALING NUTRIENTS

28. Sowers, M., et al., *American Journal of Clinical Nutrition*, vol. 42, p. 135, July 1985
29. *Documenta Geigy Scientific Tables*, 1970
30. Recker, RR, et al., *American Journal of Clinical Nutrition*, vol. 41, p. 254, Feb. 1985
31. Long, PJ, et al., *Nutrition: An Inquiry into the Issues*, p. 59, Prentice-Hall, Englewood Cliffs, NJ, 1983
32. Smith, TM, et al., *American Journal of Clinical Nutrition*, vol. 42, p. 1197, Dec. 1985
33. Jacobs, DH, *New England Journal of Medicine*, vol. 314, p. 1389, May 1986
34. Spencer, H., et al., *Archives of Internal Medicine*, vol. 143, p. 657, 1983
35. Dawson-Hughes, B., et al., *American Journal of Clinical Nutrition*, vol. 44, p. 83, July 1986
36. Gibson, RS, et al., *American Journal of Clinical Nutrition*, vol. 37, p. 37, Jan. 1983
37. Heath, H., *Journal of the American Medical Association*, vol. 254, p. 964, Aug. 1985
38. Heaney, RP, et al., *American Journal of Clinical Nutrition*, vol. 43, p. 299, Feb. 1986
39. Auckland, JN, et al., *Journal of the Royal Society of Health*, vol. 105, p. 123, Aug. 1985
40. Nordin, BE, et al., *American Journal of Clinical Nutrition*, vol. 42, p. 470, Sept. 1985
41. Avioli, LV, *Federation Proceedings*, vol. 40, p. 2418, July 1981
42. Boland, RL, *Nutrition Reviews*, vol. 44, p. 1, Jan. 1986
43. Jayson, MI, et al., *Understanding Arthritis and Rheumatism*, Pantheon Books, New York, 1974, *passim*.
44. Holvey, DN, (ed.), *The Merck Manual*, Merck & Co., Rahway, NJ, p. 1206, 1972
45. Darlington, LG, et al., *Lancet*, p. 236, Feb.1, 1986
46. Helliwell, M., et al., *Annals of the Rheumatic Diseases*, vol. 43, p. 386, 1984
47. Lee, TH, et al., *New England Journal of Medicine*, vol. 312, p. 1217, May 1985
48. Kremer, JM, et al., *Lancet*, p. 184, Jan.26, 1986
49. Ziff, H., *Arthritis and Rheumatism*, vol. 26, p. 457, 1983
50. Barton-Wright, EC, et al., *Lancet*, vol. ii, p. 862, 1963
51. *Martindale-The Extra Pharmacopeia*, p. 1752, The Pharmaceutical Press, London, 1982.
52. Annand, DL, *Lancet*, vol. ii, p. 1168, 1963
53. General Practitioner Research Group, *Practitioner*, vol. 224, p. 208, 1980
54. *Medical World News*, Oct.7, 1978
55. Niedermeier, W., et al., *Journal of Chronic Diseases*, vol. 23, p. 527, 1971
56. Simkin, PA, *Lancet*, vol. ii, p. 539, 1976
57. Chapil, HR, *Medical Clinics of North America*, vol. 60, p. 799, 1976
58. Walker, BC, et al., *Agents and Actions*, vol. 6, p. 454, 1976
59. Huber, W., et al., *Clinics in Rheumatic Disease*, vol. 6, p. 465, 1980; see also *American Journal of Medicine*, vol. 74, p. 124, 1983
60. Frank, B., *Nucleic Acid and Antioxidant Therapy of Aging and Degeneration*, Rainstone Publishing, New York, 1977
61. Johansson, U., et al., *Human Nutrition: Clinical Nutrition*, vol. 40C, p. 57, 1986
62. Spallholz, JE, in *Diet and Resistance to Disease*, Philips, M., et al., (eds.) *Advances in Experimental Medical Biology*, vol. 135, p. 43, 1981
63. Reilly, LL, in *Selenium in Biology and Medicine*, p. 343; Spallholz, JE, et al., (eds.), AVI Publishing, Westport, CT, 1981
64. *Veterinarian Medicine and Small Animal Clinician*, vol. 61, p. 986, 1966
65. Kamimura, M., *Journal of Vitaminology*, vol. 18, p. 204, 1972; see also Machety, I., et al., *Journal of American Geriatric Society*, vol. 26, p. 328, 1978
66. Balagot, R., et al., in *Degradation of Endogenous Opioids: Its Relevance in Human Pathology and Therapy*, Ehrenpreis, S., et al., (eds.), p. 207, Raven Press, New York, 1983
67. Madan, BR, et al., *IRCS Medical Science*, vol. 14, p. 288, 1986
68. *Journal of the American Medical Association*, vol. 248, p. 1369, Sept. 1982
69. Wilkins, E., et al., *Experientia*, vol. 35, no. 2, p. 244, 1979
70. Helliwell, M., et al., *Annals of the Rheumatic Diseases*, vol. 43, p. 386, 1984
71. Kaufman, W., *Connecticut State Medical Journal*, vol. 17, p. 584, 1953; see also Hoffer, A., *Canadian Medical Association Journal*, vol. 81, p. 235, 1959
72. Becker, Y., et al., *Connective Tissue Research*, vol. 8, no. 77, 1981
73. Kelley, W., et al., *Metabolism*, vol. 19, p. 1025, 1970

CHAPTER 16

1. U.S. Department of Health, Education, and Welfare, *Healthy People*, p. 101, U.S. Government Printing Office, 79-55071, Washington, DC, 1979

2. Epstein, SS, et al., *Hazardous Waste in America*, p. iv, Sierra Club Books, San Francisco, 1982. See also Regenstein, L., *How to Survive in America the Poisoned*, Acropolis Books, Washington, D.C., 1986 passim.

3. Schauss, A., *Diet, Crime and Delinquency*, p. 32, Parker House, Berkeley, CA, 1981

4. Sandler, DP, et al., *Lancet*, p. 312, Feb. 9, 1985

5. Barboriak, JJ, et al., *Journal of the American Dietetic Association*, vol. 72, p. 493, May 1978

6. U.S. Bureau of the Census, STATISTICAL ABSTRACT OF THE UNITED STATES: 1985, 105th ed., Washington, DC, 1984

7. Brody, JE, *Jane Brody's Nutrition Book*, p. 468, WW Norton, New York, 1981

8. Lucas, J., *Our Polluted Food*, John Wiley & Sons, New York, 1974

9. *Los Angeles Times*, part I, p. 3, Aug. 18, 1985

10. Sloan, AE, *Food Engineering*, vol. 57, p. 72, Sept. 1985

11. Foster, K., *American Scientist*, vol. 74, p. 163, Apr. 1986

12. Sawhney, BL, et al., *Journal of Food Protection*, vol. 48, p. 442, Apr. 1985

13. Rogan, WJ, et al., *American Journal of Public Health*, vol. 76, no. 2, p. 172, Feb. 1986

14. Kurechi, T., et al., *Journal of Food Science*, vol. 44, p. 1263, 1979

15. Tomita, I., et al., *IARC Science Publishing*, vol. 57, p. 33, 1984

16. Wagner, DA, et al., *Cancer Research*, vol. 45, p. 6519, Dec. 1985

17. Sprince, H., et al., *Agents and Actions*, vol. 5, p. 164, 1975

18. Pelletier, O., *Nutrition Today*, p. 12, autumn, 1970

19. Tewfik, H., et al., *International Journal for Vitamin and Nutrition Research*, sup. 23, p. 265, 1982

20. Ala-Ketola, L., et al., *Strahlentherapie*, vol. 148, p. 643, 1974

21. Kawai-Kobayashi, K., et al., *Journal of Nutrition*, vol. 116, p. 98, 1986

22. Huang, M., et al., *Journal of Biological Chemistry*, vol. 256, p. 1089, 1981

23. Rabinowitz, M., *Lancet*, p. 63, Jan. 1, 1983

24. Spallholz, JE, et al., *Selenium in Biology and Medicine*, Avi Publishing, Westport, CT, 1981

25. Glauser, SC, et al., *Lancet*, vol. i, p. 717, 1976

26. Chung, AS, et al., *Biochemical Pharmacology*, vol. 31, p. 3093, 1982

27. Masukawa, T., et al., *Biochemical Pharmacology*, vol. 33, no. 16, p. 2635, 1984

28. Sparnins, VL, et al., *Journal of the National Cancer Institute*, vol. 66, p. 769, Apr. 1981

29. Griffin, AC, *Advances in Cancer Research*, vol. 29, p. 419, 1979; see also Jacobs, MM, *Preventive Medicine*, vol. 9, p. 362, 1980

30. Ip, C., et al., *Carcinogenesis*, vol. 2, p. 435, 1981

31. Willett, WC, et al., *Lancet*, p. 130, July 16, 1981

32. Midander, J., et al., *International Journal of Radiation, Oncology, and Biological Physiology*, vol. 8, p. 443, 1982

33. Myers, CE, et al., *Annals of the New York Academy of Sciences*, vol. 393, p. 419, 1982

34. *Nutrition Reviews*, vol. 42, p. 260, 1984; see also Van Vleet, JF, et al., *American Journal of Veterinary Research*, vol. 39, p. 997, 1978

35. Cortes, E., et al., *Cardiac Treatment Reports*, vol. 62, p. 887, 1978

36. Bieri, JG, in *Present Knowledge in Nutrition*, p. 102, The Nutrition Foundation, New York, 1976

37. Lawson, T., et al., *Chemical and Biological Interactions*, vol. 45, p. 95, 1983

38. Patt, HM, et al., *Science*, vol. 110, p. 213, 1949

39. Williamson, JM, et al., *Proceedings of the National Academy of Science*, vol. 79, p. 6246, Oct. 1982

40. Meydani, M., et al., *Drug-Nutrient Interactions*, vol. 2, p. 217, 1984

41. Visek, WJ, et al., *Journal of the American College of Nutrition*, vol. 5, p. 153, 1986

42. Zhemkova, LN, et al., *Radiobiologiia*, vol. 25, p. 208, Mar. 1985

43. Borum, PR, et al., *Journal of the American College of Nutrition*, vol. 5, p. 177, 1986

44. Seifter, E., et al., *Journal of the National Cancer Institute*, vol. 71, p. 409, 1983

45. Bond, GG, et al., *Nutrition and Cancer*, vol. 9, p. 109, 1987

46. Micksche, M., et al., *Oncology*, vol. 34, no. 5, p. 234, 1977

47. Hendler, SS, *The Complete Guide to Anti-Aging Nutrients*, p. 88, Simon & Schuster, New York, 1985

48. Hunt, T., et al., *Annals of Surgery*, vol. 170, no. 4, p. 633, Oct. 1969

49. *Omni*, p. 38, Feb. 1983

50. Atkins, JN, *American Reviews of Respiratory Disease*, vol. 126, p. 714, 1982

51. Duncan, JR, et al., *Journal of the National Cancer Institute*, vol. 55, p. 195, 1975

52. Papaioannou, R., et al., *Journal of Orthomolecular Psychiatry*, vol. 7, no. 2, p. 94, 1978

53. *Nutrition Reviews*, vol. 40, no. 2, p. 43, 1982

54. Jackson, A., et al., *Teratology*, vol. 19, p. 341, 1979

55. Levinson, B., *Nature*, vol. 227, p. 1023, 1976

56. Kensler, HH, et al., *Science*, vol. 221, p. 75, 1983

57. Luo, X., et al., *Federation Proceedings*, vol. 46, p. 928, 1981

58. *FDA Drug Bulletin*, p. 13, 1983

59. Ershoff, BH, *American Journal of Clinical Nutrition*, vol. 27, p. 1395, 1974

60. Ershoff, BH, *Journal of Food Science*, vol. 41, p. 949, 1976

61. Nonavinakere, VK, *Nutrition Reports International*, vol. 23, p. 697, Apr. 1981

62. Roe, D., *Journal of the American Dietetic Association*, vol. 85, p. 174, Feb. 1985

63. Bamji, MS, et al., *Contraception*, vol. 32, p. 405, Oct. 1985

64. Basu, TK, *Journal of Nutrition*, vol. 116, p. 570, 1986

65. Adams, PW, et al., *Lancet*, p. 516, Aug. 31, 1974

66. Adams, PW, et al., *Lancet*, p. 7809, Apr. 28, 1973

67. Elmer, G., *Nurse Practitioner*, p. 40, Sept. 1981

68. Shojania, AM *Canadian Medical Association Journal*, vol. 126, p. 244, Feb. 1, 1982

69. *Lancet*, p. 682, Mar. 26, 1983

70. Gilbert, RM, *Journal of Studies on Alcohol*, vol. 40, no. 1, p. 19, 1979

71. Hillers, VN, et al., *American Journal of Clinical Nutrition*, vol. 41, p. 356, Feb. 1985

72. Mendenhall, CL, et al., *American Journal of Clinical Nutrition*, vol. 43, p. 312, Feb. 1986

73. Gruchow, HW, et al., *American Journal of Clinical Nutrition*, vol. 42, p. 289, Aug. 1985

74. Laposata, EA, et al., *Science*, vol. 231, p. 497, Jan. 1986

75. Pollack, ES, et al., *New England Journal of Medicine*, vol. 310, p. 617, Mar. 1984

76. Graham, T., et al., *Aviation, Space, and Environmental Medicine*, p. 793, Aug. 1980

77. *Nutrition Reviews*, vol. 24, p. 239, Aug. 1966

78. Majumdar, SK, et al., *International Journal of Vitamin and Nutrition Research*, vol. 51, p. 54, 1981

79. Fausto, N., *Biochimica et Biophysica Acta*, vol. 190, p. 193, 1969

80. Barbul, A., et al., *Federation Proceedings*, vol. 37, p. 264, Apr. 1978

81. Sprince, H., et al., *Agents and Actions*, vol. 4, p. 125, 1974

82. Edes, L., et al., *Proceedings of the Society for Experimental Biology and Medicine*, vol. 162, p. 71, 1979

83. Finkelstein, JD, et al., *Biochemical and Biophysical Research Communications*, vol. 61, p. 525, 1974

84. Branchey, L., *Alcoholism: Clinical and Experimental Research*, vol. 9, no. 5, p. 393, Sept. 1985

85. Williams, RJ, *The Prevention of Alcoholism Through Nutrition*, Bantam Books, New York, 1981

86. Lindenbaum, J., et al., *Annals of the New York Academy of Sciences*, vol. 252, p. 228, 1975

87. Thomson, AD, et al., *Journal of Laboratory and Clinical Medicine*, p. 34, July 1970

88. Rossouw, JE, et al., *Scandinavian Journal of Gastroenterology*, vol. 13, p. 133, 1978

89. Weinstein, MC, *New England Journal of Medicine*, vol. 299, no. 6, p. 307, Aug. 1978; see also Reuler, JB, et al., *New England Journal of Medicine*, vol. 312, p. 1035, Apr. 1985

90. *Lancet*, p. 1287, June 5, 1982

91. Lindenbaum, J., et al., *Nature*, vol. 224, p. 806, Nov. 1969

92. Baker, H., et al., *American Journal of Clinical Nutrition*, vol. 28, p. 1377, 1975

93. Halsted, CH, et al., *New England Journal of Medicine*, vol. 285, no. 13, p. 705, Sept. 1971

94. Bonjour, JP, *International Journal of Vitamin and Nutrition Research*, vol. 51, p. 307, 1981

95. Devgun, MS, et al., *British Journal of Nutrition*, vol. 45, p. 469, 1981

96. Middleton, HM, *American Journal of Clinical Nutrition*, vol. 43, p. 374, Mar. 1986

97. Wesselman, GD, et al., *Nutritional Reports International*, vol. 33, p. 939, June 1986

98. Fazio, V., et al., *American Journal of Clinical Nutrition*, vol. 34, p. 2394, Nov. 1981

99. Leung, FW, et al., *Annals of Emergency Medicine*, vol. 10, p. 652, Dec. 1981

100. Russell, RM, *American Journal of Clinical Nutrition*, vol. 33, p. 2741, 1980

101. Leo, MA, et al., *New England Journal of Medicine*, vol. 307, p. 597, Sept. 1982

102. Dinsmore, WW, et al., *American Journal of Clinical Nutrition*, vol. 42, p. 688, Oct. 1985

103. *Nutrition Reviews*, vol. 43, p. 158, May 1985

104. Herlong, HF, *Hepatology*, vol. 1, p. 348, July 1981

105. Morrison, S., et al., *American Journal of Clinical Nutrition*, vol. 31, p. 276, 1978

106. Sclafani, L., et al., *Journal of Parenteral and Enteral Nutrition*, vol. 10, p. 184, 1986

107. Dworkin, B., et al., *Digestive Diseases and Sciences*, vol. 30, p. 838, Sept. 1985

108. Kuksis, A., et al., *Nutrition Reviews*, vol. 36, p. 233, 1978

109. Kuksis, A., et al., in *Present Knowledge in Nutrition*, ch. 27, The Nutrition Foundation, Washington, DC, 1984

110. Rudman, D., et al., in *Carnitine Biosynthesis, Metabolism, and Functions*, Frenkel, R., et al., (eds.), p. 307, Academic Press, New York 1980

111. Crownover, BP, et al., *Journal of Pharmacology and Experimental Therapeutics*, vol. 236, no. 3, p. 574, 1986

112. Gershbein, LL, et al., *Research Communications in Chemical Pathology and Pharmacology*, vol. 28, no. 3, p. 457, June 1980

113. Nakagawa, S., et al., *Hiroshima Journal of Medical Science*, vol. 34, p. 303, Sept. 1985

114. Newman, RA, et al., *American Journal of Physiology*, vol. 164, p. 251, 1951

115. Visek, WJ, et al., *Journal of the American College of Nutrition*, vol. 5, p. 153, 1986

116. McCarty, M., *Medical Hypotheses*, vol. 7, p. 515, 1981

117. Glen, I., et al., paper presented at the International Conference on Pharmacological Treatments for Alcoholism Institute of Psychiatry, University of London, England, Mar. 29, 1983

CHAPTER 17

1. Geissler, C., et al., *American Journal of Clinical Nutrition*, vol. 39, p. 478, Mar. 1984

2. Sreebny, LM, *Community Dentistry and Oral Epidemiology*, vol. 10, p. 1, Feb. 1982

3. *Lancet*, p. 117, July 12, 1986

4. Shaw, JH, *American Journal of Clinical Nutrition*, vol. 41, p. 1117, May 1985

5. Sheiham, A., *Lancet*, p. 282, Feb. 5, 1983

6. Bibby, BG, *Cereal Foods World*, vol. 30, p. 851, Dec. 1985

7. *Nutrition Reviews*, vol. 44, p. 233, July 1986

8. Alavrez, JO, et al., *Lancet*, p. 91, Jan. 11, 1986

9. Dannenberg, JL, *Journal of the American Dental Association*, vol. 105, p. 172, Aug. 1982

10. Robinson, CH, *Fundamentals of Normal Nutrition*, p. 10–11, Macmillan, New York, 1978

11. *American Health*, p. 31, Sept. 1983

12. Wilkinson, EG, et al., *Research Communications in Chemical Pathology and Pharmacology*, vol. 12, p. 11, 1975

13. Vogel, R., *Journal of Oral Medicine*, vol. 33, p. 20, 1978

14. Henkin, B., et al., *Annals of Internal Medicine*, vol. 99, p. 227, 1983

15. Gibson, RS, et al., *American Journal of Clinical Nutrition*, vol. 37, p. 37, Jan. 1983

16. Krebs, NF, et al., *American Journal of Diseases of Children*, vol. 138, p. 270, Mar. 1984

17. Larsson, LG, et al., *Cancer Research*, vol. 35, p. 3308, 1975

18. Combs, GF, *Proceedings of the Nutrition Society*, vol. 40, p. 187, 1981

19. Patty, I., et al., *Lancet*, vol. ii, p. 876, 1982

20. Frommer, DJ, *Medical Journal of Australia*, vol. 2, p. 793, 1975

21. Sanderson, CR, et al., *Gut*, vol. 16, p. 177, 1975

22. Kumar, N., et al., *British Medical Journal*, vol. 288, p. 1803, June 1984

23. Brender, JD, et al., *American Journal of Public Health*, vol. 75, p. 399, Apr. 1985

24. Hobbs, B., *Food Poisoning and Food Hygiene*, 2nd ed., Edward Arnold Ltd, London, 1968

25. Archer, DL, et al., *Journal of Food Protection*, vol. 48, p. 887, 1985

26. Chasnoff, IJ, et al., (eds.), *Family Medical and Health Guide*, p. 240, Publications International, Skokie, IL 1984

27. Painter, J., *British Medical Journal*, vol. 2, p. 156, 1971

28. Eastwood, MA, et al., *American Journal of Clinical Nutrition*, vol. 43, p. 343, Mar. 1986

29. Bass, L., *American Journal of Nursing*, p. 254, Feb. 1977

30. Andersson, H., et al., *Human Nutrition: Applied Nutrition*, vol. 39A, p. 101, Apr. 1985

31. Anderson, JW, *Federation Proceedings*, vol. 44, p. 2902, Nov. 1985

32. Burkitt, DP, et al., *Lancet*, p. 880, Oct. 19, 1985

33. Dickerson, JW, et al., *Journal of the Royal Society of Health*, vol. 105, p. 191, Dec. 1985

34. Davies, GJ, et al., *Human Nutrition: Applied Nutrition*, vol. 39A, p. 139, Apr. 1985

35. Southgate, DA, *American Journal of Clinical Nutrition*, vol. 31, p. S107, Oct. 1978

36. Trainanedes, K., et al., *American Journal of Clinical Nutrition*, vol. 44, p. 390, Sept. 1986

37. Fleming, SE, et al., *American Journal of Clinical Nutrition*, vol. 41, p. 909, May 1985

38. Gilliland, SE, et al., *Applied Environmental Microbiology*, vol. 49, p. 377, Feb. 1985

39. *Nutrition Reviews*, vol. 42, p. 374, Nov. 1984

40. Gregori, G., et al., *Acta Biomedica Ateneo Parmense*, vol. 56, p. 23, 1985

41. Alm, L., *Nahrung*, vol. 28, p. 683, 1984

42. Thornton, JR, et al., *British Medical Journal*, vol. 290, p. 1786, June 1985

43. Van Ness, MM, et al., *American Family Physician*, vol. 31, no.4, p. 198, Apr. 1985

44. Yatzidis, H., *British Medical Journal*, vol. 4, p. 51, 1972

45. Hall, RG, et al., *American Journal of Gastroenterology*, vol. 75, p. 192, 1981

46. Gupta, AK, et al., *IRCS Medical Science*, vol. 14, p. 212, 1986

47. Mann, J., *Journal of the American Medical Association*, vol. 255, p. 666, Feb. 1986

48. Bennion, LJ, et al., *Journal of Clinical Investigation*, vol. 56, p. 996, Oct. 1975

49. Toouli, J., et al., *Lancet*, p. 1124, Dec.6, 1975

50. Ginter, F., *World Review of Nutrition and Dietetics*, vol. 33, p. 104, 1979

51. Thomassen, MS, et al., *British Journal of Nutrition*, vol. 51, p. 315, May 1984

52. Gupta, AK, et al., *op.cit.*

53. Tanimura, H., et al., *Annals of the New York Academy of Sciences*, vol. 393, p. 214, Sept. 1982

CHAPTER 18

1. Moffatt, RJ, *Journal of the American Dietetic Association*, vol. 84, p. 1361, Nov. 1984

2. Nickerson, HJ, et al., *American Journal of Diseases of Children*, vol. 139, p. 1115, Nov. 1985

3. *Dairy Council Digest*, vol. 51, no. 3, p. 15, May 1980

4. Keys, A., et al., *Journal of Nutrition*, vol. 26, p. 399,1943

5. Anderson, RA, et al., *Biological Trace Element Research*, vol. 6, p. 327, 1984

6. Handing, A., et al., *Acta Medica Scandinavica*, vol. 209, p. 315, 1981

7. Guthrie, H., et al., *Journal of Nutrition Education*, vol. 13, no. 2, p. 46, 1981

8. *Proceedings of the New York Academy of Sciences*, vol. 33, no. 6, p. 625, 1971

9. Hendler, SS, *The Complete Guide to Anti-Aging Nutrients*, p. 275, Simon & Schuster, New York, 1985

10. Ushakov, A., et al., *Aviation, Space, and Environmental Medicine*, vol. 49, p. 1184, 1978

11. Evans, WJ, et al., *American Journal of Clinical Nutrition*, vol. 41, p. 1146, May 1985

12. Koivisto, VA, et al., *Journal of Applied Physiology*, vol. 5, p. 783, 1981

13. Foster, C., et al., *Medicine and Science in Sports and Exercise*, vol. 11, no. 1, p. 1, 1979

14. Bicknell, F., et al., *The Vitamins in Medicine*, Heinneman, London, 1945

15. Nijakowski, F., *Aviation, Space, and Environmental Medicine*, vol. 17, p. 397, 1966

16. Belko, A., et al., *American Journal of Clinical Nutrition*, vol. 37, p. 509, 1983

17. Ajayi, OA, et al., *American Journal of Clinical Nutrition*, vol. 39, p. 787, May 1984

18. Tremblay, A., et al., *Nutrition Research*, vol. 4, p. 201, 1984

19. Jette, M., et al., *American Journal of Clinical Nutrition*, vol. 31, p. 2140, 1978

20. Costill, DL, et al., *Medicine and Science in Sports and Exercise*, vol. 10, no. 3, p. 155, 1978

21. Ivy, J., et al., *Medicine and Science in Sports and Exercise*, vol. 11, no. 1, p. 6, 1979

22. Folkers, J., et al., *Journal of Molecular Medicine*, vol. 2, p. 431, 1977

23. Hornsby, JL, et al., *Journal of Cellular Physiology*, vol. 112, p. 207, 1982

24. Howald, H., *Annals of the New York Academy of Sciences*, vol. 258, p. 458, 1975

25. Suboticanec-Buzina, K., et al., *International Journal for Vitamin and Nutrition Research*, vol. 54, p. 55, 1984

26. Schrauzer, G., et al., *Annals of the New York Academy of Sciences*, vol. 258, p. 377, 1975

27. Wilbur, V., et al., *Nutrition Reports International*, vol. 17, p. 156, 1978

28. Barzani, V., et al., *Bollettino-Societa Italiana Biologia Sperimentale*, vol. 55, p. 190, 1981

29. Weidemann, MJ, et al., *Biochemical Journal*, vol. 111, p. 69, 1969

30. Kamikawa, T., et al., *Japanese Heart Journal*, vol. 25, p. 587, 1984

31. *Nutrition Reviews*, vol. 43, p. 220, July 1985

32. Visek, WJ. *Journal of Nutrition*,vol. 116, p. 36, Jan. 1986

33. Robinson, C., *Fundamentals of Normal Nutrition*, p. 63, MacMillan Publishing, New York, 1978

34. Williams, M., *Nutritional Aspects of Human Physical and Athletic Performance*, C.C.Thomas, Springfield, IL, 1976, *passim.*

35. *Physician and Sports Medicine*, p. 43, Aug. 1975

36. Grandjean, AC, *Cereal Foods World*, vol. 30, p. 848, Dec. 1985

37. Costill, DL, et al., *Journal of Applied Physiology*, vol. 40, no. 1, p. 6, Jan. 1976

38. McBolet, S., et al., *Clinical Medicine*, vol. 47, p. 280, 1976

39. Olsson, KE, et al., *Scandinavian Journal Rehabilitative Medicine* , vol. 3, p. 31, 1971

40. Frizzell, RT, et al., *Journal of the American Medical Association*, vol. 255, p. 772, Feb. 1986

41. Consolazio, CF, et al., *American Journal of Clinical Nutrition*, vol. 28, p. 29, 1975

42. Lemon, PW, et al., *Journal of Applied Physiology*, vol. 48, no. 4, p. 624, 1980

43. Miller, LT, et al., *Journal of Nutrition*, vol. 135, p. 1663, Dec. 1985

44. Richardson, J., et al., *Journal of Sports Medicine*, vol. 21, p. 119, 1981

45. Ershoff, B., *Proceedings of the Society for Experimental Biology and Medicine*, vol. 78, p. 385, 1951

46. Orndahl, G., et al., *Acta Medica Scandinavica*, vol. 211, p. 493, 1982

47. Gebre-Medhin, M., et al., *Acta Paediatrica Scandinavica*, vol. 74, p. 886, 1985

48. Williams, M., *Drugs and Athletic Performance*, C.C.Thomas, Springfield, IL, 1974

49. Isidori, A., et al., *Current Medical Research Opinion*, vol. 7, no. 7, p. 136, 1981

50. Richardson, J., et al., *Journal of Sports Medicine*, vol. 19, p. 133, 1979
51. Strydom, N., et al., *Journal of Applied Physiology*, vol. 41, no. 2, p. 202, Aug. 1976
52. Lotzof, L., *Medical Journal of Australia*, vol. 1, no. 24, p. 904, June 1977
53. Handing, A., et al., *Acta Medica Scandinavica*, vol. 209, p. 315, 1981
54. Nickerson, HJ, et al., *American Journal of Diseases of Children*, vol. 139, p. 1115, Nov. 1985
55. Ohira, Y., et al., *Journal of Nutrition*, vol. 111, p. 17, 1981
56. Bowering, J., et al., *Journal of Nutrition*, vol. 111, p. 1648, 1981
57. Finch, CA, et al., *Journal of Clinical Investigation*, vol. 58, p. 447, 1976
58. Ohira, Y., et al., *British Journal of Haematology*, vol. 41, p. 365, 1979
59. Brune, M., et al., *American Journal of Clinical Nutrition*, vol. 43, p. 438, Mar. 1986
60. Dillard, C., et al., *Journal of Applied Physiology*, vol. 45, p. 927, 1978; see also Brady, P., et al., *Journal of Nutrition*, vol. 109, p. 1103, 1979
61. Powers, HJ, et al., *Human Nutrition: Clinical Nutrition*, vol. 39C, p. 427, Nov. 1985
62. Ahlborg, B., et al., *Acta Physiologica Scandinavica*, vol. 74, p. 238, 1968
63. Richardson, J., *Journal of Sports Medicine*, vol. 20, p. 150, 1980
64. Saxena, OA, et al., *Indian Journal of Physiology and Pharmacology*, vol. 24, p. 233, 1980
65. Dorling, E., et al., *Notabene Medici*, vol. 10, no. 5, p. 241, 1980
66. Forgo, I., et al., *Medizinische Welt*, vol. 32, no. 19, p. 751, 1981
67. Forgo, I., et al., *Arztliche Praxis*, vol. 33, no. 44, p. 1784, 1981
68. Forgo, I., et al., *Notabene Medici*, vol. 12, no. 9, p. 721, 1987

CHAPTER 19

1. Neldner, KH, *Geriatrics*, vol. 39, p. 69, Feb. 1984
2. Downing, DT, et al., *Journal of the American Academy of Dermatology*, vol. 14, p. 221, 1986
3. Nassar, BA, et al., *Nutrition Research*, vol. 6, p. 1397, 1986
4. Galland, L., *Journal of the American College of Nutrition*, vol. 5, p. 213, 1986
5. Wright, S., et al., *Lancet*, p. 1120, Nov.20, 1982
6. Manku, MS, et al., *Prostaglandins, Leukotrienes, and Medicine*, vol. 9, p. 615, 1982
7. Voorhees, JJ, et al., *Archives of Dermatology*, vol. 119, p. 541, 1983
8. Cunnane, SC, *Pediatric Research*, vol. 16, p. 599, 1982
9. Haboubi, NY, et al., *Journal of Clinical Pathology*, vol. 38, p. 1189, 1985
10. Schachner, L. *Pediatric Clinics of North America*, vol. 30, p. 501, June, 1983
11. Cunliffe, J., *British Journal of Dermatology*, vol. 101, p. 321, 1979
12. Verna, KC, et al., *Acta Dermatovener*, vol. 60, p. 337, 1980
13. McCarty, M., *Medical Hypotheses*, vol. 14, p. 307, 1984
14. Rollman, O., et al., *British Journal of Dermatology*, vol. 113, p. 405, 1985
15. Elias, PM, et al., *Archives of Dermatology*, vol. 117, p. 160, Mar. 1981; see also *International Journal of Dermatology*, vol. 20, p. 278, 1981
16. Bollag, W., *Lancet*, p. 860, Apr. 16, 1983
17. Michaelsson, G., et al., *Acta Dermato-Venereologica*, vol. 64, p. 9, 1984
18. Tanaka, K., *New England Journal of Medicine*, vol. 304, p. 839, Apr. 1981
19. McClain, CJ, et al., *Journal of the American Medical Association*, vol. 247, p. 3116, June 1982
20. Bonjour, JP, *International Journal of Vitamin and Nutrition Research*, vol. 47, p. 111, 1977
21. Shelley, WB, et al., *Journal of American Academy of Dermatology*, vol. 13, p. 97, 1985
22. Elmer, G., *Nurse Practitioner*, p. 40, Sept. 1981
23. Shelley, WB, et al., *Lancet*, p. 576, Sept. 8, 1984
24. Worobec, S., et al., *Journal of the American Medical Association*, vol. 251, p. 2348, May 1984

Endnotes 431

CHAPTER 20

1. Nepper, H., et al., *Digestion*, vol. 22, p. 255, 1981
2. Blacklock, N., in *Western Diseases: Their Emergence and Prevention*, p. 60, Trowell, HC, et al., (eds.), Harvard University Press, Cambridge, MA, 1981
3. Johnasson, G., et al., *Journal of the American College of Nutrition*, vol. 1, p. 179, 1982
4. Yendt, ER, et al., *New England Journal of Medicine*, vol. 312, p. 953, Apr. 1985
5. Pru, C., et al., *Nephron*, vol. 39 p. 112, 1985
6. Prickett, J., et al., *Journal of Clinical Investigation*, vol. 68, p. 556, Aug. 1981
7. Borum, PR, et al., *Journal of the American College of Nutrition*, vol. 5, p. 177, 1986
8. Kleiner, MJ, et al., *American Journal of Clinical Nutrition*, vol. 33, p. 1612, July 1980
9. Twelves, CJ, *Lancet*, p,.737, Mar. 29, 1986
10. Fahim, M., et al., *Federation Proceedings*, vol. 35, no. 3, p. 361, Mar.1, 1976
11. Kinney, AB, et al., *Nursing Research*, vol. 28, no. 5, p. 287, Sept. 1979
12. Brody, J., *Jane Brody's Nutrition Book*, p. 227, WW Norton, New York, 1981

CHAPTER 21

1. Burr, ML, et al., *Human Nutrition: Applied Nutrition*, vol. 39A, p. 349, Oct. 1985
2. Pelikan, Z., et al., *Annals of Allergy*, vol. 58, p. 164, Mar, 1987
3. Koepke, JW, et al., *Annals of Allergy*, vol. 54, p. 213, Mar. 1985
4. Martin, LB, et al., *Journal of Food Protection*, vol. 49, p. 126, Feb. 1986
5. Folkers, K., et al., *IRCS Medical Science*, vol. 9, p. 444, 1981
6. Folkers, K., et al., *Hoppe-Seyler's Zeitschrift Physiologische Chemie*, vol. 365, p. 405, Mar. 1984
7. Reynolds, RD, et al., *Federation Proceedings*, vol. 43, p. 470, 1984
8. Reynolds, RD, et al., *American Journal of Clinical Nutrition*, vol. 41, p. 684, Apr. 1985
9. Mohsenin, L., et al., *American Review of Respiratory Disease*, vol. 127, p. 143, 1983
10. Spannhake, R., et al., *American Review of Respiratory Disease*, vol. 127, p. 139, 1983
11. Okayama, H., et al., *Journal of the American Medical Association*, vol. 257, p. 1076, Feb.27,1987

CHAPTER 22

1. Goodman, DS, *New England Journal of Medicine*, vol. 310, p. 1023, Apr. 1984
2. Vijayaraghavan, K., et al., *Lancet*, p. 149, July 21, 1984
3. Vijayaraghavan, K., et al., *Nutrition Reports International*, vol. 25, p. 431, Mar. 1982
4. Robinson, CH, *Fundamentals of Normal Nutrition*, p. 11, Macmillan, New York, 1978
5. Dhanamitta, S., et al., *Nutrition Reports International*, vol. 27, p. 67, Jan. 1983
6. Sommer, A., et al., *American Journal of Opthalmology*, vol. 93, p. 84, Jan. 1982
7. Varma, S., et al., *Photochemistry and Photobiology*, vol. 36, no. 6, p. 623, Dec. 1982
8. Parkit, M., *Los Angeles Times*, part 5, p. 1, Aug.31, 1986
9. Skalka, HW, et al., *American Journal of Clinical Nutrition*, vol. 34, p. 861, May 1981
10. Damodaran, M., et al., *British Journal of Nutrition*, vol. 41, p. 27, 1979
11. Crary, EJ, et al., *Medical Hypotheses*, vol. 13, p. 77, 1984
12. Gunby, P., *Journal of the American Medical Association*, vol. 243, no. 10, p. 1021, Mar. 1980
13. McIntosh, EN, *American Journal of Public Health*, vol. 72, p. 1412, Dec. 1982
14. Yan-You, W., et al., *Lancet*, p. 518, Sept.7, 1985

15. Ziporyn, T., *Journal of the American Medical Association*, vol. 253, p. 1846, Apr. 1985

16. Bryce-Smith, D., et al., *Lancet*, p. 350, Aug.11, 1984

17. Krebs, N., et al., *American Journal of Diseases of Children*, vol. 138, p. 270, Mar. 1984

18. Sayetta, RB, *American Family Physician*, vol. 33, no. 5, p. 181, May 1986

19. Pangborn, RM, et al., *Food Technology*, p. 75, Aug. 1975

20. Hutton, CW, et al., *Journal of the American Dietetic Association*, vol. 82, p. 148, Feb. 1983

21. Mowrey, DB, *Lancet*, p. 655, Mar.20, 1982

INDEX

433